128 Days and Counting

A 28-Year-Old Caregiver's Memoir

Honore Nolting

ISBN (978-0-692-95970-1)

Book Design by Caitlin Cave

Printed in the United States of America

www.128daysandcounting.com

To my parents, Joe & Marye Beth, thank you for all the sacrifices you made so I could become the person I am today.

To Denny & Dorinda, thank you for loving me like one of your own.

To our family and friends who supported us and took care of us so we could focus on our cancer fight, we are forever grateful for your love and support.

To our doctors and nurses, you are angels on earth.

And to Tom, thank you for being vulnerable and agreeing to share our story. You create so much of the laughter in my life, and joy in my heart. Thank you for being you.

Prologue

If you are fighting cancer... I hope this memoir gives you hope and reminds you that what you and your body are doing are incredible. I hope that on the darkest days of your fight, this book reminds you that you can beat your diagnosis and make it through the aftermath of cancer.

If you are a caregiver... I hope this memoir gives you power, and is a reminder that you are not alone. The sacrifices you are making are the greatest gifts you can give someone fighting cancer. It's a tough role, and dangerously lonely some days, but the greatest honor too. I'd also recommend a box of Kleenex.

For the curious reader... these are layers of stories that bounce back and forth around our lives, which I hope will bring you laughter, curiosity, and perhaps a new perspective.

If you are hopeless romantic... this is the most wonderful love story. It may not be traditional, but it's an incredible few chapters of an extraordinary love.

*For everyone else...*this is our heart on paper, and like any good book, I hope it inspires you.

PART 1
Frasier Crane

"What's your husband's name?" he asked.

"Tom," I replied.

"Does he know you are here?"

"Yes, he thought it was a good idea. I called you in a moment of weakness. I almost canceled four times. I'm only here because I promised him I would come at least once."

"So on the phone, you mentioned this is your first time speaking with a therapist, correct?"

"You've got that right," I bluntly answered.

The last thirty minutes had been a little blurry, and I didn't remember driving to his office. I remember packing up at work, and then I seemed to have magically appeared here. I looked across at this stranger talking to me. I hadn't even known what he looked like ahead of time because apparently in this digital age someone can still not have a picture online. How is that even possible? Luckily for him, he had great ratings online as a therapist, so I took a chance on not being able to see if he had trusting eyes, which I wouldn't normally do. Perhaps I should see it as a positive, though, I thought - maybe this guy will work some magic if he's managed to be anonymous this long.

I didn't take my coat off. That seemed too personal, and despite the word vomit of personal topics I was about to discuss with this guy, it felt like too much too soon. I sat on his couch, a wooden coffee table between us, and he sat on the other side in his office chair, pushing himself back and forth with his foot on the edge of the table. I liked his juju – his voice was calm – though I felt a bit gypped that he didn't have more of a Morgan Freeman vibe in his voice. His eyes were trusting – thank goodness - and I liked his smile, but he seemed to smile with a purpose or to be thought-provoking. I needed to get to the bottom of that because I had plenty of thoughts without adding his sneaky smile to the mix.

"So I'll let you start. I will take some notes as we talk, but for now why don't you tell me why you came here," he said.

I snapped back to reality and stopped analyzing him as I took a deep breath.

"Well, I guess that's a loaded question…I'm twenty-eight years old, my husband is thirty and was diagnosed with late stage-three cancer. We have been fighting it for four months, and I'm terrified he's going to die."

This therapist had no idea what he signed up for when he agreed to see me.

C Day

Tom had been rolling around most of the night thanks to our cheap mattress, and that meant I had been up most of the night too. The night before he had started a strange cough and had chest pain but we hadn't thought much of it. We were in the process of training for a 5K, because sadly for us, our non-running bodies actually needed to train for a 5K. He figured he was just a little sore from getting back into running and that he had pulled a muscle in his side. I wouldn't say he's the most gazelle-like runner, so a pulled muscle from this arm-pumping thing he does when he runs wasn't completely out of the question.

At five-thirty in the morning, I rolled over to see him putting on clothes.

"Babe, I'm going to run to the ER to get this checked out; the pain has gotten worse."

"Let me get dressed. I'm taking you," I replied.

"No, really; I'm sure it's nothing. I'll call you in a bit. Please just catch up on sleep," he said.

There was hardly any light coming in the bedroom, but I could tell this was something.

"No, I'm coming."

"I'm already leaving," he said as he marched down the stairs to the garage.

He had forgotten that it doesn't take much for the stubborn Irish girl in me to come out. I got up, got dressed for work, tossed on some makeup, grabbed my work bag and headed towards the car. I was only about five minutes behind him, so we would get this cleared up and then we could both head to work from the hospital. We had unintentionally planned this well.

It was a crisp late-summer morning. The windows were down and the radio was on as I drove to the hospital, hoping that this was nothing serious because we had busy few weeks ahead. We were about to embark on a fall full of trips, parties, and fun adventures. The sun was peeking above the trees and the colors were just starting to change. It was beautiful; the day seemed quite perfect, minus this quick trip to the ER.

I parked next to his car and walked into the waiting room where he was about to sit down. I crossed the waiting area and sat down next to him with a smile on my face.

"I told you not to come," he said, pretending to be mad, but I knew he was glad I was there.

"I tell you not to root for the Bears all the time. You don't listen to me either," I replied.

He shook his head as he leaned over and kissed me on the forehead and grabbed my hand.

2

The waiting room wasn't too full, so I hoped it wouldn't take long for us to see a doctor. In the meantime, I pulled up WebMD to see if I could figure out the mysterious pain.

"Tell me more about the symptoms. Have they changed from last night?" I inquired.

"Yes, but the pain got worse and worse overnight. Maybe it's something with my heart," he replied as he reached up to his chest.

I did some searching and narrowed down the WebMD results.

"According to my lack of medical degree and WebMD it's either a small tear in the lung, heart palpitations, or a pulled muscle."

"None of those sound too terrible. Usually when I check WebMD, I have all the symptoms of cancer," he joked.

"Isn't that the truth?" I said as I snickered. "I remember using WebMD in college and I convinced myself that I had a rare genetic disease. Thirty minutes into my self-diagnosis I realized that it's only found in males."

As Tom's patience with my diagnostic skills was about to run out, we were ushered back to a room. Tom put on a gown and got comfortable on the hospital bed. Behind the bed was a wall of gadgets and gizmos and the only one recognizable to me was a clock. We waited patiently, chatting with each other - trying to figure out how long it would take and guessing what tests they would run. Given my lack of knowledge about the gizmo wall, I probably wasn't the best person to be hypothesizing.

While we were waiting, I knew I had to call my mother-in-law, Dorinda. I had promised her long ago that if ever we were in the ER, I would call her. Tom tended to err on the side of not wanting his mom to worry, so he often tried to hold out until after he knew more before bringing her into the loop. I persuaded him to let me call her.

"What's wrong?" she replied as she picked up her work phone. This wasn't an unusual since she is a worrier. Tom and I laughed, knowing that would be her greeting.

"Hi there. First of all, nothing is wrong, but we are at the ER right now. Tom was having some weird side and chest pain, and so we figured we would be better to be safe than sorry and get things checked out," I replied.

"Let me guess, my son told you not to call me?" she asked.

"Yup!" I replied, laughing.

After filling her in, she offered to come to the hospital, which we told her wasn't necessary. As we wrapped up we told her we would call her when we knew what was happening and let her know what aliment he had managed to get from his 5K training.

Shortly after, the doctor came in and talked through Tom's symptoms, looked at his chest to see if there were any protrusions, and told us he was going to run some bloodwork and do a chest x-ray. It seemed simple enough and moments later the nurse came in to take Tom for his chest x-ray. I was left behind in the room, so I called my mom to let her know we were at the hospital. I was trying to keep busy because the time felt slow when he was away. I'm sure it was only about fifteen minutes, but I was excited to see his bed getting wheeled back into the room.

It was at this point that time started to stand still. After a brief wait, the doctor came back into the room. There seemed to be a shadow of some sort near his lung and they wanted to do a CT scan of his chest. We were not sure what he meant by shadow, but he informed us that it could be a mass of some sort or an infection in his lung. The doctor was very serious and seemed concerned; we knew something wasn't right. As he walked out of the room, I turned my head towards Tom and lifted my eyebrows up high.

"I wonder what it could be," I remarked, trying to keep my mind away from the worst-case scenario.

"This has to be a joke – watch me have cancer or some bullshit like that," Tom replied, clearly caught off guard by what the doctor had just told us.

"Oh stop, let's see what the scans say before we jump to any conclusions," I replied, trying to keep my composure. "Should I call your mom?"

"No, let's wait until we actually have some answers," he replied.

We stared at each other. Neither of us knew what to say, but we were quickly interrupted by the nurse, who had previously been so upbeat. She was very somber and took Tom away again for the CT. I squeezed Tom's hand as they pulled him away in his hospital bed for the tests. I went back to my chair and stared at the floor. I had no idea what was happening, but knew that the direction we were headed couldn't be good. A thousand distractions plowed through my mind, people I should call, sending a note to my boss, doing more research online, but none of it processed – I was paralyzed. I stared. I didn't move the entire time he was getting his scan done; I didn't touch my phone; I didn't move a muscle. I sat there and stared. Thirty minutes had gone by when, once again, Tom's hospital bed reappeared in the doorway of his room. If I had felt paralyzed for the past half hour, I couldn't imagine what he had been feeling. I knew right then that my only time to be paralyzed had just passed.

The doctor came in an eternity later, though realistically it was only about thirty minutes. There was a tumor in Tom's chest and they were going to admit us to the hospital and complete a biopsy. It was too soon for them to give us more information, but they would tell us more once we did some additional tests. The doctor walked out and Tom and I looked at each other. Tom quickly looked away and looked up to the ceiling trying to avoid tears.

"We don't know anything for sure yet," I replied, choking back tears, though I, too, feared the worst.

I'm not sure how long we sat there, staring at each other. I had moved from my chair to his bed and was sitting off the side, holding his hand.

Eventually, I reached for my phone. I flipped around my phone as he watched me. He started shaking his head when he saw me select his mom's contact. I was shaking.

"Hi, Honey, how's it going?" she asked as she picked up the phone.

"I think you should probably come to the hospital if you can," I replied in a monotone voice.

"What's wrong?" she asked.

"There's a mass in his chest, we are being admitted to the hospital," I replied, holding back tears once again.

"I'm on my way – where are you?"

"We are still in the ER right now, but the plan is to move us. Come to the ER unless you hear from me otherwise," I said.

"Okay, bye," she quickly replied as she hustled off the phone.

Tom was upset hearing his mom's panic and squeezed my hand.

"A lot of times a tumor is benign," I said.

Tom kept staring at me, trying to not get upset, and made random comments to my ramblings.

"Whatever this is, we can figure it out," was my final thought as the nurse came into the room.

She told me to gather up our things and that we would be moving down the hall to free up the ER room while we were waiting for a room to be available upstairs. I grabbed our stuff and followed Tom as they started to push his bed out of the room.

When they had pushed the bed out of the room completely, Tom heard his name and saw his parents coming down the hall. My mother-in-law had called my father-in-law to meet her. His mom gave me a hug, and thanked me for calling her. My father-in-law, Denny, reached in and gave me a hug too, I could see in his eyes he was concerned. My father-in-law has a very particular kind of hug; he puts one hand on the side of your face, kisses the other side and gives a tight squeeze. In that moment, I didn't want him to let go.

We followed the bed down the hall and explained how we had ended up in this situation. Tom's mom was walking next to the bed, and my father-in-law and I followed. As we were approaching the room, the nurse from the ER tapped me on my shoulder and summoned me to chat with her. My father-in-law proceeded into the hospital room while I stopped to answer her questions. She had been so kind to us and had made us feel so incredibly comfortable. She asked me a few additional things about Tom's health for the records, which I answered, followed by a few questions of my own.

"I know you can't say anything, but is this bad? Are we about to get the rug pulled out from under us?" I asked, looking her straight in the eye.

"You two are a wonderful couple. I really don't know much, but I will be thinking of you both and hope it's the best possible outcome," she diplomatically replied.

"Can you at least tell me where they are admitting us?" I asked.

"2 East South," she replied.

"And what is that floor?" I asked; medically savvy enough to know that it should help give me a hint.

"Oncology and Geriatric," she replied, looking me straight in the eye.

"Given our age, I'm going to go ahead and assume we are headed to oncology?" I said, though it really wasn't a question.

She put her hand on my shoulder, rubbed it up and down on my arm and wished us the best as she walked away. Still holding the heaps of our stuff, I turned my head the other way and looked at the door frame where I had seen them wheel Tom's bed.

"It could still be benign," I softly said to myself as I took a deep breath and walked the few steps down the hall to our new room.

Tom was filling his parents in and I let him hit the high points before suggesting that we take a quick minute to let our bosses know we wouldn't be coming in. We knew we would be at the hospital for at least one night considering he was getting admitted. In addition, I needed to clue in my parents to what was going on. I had also been texting my sister and my best friends during the morning, but I didn't know where to begin.

I stepped out of the room while Tom chatted with his folks. I don't remember whom I called; I think I called my mom first to fill her in since she knew we were at the hospital. I felt terrible calling her back with such bad news and with no answers to provide.

"We are being admitted," I said as she picked up the phone, forgetting to include any sort of pleasantry.

"What for?" she asked with concern in her voice.

"They found a mass of some sort in his chest; we are being admitted for them to take a further look and get a biopsy. They really don't have much else to tell us, but this isn't looking good," I replied, attempting to be calm.

"Who said this isn't looking good, you? Or a doctor?" she asked, having always been quite rational in her approach to these types of situations.

"Well, the doctor didn't seem to be too excited," I sarcastically replied. "We are being admitted to the oncology floor too, which I predict isn't the best sign."

She asked more questions, including the typical mother question of inquiring if she should come to the hospital. I told her not to come down for now, and that I'd keep her up to date.

I called my dad next and filled him in, minus the oncology floor part. Where my mom had taken the rational approach, my dad was a worrier. I'm very close with both of my parents, but because of a medical diagnosis that my dad had years back, he and I are especially close. I didn't cry, I just told him the facts and that I would call him as soon as we knew more. However, he was no fool, he knew full well that I was falling apart on the inside and scared. My dad worked as a PET scan driver and assistant. Positron Emission Tomography is a kind of cancer-scanning technology that many hospitals rent but don't purchase due to the expense of the machine. He's far too familiar with cancer due to his work, and was still angry about the loss of his only brother to esophageal cancer just seventeen months earlier.

Lastly, I filled in my sister. She too was completely puzzled as to what was happening, how this had happened so fast, and when we would know more. I called and chatted with all of three of them in less than ten minutes because I wanted to get back to Tom.

I sat near the head of Tom's bed and we chatted with his parents. My father-in-law kept saying he was sure this was nothing; I was hoping he was right, but the nurse had given me little hope. It seemed like hours, but it wasn't long before they were moving us to his room. We settled into the last room at the end of a hallway right near the elevators. Room 240. Add that to the list of things I will never forget.

The room was white, very asylum-like, not that I've ever been in an asylum, but I think I've seen enough movies to know they are not fun places to be. Even a throw pillow would have made a world of difference for the room. There was a couch against the windows, which was right next to a pseudo recliner-type chair, both made of a plastic material. We had a small closet and a bathroom in the room. I could take ten normal-sized steps and be at the other side of the room, and that was being generous. We dropped our stuff and nurses surrounded us. A woman walked in to take Tom's vital signs, but luckily didn't take mine because I was pretty close a flat line at that point.

A few minutes later a nurse peered around the curtain and said hello.

"Hi, I'm Nancy; I'm going to be your nurse. It sounds like you guys have had quite the morning. We are going to get you settled in and hopefully you will have some answers soon," she said with a smile on her face. She looked young, with a big blonde ponytail and had a soft demeanor. She asked us some questions about everything that had happened that morning, but it was a blur.

I was sitting on the chair, helping to answer questions, and I kept getting things handed to me. A folder was shuffled my way with a hospital map, finance information, staff information, a cafeteria and room service menu, and a note pad. As I flipped through the material I couldn't process what I was seeing. The gravity of the situation hadn't scratched the surface of my brain.

So many tests happened between when we got into that room to four hours later when our oncologist peeked her head around the curtain. We had been randomly assigned the on-call oncologist associated with the hospital – I would later find out that this was our first "everything happens for a reason" moment. She was a pretty Polish woman, who also looked very young. She immediately had a calming bedside manner and introduced herself.

On the wall closest to the door was a computer that she turned toward us as she pulled up Tom's records. We all stood on the other side of the bed looking at her and the screen. I was closest to Tom's head, with my father-in-law next to me, and my mother-in-law next to him, toward the foot of the bed. The doctor started talking about what she saw in the scans and blood work and showed us imagines from the CT. A 5x4x4 inch tumor was in Tom's chest, it was a monster. Without further analysis they had narrowed it down to three types of potential cancers, but were quite confident that it was a rare form of testicular cancer. This was when my naivety appeared for the first and last time.

"So there is no chance this tumor could be benign?" I asked.

"No, we are certain of the cancer due to his blood work; it's just a matter of what type of cancer we are dealing with," she replied.

I suddenly had tunnel vision and heard random words for a few minutes.

"Chemo treatments, each lasting five days," "Testing," "Surgery," "Blood," "Mediastinal," and "Germ Cell Tumor" are all things I heard her say; I just wasn't quite sure what order to put them all in. I snapped back to reality as she shut down the computer and pushed it back against the wall.

"I'm so sorry; I know this has been a really hard day. Is there anything else I can help with right now? If not, let's plan to get the additional tests done in the morning and I'll come back in the afternoon," she said.

That's when I lost it. I cried. Oprah cried. The kind of crying where you wake up the next day still red and you have a headache. Tom had been looking at the doctor and turned his head to me when he heard my first sniffle. The look he gave me will forever be in my mind. It was complete fear. He reached up and grabbed my hand. I felt my father-in-law's hand on my back for comfort as he also tried to comfort my mother-in-law. The doctor walked out of the room, and we all looked at each other. There were so many feelings in that moment. I wondered if it was real; I hoped I was dreaming, and I suddenly had morbid thoughts pop into my mind. I sat on the side of the bed and looked at Tom who was also choking back tears but was surprisingly calm. He held my hand and we stared at each other as I attempted to not cry too hard.

"Why don't we go for a walk and give these two some time," I heard my father-in-law say. His parents left the room so we could process everything we had just heard – how foolish of us to think that task would ever be complete.

The Hangover

It was 5:30 a.m. the morning after the diagnosis and I hadn't slept much. I had stayed on the couch next to Tom. My mind was tortured, and the uncomfortable beds weren't helping. I hadn't left Tom's side except for an hour the night before to run home and grab stuff for our hospital stay. I kept tossing and turning, and nurses had been in and out all through the night. At random times during the night, as we turned back and forth, we would look up at each other to see if the other was awake.

The night before, Tom's Aunt Paula and Uncle Rick had come up to visit. His aunt and uncle were like his second parents – Tom often joked that they had used him as their test child. Their two children, Stephen and Kailee, were like Tom's younger siblings. They grew up together and were very close. The emotions were high when his aunt and uncle arrived, but we managed to have some dinner and tried to process it all. Again, foolish. Since he was surrounded by his family, I had seized the opportunity to run home. Aunt Paula came with me, clearly nervous about me being alone at a time like this, and helped me drag everything back to the hospital. I distinctly remember walking to the car and telling her we would have so much to be thankful for at Thanksgiving. Why that popped into my head, I have no idea, but I already knew we were going to be very thankful. She was patient, listened and assured me everything would be okay – she too was coming off quite a stressful year and told me that if you had told her a year ago what would transpire in her life, she would have told you it wasn't possible. I knew she was right, but it was hard to look past an hour, much less think about a year from now. It was too scary.

I was awake thinking about that conversation with her when I realized that at 5:45 a.m., I was likely done sleeping for the night. I saw I had over twenty texts on my phone. News had traveled with friends and family, and the support was already flooding in. I peeked up to see if Tom was sleeping before I moved too much. He was fast asleep, which made me happy; he needed rest. I rested on the pillow, wiping away tears as I read the messages from family and friends.

At about 6:00 a.m. I started to hear Tom moving, but I didn't move in case he fell back asleep. About a minute later, I heard a gasp. I quickly popped up and turned towards Tom. His eyes met mine right before his hands met his face. He covered his face and sobbed, "I thought it was a dream; I thought it was a dream. How is this not a dream?!" My heart broke. I jumped up, went to his bed and literally moved him over and laid on my side next to him. He rolled into me and cried as I squeezed him. I knew this was a moment that he might be coming out of shock. I squeezed him hard because I was trying my hardest not to cry too. I teared up but at that moment managed to keep it together.

"We've got this, we've got this," I kept telling him as I rubbed his back. I believed 98 percent in my own statement, and I would worry about the other 2 percent later. Minutes passed, and I kept saying things that I thought would calm him down. As I squeezed less, Tom squeezed harder. We laid in that small bed clutching each other for over half an hour, crying and trying to convince ourselves we could deal with the nightmare that had unfolded.

We knew we had a long day of testing ahead including the biopsy, an MRI, and ultrasounds to get a final diagnosis. As we were calming down, Nancy came in to check on his vitals and say good morning. I awkwardly flopped out of the tiny hospital bed and started cleaning up the room a bit as we chatted with Nancy. She had quickly become close to us and had been so helpful during our admission day. She exuded a confidence that we both appreciated and made us feel comfortable. She also was savvy enough to immediately know we were having a rough morning. We got a plan for his medication for the day and an idea of the testing schedule. It was going to be a busy day and people would pick him up throughout the day for the tests. We would see the oncologist in the afternoon once all the testing was done so she could provide her final diagnosis.

Nancy walked out, encouraging Tom to try some breakfast, and said she'd be back with medicine. We had a few moments before Tom's mom walked in. She was prepared for another day at the hospital and came with Starbucks, a cooler of drinks and bags of snacks. She hadn't slept either and was eager to see us both, but it was going to be a hurry-up-and-wait kind of day.

Tom was having a rough morning and throwing up, which was making the situation even more challenging. Our first big test was his biopsy. The technician came to get him and said I should come with Tom; I needed to sign off on the procedure because he had been given heavy narcotics. I walked behind as the transport person rolled his bed through a maze of hallways and elevators until we ended up in the basement of the hospital. The transport person looked shocked to be taking a couple so young to a test like this and struck up a conversation with us. We told him the saga of the last twelve hours, and he shook my hand as he dropped us off and wished us the best.

We got rolled into a dimly lit room with scanning equipment where the nurses were preparing for the biopsy. The doctor came in and, as we had experienced far too often in the past day, was taken aback by the youth of the people looking back at him. He was a very sweet man and explained exactly what he was going to do. Tom was going to be put in a bit of a twilight, but they couldn't put him completely under since they needed to talk with him during the procedure. In addition, they would use a topical numbing agent on his chest. Essentially, they were putting a big needle into his chest, and then putting a second needle within that needle to get the tissue from the tumor.

They would immediately hand it off to the nurses who would put it under the microscope over in the corner of the room. Once they had enough tissue they would be done. With that, I signed off, and they escorted me to a small waiting area.

The waiting area had no cell reception because of all the equipment in the area, so I sat and stared at the clock. The doctor said it would be about twenty to thirty minutes. I was so antsy and was getting lost in my thoughts and only catching myself once I started to choke up and get teary-eyed. I figured I could distract myself as I pulled up the photo album on my phone. The last picture I took was from Sunday and was a picture of Tom helping an old man in our neighborhood.

We had been driving down the street and saw our elderly neighbor kicking two boxes up to his door while using his walker. He would push the boxes a bit with his foot and then move the walker about an inch. I immediately pulled over, and without words, Tom jumped out of the car and offered to carry the boxes in for the old man. Our neighbor was delighted. Tom grabbed the boxes and took them to the door as the man slowly followed. He thanked Tom with a wave as he headed back to the car.

"Good work," I said as he jumped back in the car.

"That would have taken him hours if someone hadn't stopped," he replied.

As we drove down the street to our house, I smiled as I looked at him and said, "I love you." I was so glad that I was married to someone who didn't think twice about stopping to help a stranger. Even more, this was the morning of the Bears/Packers matchup, a usually heated day in our household since I was born and raised in the great state of Wisconsin, and he is from Illinois. Perhaps I'm a bit biased in my descriptions of our home states, but our rivalry was strong.

The next picture was of Lake Michigan from Evanston, IL. I had been down by the water and a storm was coming in - the photo I captured was unique with circling clouds. I had been in Evanston to meet a friend for lunch but went to the lake after lunch on my own. Water has always been my happy place, common for my Cancer zodiac sign, and in the weeks prior to his diagnosis we were already in the midst of medical chaos. After a year and a half of trying for a baby, we were in the process of getting a series of tests done. We were a bit down about the fertility nightmare, and I had gone to the water to just breathe in some of the Great Lakes air before heading back home. The photo calmed me, and I took in a deep breath and looked up as someone walked by. Every time someone came around the corner, I would snap my head up to see if it was the doctor.

The next picture was from the previous week, a screen shot of a quote that I had seen online at some point. It read:

"Before you speak to me about your religion, first show it to me in how you treat other people; before you tell me how much you love your God, show me in how much you love all His children; before you preach to me of your passion for your faith, teach me about it through your compassion for your neighbors. In the end, I'm not as interested in what you have to tell or sell as I am in how you choose to live and give." – Cory Booker

In hindsight, the quote was an interesting precursor to Tom helping our neighbor. It obviously struck me at the time, but I didn't distinctly remember reading this quote or saving it. It reminded me of my dad. A Vietnam veteran, he wasn't always overly religious despite our Catholic upbringing. We went to church every Sunday with my mom, and it was normal for Dad to stay back. He would attend some days, and was always there for any sacrament or holiday, but most days he would say, "I'll see you at church if you sit by the window!" as we walked out the door. It never bothered me, and for some reason I never questioned it, but the Cory Booker quote embodied all of who my father is as a person. He lives his life a certain way instead of talking about how he lives his life. I know plenty of people who don't miss a Sunday in the pew but are the least-Christian people I know when it comes to how live their lives the rest of the week. My dad was the opposite; he didn't sit in a pew every Sunday, but he would go to bat for any person he met, help anyone he could and is one of the most genuine souls in the world. The thought of him made me want to cry as I knew he how upset he and my Mom were about Tom's diagnosis.

It felt like I had already been waiting for an hour as I looked up to the clock. Only twenty minutes had passed. As I swiped to the next photo, I saw another quote; clearly I had been in quite the reflective mood that week. In the background of the photo was a long table with people eating and the overlay quote read, "When you have more than you need, build a longer table not a higher fence." I remembered taking a screen shot of this one because it's the epitome of how I strive to live my life. Suddenly my mind raced to what we would need and what might happen with everything that seemed to be lying ahead for us. I wondered how bad the medical bills would be, if we would need to sell our house, if Tom could go on disability, or if I would need to take a leave from work. I started feeling myself get overwhelmed again and tears welled in my eyes.

I snapped back to reality as the doctor came around the corner. I jumped up and he told me it went well, but that he hadn't actually put Tom under since the tumor was so close to the surface. The craziness of that didn't process as I immediately asked him how long until the results would be back. He told me Monday, depending on what exactly the oncologist needed to validate. It was Thursday. Cue the emotions; cue the overwhelmed mind, and this poor doctor suddenly had a sobbing wife begging him to do something faster because we needed answers so we could try to regain control of our lives.

The doctor calmly walked over to a desk area and grabbed a tissue, took a few steps, turned around and grabbed the entire Kleenex box, then walked back to me. Clearly, this wasn't his first rodeo.

"I'm so sorry; I can't imagine what a rollercoaster the last twenty-four hours has been. I will see what I can do, but some of these tests require time and there isn't much we can do to speed that up," he calmly replied as he reached out and put his hand on the side of my arm.

"I know. I'm sorry, I really haven't cried this hard yet; I think I've been in shock," I replied as I tried to pull myself together.

"Please don't apologize. You're a young couple and your husband is ill," he said as he motioned for me to walk with him back to the room.

I followed him and took a few deep breaths as he walked me back down the hall to see Tom. I turned the corner to a horrifying scene. Tom was in his hospital bed, gripping the sides of the bed and shaking in pain.

His eyes welled with tears as he stuttered out, "They didn't put me under. I felt most of it."

I looked up at the doctor who again reminded me that he had decided to not put Tom under and only use the topical numbing agent. Tom had laid on a cold piece of metal as he saw a large needle go into his chest, and then heard the extraction of the tissue. Each time they took a sample it sounded like a gunshot and Tom wasn't aware that they deliberately weren't putting him under – he was clearly traumatized. The worst part was that we were now sitting and waiting for a transport person to come and take us back to his room with no access to pain medications until we were back upstairs.

I wrapped my hand around his hand clutching onto the bed as he shook in pain. My eyes welled up again as I stared at him and told him I loved him. The nurses and doctors kept calling the transport and even were kind enough to call up to Nancy and let her know to have his medication ready and that we should be back soon. This was the first of many times that I felt completely helpless. There was nothing I could do to make the pain go away; I had already put pressure on the nurses to call again, and we were at the mercy of time. Finally, our transport person showed up and took us back to our room. I never let go of his hand the entire walk back.

As we were coming down the hall, Nancy was coming towards his room with the pain medicine and looked at me, surprised and curious as to why they wouldn't have put him under for his biopsy. As we told Nancy what happened and filled in his mom, Tom started to throw up again. Tom's mom jumped up to get a cold cloth, and I quickly handed him a puke bag and got a towel to wipe his face. It all felt like a nightmare. Nancy stuck it out with us and didn't leave our room for almost forty-five minutes. She made sure we got him comfortable, got his pain under control and that the vomiting had stopped.

A while later, just as Tom was dozing off, we heard a knock on the door as a woman came in to take Tom for his testicular ultrasound. I couldn't look at Tom and I was trying not to laugh as she walked in the room and introduced herself. She was young, perhaps a few years younger than me, and stunningly gorgeous. I'm confident in my looks, but she was a ten, off the runway beautiful and made me do a double take. I smiled as I looked over at Tom, who looked at me with the funniest face I'd seen in the past two days.

"That's a joke, right?" he softly said to me, knowing that I knew exactly what he was talking about.

I smiled. "Who knows, maybe just transport?" I softly replied as the nurse was validating his name and birthdate.

For this test Tom was on his own, and my mother-in-law and I had to stay back in the room. I gave him a kiss as he walked to the transport bed in the hall.

A short while later Tom was wheeled back to the door of the room. I got up to help him to his bed and asked him what happened. Tom, always comedic in his delivery, was laughing as he replied.

"Oh yeah, that woman just did the ultrasound. I've never tried harder in my life to not make eye contact with somebody. That was awful," he said while shaking his head and walking back to his bed.

I couldn't stop laughing; I wanted to know more but couldn't pull the words together in my laughter. Tom couldn't stop laughing either as he watched me laugh. Tom has always prided himself on being able to make me laugh hard and tries to get me to a point where I can't control my laughter.

"It was just long enough that I will be traumatized for life," he said, laughing, as he climbed back into bed. I had officially caught the giggles but got myself calm to see what he wanted for lunch since my sisters-in-law were bringing food to the hospital. He wasn't in the room longer than ten minutes before they took him away again for an MRI. It wasn't even 11 a.m., and he had already been poked, prodded, jellied, and scanned more than any person would desire in a week, much less a few hours. I kissed him goodbye again as they wheeled him away.

A short while later we heard another knock on the door as Tom's two step-sisters, Staci and Christina, arrived with food. I was supposed to have dinner with them the night before but had canceled mid-morning when we were admitted to the hospital. We usually catch up with dinner and lots of wine, and they too had been in shock to find out about Tom's preliminary diagnosis. They had texted me throughout the evening to see what they could do and were eager to see us. They arrived, with my fifteen-month-old niece and a lot of food. We were all hugging as tears rolled down my face; they were in as much shock as everyone else and wanted to know what had been happening – and where Tom was. About fifteen minutes into our conversation, I heard the transport bed wheel up to the door. I jumped up and helped Tom get out of that bed and back into the room.

He said hello to everyone and got in his bed. I could tell something was wrong. He looked up at me; I grabbed the puke bag, and sure enough, he started throwing up again. My mother-in-law grabbed a cold towel and went to get Nancy as I rubbed his back and assured him that the tests were over for the day. He had just finished the last one, and he would be able to rest all afternoon. I rubbed his back and tried to calmly talk to him as he continued to throw up. I looked up at Christina, who was on the other side of the bed, holding a napkin for his face for when he was done throwing up. I'll never forget the look on her face; she looked confused, sad and helpless all at once. For everyone, seeing him so sick just didn't seem possible. He was fine a few days ago and suddenly he had a cancerous tumor in his chest. She looked me straight in the eye, and I could feel her hurt for us. We both looked down at him as he finished throwing up.

Never wanting anyone to know he wasn't feeling great, he smiled as he looked around.

"Thanks for coming," he joked, "I think I'm going to hold off on lunch for a bit."

Tom never wants to inconvenience anyone; he goes out of his way to not be a bother to people, so I knew this was tough for him. It was something we were going to have to get used to if we were going to make it through the days ahead.

After visiting for a while, I walked Staci and Christina out to the elevator and they both gave me a hug. We were discussing all the ramifications of this diagnosis and what it meant for Tom and I having a family that we both had wanted for so long. I looked up at them and burst into tears again as I pulled the neck of my hoodie up to my face. The shock had begun to wear off, and the emotions were more than I could handle. They hugged me; my little niece looking shocked on the hip of Christina, and assured me everything would be okay. I hoped they were right.

Late afternoon, our oncologist came back into the room with her official diagnosis. Tom had a mediastinal nonseminomatous germ cell tumor that was shaped so strangely that it was touching his heart, lung and liver. This tumor was a force to be reckoned with, and the treatment was going to be quite the battle. She was recommending four treatments of chemo that each lasted three weeks. The first week was five consecutive days of chemo treatments in the hospital. One of the drugs that he would need required a twenty-four-hour drip of a medicine to manage the potential effects on his bladder, so it was recommended that we do treatment as patients of the hospital versus outpatient. After the five days of chemo, we would then have the next two weeks "off" and then repeat the cycle. Twelve weeks of chemo with twenty chemo treatments total. I immediately started doing the math in my head; twelve weeks put us in December. This was going to be a long few months. After the treatment, they would do surgery to remove the tumor from his chest. Once they got the tumor, they would see if there was any remaining active cancer inside it. If there was, we would have to do two more rounds of chemo, tacking on ten more chemo treatments and six more weeks of chemo post-surgery. If not, we would be done after surgery.

I remember her talking through the recommendations and feeling like I was hearing nails on a chalkboard every time I heard the word "if". How could so much of medicine be an "if"? I get it; humans are like snowflakes, no two are alike, but could there really be this many variables and "ifs" in such a serious situation? Our doctor patiently answered all our questions and said that she wouldn't recommend us for discharge until Tom's vomiting and medicine regimen was under control, most likely the next day. She asked us to schedule an appointment to see her the next week and she would walk us through the details of the treatment and what our options would be for injection sites, etc. In the meantime, she said we should get a second opinion. In hindsight, it takes a very special doctor to look at your patient and tell him to get a second opinion. She was one of the most qualified doctors I've ever worked with, completely immersed in her field, and yet she recommended that we get all the facts checked and seek other opinions so we could be as comfortable as possible with whatever decisions we had to make – what a gift.

She walked out of the room, and within minutes Tom was throwing up again. I was starting to think the throwing up was less about the medications and more about how he was reacting to hearing all the information we had been hearing in the past twenty-four hours. Nancy came in to help and asked how our conversation with Dr. Sobol had gone – she could see in my eyes that I was lost. I sat on the end of Tom's bed, she sat in the visitor's chair, and my mother-in-law was on the couch. I asked Nancy about our doctor – considering she had been randomly assigned to us – and wanted to know what she thought about getting a second opinion. She told me about how fast cancer treatments are evolving and that she thought it was a good idea but that Dr. Sobol was one of the best doctors. Strangely enough, I felt close enough to Nancy in the twenty-four hours that I had known her that I asked her one simple question.

"Nancy, if your husband had just been diagnosed with cancer, who would you take him to see?"

"Dr. Sobol would certainly be at the top of my list – they are a great team of doctors – you would be in great hands," she replied.

We already loved Dr. Sobol and felt so comfortable with her that we were planning on working with her, but did think it was in our best interest to see other doctors too, considering how rare Tom's cancer was – there were less than a few hundred cases a year in the U.S. We needed to get as many opinions as possible from anyone who had seen one of these tumors before. I had my work cut out for me.

Tom continued to be sick through the early evening and eventually fell asleep around 6 p.m. My mother-in-law was still there, so I stepped out to make a few phone calls to my family and fill them in about everything I had learned. While I had been texting them updates, the autocorrecting on my iPhone with medical terms was at the point where I was about to throw my phone out the window. I made several calls, the last of which was coordinating with my mom on how she would get to us tomorrow. She insisted on coming and as much as I felt guilty that she was driving down, I wanted to see my mom. My family was in Milwaukee, only about eighty miles away from us in the suburbs of Chicago, so it wasn't too long of a drive, but I knew she was eager to see me. When I walked back to the room, it had gotten dark. The only light in the room was from the TV and my mother-in-law's laptop.

She whispered to me, "I think I'm going to go home since he's been sleeping." She had been a trooper all day, hanging with us at the hospital.

"Sounds good," I replied, planning to close my eyes too and try to sleep for a while, not knowing what the night could bring. I helped her pack up her things in the dark and walked her to the door. I stepped out into the hallway and gave her a hug goodbye – she said she would be back first thing in the morning but to call if I needed anything. The morning seemed so far away.

I snuck back into the room and realized I was foolish to think I was going to be getting sleep anytime soon. It was time for me to do some research on for second opinions, and more importantly, now that we knew what he had, learn as much as possible about his type of cancer. I pulled up my laptop and started to do my research. After about an hour and a half, a nurse tech came in to get Tom's vitals, and he woke up. He felt one hundred times better since he hadn't been throwing up for a few hours and had gotten some sleep. His color looked better; his eyes looked better, and he was a bit more like his usually bubbly self. He was hungry for the first time in days. I looked at the clock. It was 8:30 p.m., thirty minutes past the cafeteria closing. I jumped up and walked down the hall to find our night nurse, Julie, who we also already adored. I asked if there was any way we could get some food since Tom had woken up and had an appetite. Julie dropped what she was doing and went down to the cafeteria to see what she could find.

A few minutes later she peered around the corner of our door with a tray of random foods – she had convinced them to let her take what was left. We had some broth, Jell-O, a roll, two Italian ices, and one unknown substance in a bowl. Tom sat up and crossed his legs on his bed, and we put the tray across the bed perpendicularly. I sat with my legs crossed at the foot of the bed on the other side of the tray – it was our first official hospital bed picnic.

We sat on his bed, eating Italian ices and chatted. It was such a shift from where we had been the last twenty-four hours. The shock had worn off; he was starting to feel "better," and we sat there eating our treats and getting a plan. I filled him in on all the messages we had gotten since he'd been sleeping and what I had found in my research. We laughed, we cried, we both admitted we were scared, but we knew we could do this together. It was a strangely special moment for us, having a goofy picnic in a hospital bed, but we felt like we were regaining control and knew that our relationship could make it through this.

Nobody Likes a Two-Day Hangover

Despite a night that was constantly interrupted by nurses and doctors, Tom was starting to feel better, meaning we would likely be able to head home. The hardest part of every morning was waking up and readjusting to our reality, because it still felt like a dream. Tom got emotional again and cried out, "I'm sorry, I'm so sorry" when he woke up. I burst into tears as I went to his bed and told him he should never apologize for what had happened. He didn't choose to get cancer or plan this to make our lives harder. His guilt had already started to consume his mind. I knew it was normal but still so hard to hear.

Shortly after we composed ourselves, my mother-in-law appeared bright and early with Starbucks in tow and was thrilled to see how much better Tom looked. Even though he looked better, there were still heavy hearts and a strange, unspoken acknowledgment that any laughter was just trying to avoid the tears and sadness. A while later I got up to stretch a bit and peeked into the hall – lo and behold, my mom was walking down the hall. I gave her a big hug as she approached the door I was so happy she was there, and I could tell she was happy to be with me too.

As she walked into the room, Tom had gotten up from the bed to give her a hug with a huge smile on his face. The smile, however, is not what most people would be smiling about. My mom isn't a big hugger and for many years had always despised when her sons-in-law would hug her. Her disdain for hugs had only made it more fun for my brother-in-law, Andy, and Tom to attack her and not let go when they see her, usually resulting in her groaning and saying "Let go of me!" As my mom came around the corner, she chuckled to see Tom up from the bed, his arms stretched out, and a smile on his face.

"I think I deserve a hug!" he proclaimed as she was already tucking in her shoulders to avoid the hug.

"I suppose I can't say no, can I?" she answered, laughing and looking at Tom's mom for an excuse as she gave him a hug.

"I had to get cancer to get a hug from you – that's pretty extreme, don't you think?" he joked.

We visited for a bit and then I went to the cafeteria to grab some breakfast with my mom. Tom's mom was there with him, but it made me so nervous to leave him because I hadn't left his side other than to run home and grab our things. They promised to text me if the doctor came in. Mom and I grabbed some food from the cafeteria and sat down. She was calm and wanted me to fill her in on how the night went, how we were holding up, and what my parents could to do help. I kept it together for the beginning of our conversation, but as I began telling her that Tom was apologizing this morning, I fell apart again, crying.

My mom was sitting across the table from me, and the tears started coming down her face too. I can't imagine how difficult it was for her to sit across from her daughter and not be able to help fix the problem – the thing moms typically do best. The last thing I wanted was for her to be upset too, but it was the first time I could truly let my guard down. My mom is a trained trauma specialist, so she has quite a bit of experience in what we were going through – trauma comes in all shapes and sizes, and this life-altering event certainly qualified as a big one.

We sat there for a while, and she helped me organize my thoughts and put together a plan for updating the family. I was getting antsy to get back to Tom, so we headed back up to the room so she could visit a bit more before saying her goodbyes. Seeing my mom had recharged me – I was raised by amazing parents and a strong woman for a mother; I knew I could do this. A few hours later, we officially got approved for discharge. Our oncologist had told us all the appointments we would need to schedule in the upcoming week and stressed that it was important that we start treatment as soon as possible. As they were preparing our discharge paperwork, I made the appointments for the following week – it was going to be a long haul, but the thought of being comfortable with our treatment plan was going to power us through.

I headed out to pull the car around for Tom as he was prepped to leave and settled in a wheelchair. I walked to the car, and in those moments of solitude tried to process what was happening. I was eager to be home but also a bit scared to leave the hospital in case he started getting sick again. I didn't want him to know I was worried, so I convinced myself I had seen enough medical shows to at least fake that I knew what I was doing and that I was capable of taking care of him. I pulled the car around as Tom's folks walked next to his wheelchair. We got things settled in the car and got Tom in the passenger seat. Tom's parents closed the door and peeked their heads in.

"What can we do?" they asked.

"I think we are okay for now. I'll let you know if we need anything though," I replied, truly puzzled as to what we would need.

I remember their faces looking back at us – wanting to help but having no idea how. We were in a bit of a strange place and a holding pattern. Other than Tom resting and taking his medicine, there was very little to do until we got second opinions and got a plan together. I too felt as helpless as they did.

As we drove home, Tom and I talked about how we both were in desperate need of a shower and how nice it was to be out of the hospital. We had our windows down and the air was full of the scents of fall. The trees had just started turning colors and despite everything going on, we appreciated how nice it was outside and how gorgeous everything looked. At a stoplight, I looked over at Tom. He had lost quite a few pounds in the past three days; his beard was starting to grow in, and he looked exhausted. Every ounce of my being just wanted to make him feel better, or do this for him. We had a long road ahead.

Later that evening, we were waiting for Tom's aunt, uncle and cousin to come by. They were coming with dinner, which was such a help on an emotional day – if I had been meal planning, we would have stress-eaten a pint of ice cream. Twenty minutes before they showed up, we got a phone call. I picked up the phone and heard a familiar voice.

"Honore, I'm so sorry. It's Doctor Feinberg." I felt a bit frozen, knowing what she was calling about.

"Hi, Doctor Feinberg, thanks for calling us back. I believe Dr. Sobol has filled you in on the situation?" I asked.

"Yes, I'm so sorry. He looked so great in the office last week. How are you two holding up?" she asked.

Dr. Feinberg was a new friend to both of us; she was our fertility doctor who had seen us several times in the weeks leading up to Tom's diagnosis. After a year and a half of unsuccessfully trying to get pregnant, we had been seeing her to figure out what was holding us up from having a family. We had reached out to her to see what, if anything, we should do prior to his chemo.

"We are okay," I replied, trying to hold it together as I put her on speaker. "We just wanted to touch base with you and see what thoughts you had on the situation and if there is anything we should do before we start chemo. Our doctor said we need to move fast, so if we need to do anything, it would need to be next week."

"I've been trying to track down a urologist that specializes in these types of situations, but I can't seem to get a hold of him. I'm going to keep trying, but based on some other calls I've made, I think that the likelihood of you being able to have kids naturally probably is no longer an option, and it wouldn't be safe to bank anything right now. At this time, I would recommend that you focus on getting Tom healthy. I'm so sorry to have to tell you this. I know it's been a rough few days."

I looked over at Tom as tears welled up in my eyes. He squeezed my hand as I tried to get the doctor to change her answer. "So, there is no chance or just a low chance?" I asked.

"I would leave that up to a urologist for a definitive answer, but I do think its single digit odds, if at all," she replied.

I didn't know what to say.

"I'm so sorry, Honore. I'm going to keep trying the urologist tonight and will let you know if I hear anything different. If you need anything, don't hesitate to reach out. If there is anything I can do to help, I'm here."

I knew she meant what she was saying, but I felt like we had just gotten the final punch in an already crushing week.

"Thanks, Dr. Feinberg, I really appreciate that. Thanks for calling." I hung up the phone.

For the second time that week, my floodgates broke, and I sobbed. Tom was equally as upset. We knew we only had a few moments before his family was going to show up with dinner. I'm not sure who took the lead, but we got ourselves calmed down and agreed that we were going to have a family somehow, some way, and that we would focus on that once he was cancer free. In a strange way, we had been so focused on getting pregnant for so many months that there was an element of relief when we knew we wouldn't have to think about it for a while.

We heard car doors shut in the driveway and knew our visitors were here with dinner. I still lacked an appetite but knew that food was needed. I walked down and let them in and then looked away for a few moments. I couldn't stomach watching Tom see his cousin Stephen for the first time since the diagnosis. They were like brothers, and I knew I would cry if things got too emotional. We sat at the table and filled everyone in on how things had gone and Tom's harrowing tale of the smoking-hot nurse doing his ultrasound. Their company helped distract us until I looked down and saw my phone ringing again. I excused myself from the table because I recognized the number. I was a bit surprised she was calling back so late and I snuck into the bedroom as I answered.

"I managed to get a hold of the specialist I had mentioned," Dr. Feinberg said. "He assured me that we are right in not taking any interventions right now but that you should have hope that things can be done to help on the other side of Tom's cancer. It's single-digit odds, but there have been lots of advances in this area, and he's eager to meet you both when you beat this," she said as I heard a smile on her face.

"Oh wow, that's awesome. Thank you so much!" I replied. I was on the world's worst rollercoaster of emotion, but I felt like this was a moment to breathe at the top of the next dip. As we finished chatting, I hung up the phone and looked into the mirror on our dresser. I felt like I didn't recognize myself; the person in the mirror didn't look like how I felt. That girl looked like she was somewhat put together and living life. The person I was right now felt like she was clawing her way out of hell and trying to carry her husband along with her. I stared for a moment and snapped back to reality when I heard laughter coming from the kitchen. I walked back to the table. Tom asked who had called.

"Dr. Feinberg called back. All good; we can discuss later," I said as I squeezed his hand. We continued eating – if you didn't know what had happened, you would never know that Tom was as sick as he was. If there were a snapshot of this moment, you would see a family around the table chatting.

Later, after his family had left, I told Tom about the second phone call and he too was optimistic, but feeling like we were on a rollercoaster of emotions with no control. We were hanging out in the living room, I was reading him messages I had received, and we were waiting for one more visitor. Tom's best friend, Greg, and his wife happened to be in the area that night and wanted to swing by and see us. Greg and Tom have been friends since birth. They lived on the same street; Greg was born a few months after Tom and was his "first friend". They grew up as partners in crime and had a bond that was very special. This was another greeting at the door that I was nervous to see unfold because the emotions were potentially more than I could handle. His wife, May, was an oncology nurse and eight months pregnant.

The doorbell rang, and their faces appeared at our door. I was so happy to get hugs from them both, and immediately started asking May questions about some of the different medicines that they had given us. I was trying to get it all in order and felt completely incompetent. We visited with them for a while and for the most part had light-hearted conversations that kept our spirits up despite the day we'd had. I remember looking at May and her pregnant belly. I knew that would be me someday, but that the someday would need to be farther in the future than we had planned. We were genuinely excited for them to have this baby, but all I could hear in my head is our fertility doctor saying "single digit odds." We would just have to spoil their baby boy until we had our own – and Uncle Tom and Aunt Honore were great at spoiling kids.

Later that night as we closed the door behind our visitors, Tom and I grabbed each other for a hug. We stood on the carpet in front of the door and just hugged. Neither of us attempted to let go.

"Thank you," I heard Tom mutter over my shoulder.

"For what?" I asked.

"Being the best wife in the world. I love you so much," he said as he took in a deep breath.

"I love you more," I said as I pulled back to give him a kiss.

Our wedding rings were both engraved with "I love you more" on the inside of the band. Our ever-competitive relationship included who loves the other most.

"Impossible," he replied.

"Trust me, I love you more...but I hate cancer even more than that," I quipped as I gave him a kiss.

The Web of Support

Saturday morning, we were so exhausted, and we had been up throughout the night. Tom was in quite a bit of pain, and the cough he had from the tumor was terrible. All night I would get up and make sure he had the right medicines and water by his bed. I was so concerned that I was in a sleepy daze, so I would check the prescription bottle over and over to make sure he wasn't getting too much of something or the wrong medication.

It was a beautiful Saturday in late September. The leaves were changing colors; you could hear the neighbors mowing their lawns or bustling their kids around for activities. Our biggest activity so far had been moving from the bedroom to the couch. We were having a lazy day but had every window in the house open. A few days cooped up in a hospital room had provided a reminder of how wonderful it is to have fresh air flowing through our living space.

My phone was buzzing all day. Family and friends were asking what they could do for us and wanted to find out more about what had happened. I knew we were incredibly lucky to have this support network, but I started getting a bit anxious that all of the updates and messages would likely be flowing through me, given Tom's upcoming treatments. I figured it was best to blog our updates to keep everyone informed about what was going on – and keep it consistent. I had already received messages that made it clear information wasn't getting around accurately. It's like the game of telephone where one person starts the phrase and whispers to the person next to them. It's almost always transformed into something that makes no sense by the time it gets around the circle. It was never ill intended; it happens when things get relayed through people, especially when it comes to medical terms.

I was on the couch watching a movie with Tom when I created the blog. I couldn't figure out what to name the blog – I wanted to be clever but not insensitive. Tom and I came up with a bunch of different names, and we changed the title almost ten times until we landed on Life's Adventures: Cancer Edition. It seemed to put our situation simply: it was a life adventure, not one we had ever hoped for or wanted but an adventure nonetheless. I had to add the Cancer Edition partly because an edition implied that there would be a beginning and an end. We were going to beat this thing. The cancer adventure would end with a cancer-free diagnosis; that was our intent from the beginning.

The blog was empty and there was a placeholder that showed where the first post would be located. On the bottom right was a big blue button that said "New Post" – the pressure was on. I wrote a few things, then deleted them, then wrote again and continued this back and forth. A writer's block wasn't the greatest start to my blogging career, but I realized why it was difficult. I needed to write a letter to our friends and family first that shared the news and then guide them to the blog. I wrote the basics on the blog post and then focused on writing the email. Each name I put in the "To" made me more grateful for the amazing group of friends and family that I knew would have our backs. Then the hard part came, writing the message. It took a few versions before I read it out loud to Tom to get his thoughts.

Hi, Everyone,

As many of you may or may not know, our life took an unexpected turn when Tom was diagnosed with cancer this week. We had an incredible forty-eight hours of life that changed Tom from a healthy thirty-year old on Tuesday to a cancer patient by Friday. We have been so touched and overwhelmed by everyone's support and are confident that we can beat this thing. Tom and I are incredibly fortunate to have an amazing group of family and friends and have created the blog below so that we can keep people updated instead of the mass communications that would be required to keep everyone in the loop. We want our focus to be on Tom, and his recovery as much as possible and less on making tons of calls, etc. Please know in our perfect world we would be able to call each of you individually, but that is just unrealistic for what lies ahead for us.

So many people have asked what they can do to help. We are SO SO SO appreciative, and we certainly may take you up on that when we know what help we need as we get more answers about the upcoming treatment rigor, etc. For now, we have two things that would be incredibly helpful:

1. Please feel free to forward the link below on to others via email that you think may care or want to know but please keep this situation, and the link to the site, off all social media. In the extensive research that we have been immersed in over the past few days we have found several reasons for this, the most important being that there are some very mean people in the world that then know when we are away from the house for treatments, etc. and we come become a target for more chaos. We certainly don't want to add to this equation. I personally have faith in humankind, but again, to limit our risk would be our ideal situation.

2. For local folks, if you could please call or text before you come by we would be forever grateful. We will be on a funky schedule, trying to catch sleep when we can, have good days and bad days, and managing some gnarly symptoms so this will be incredibly helpful and super important for what will be a long few months. We will find more about the chemo treatments this week, but we do know he is going to need to have very limited exposure to people/crowds/etc. during certain stages of his treatment due to his weakened immune system. We certainly want all the love around us, but we just want to make sure we keep everyone safe and ensure he is staying on track with the recovery process.

26

So in advance, THANK YOU. We already feel like those two words don't even convey what we feel for all the support we have received. Thank you for the love, your understanding and your prayers.

xoxo, Honore and Tom

"Wow, babe – that's really good," Tom replied.

"Are you good if I send?" I asked.

"Yup – go for it. This should be interesting," he replied.

There were several people that were on this email that we knew would be hearing this news for the first time. I wish I could have called every single one of them, but I knew that wasn't reasonable, and quite frankly I could still hardly talk about it without choking up. Before I sent it, I also wanted Tom to hear what I had posted on the blog. He liked the first post, and we agreed that he would be my unofficial editor and that I wouldn't post anything unless we both agreed that we were comfortable posting it.

"Sent," I stated as I looked over to Tom and let out a sigh.

I started wondering what people would think when they opened the email. It was late on a Saturday night by the time I sent it, so I figured some people would likely not read it until Sunday or Monday. Tom forwarded the email on to some of his friends and his coworkers, and we sat on the couch reading out loud the different replies. We eventually went to bed and were lying in bed chatting.

"What was the blog post again? Sorry, I know you just read it to me," he asked. I pulled it up on my phone and read it out loud to him:

9.19 - And So We Fight

What we know so far: (1) Tom has been diagnosed with cancer. (2) We have an amazing network of friends and family that have got us in contact with some of the best doctors in the US. (3) We will absolutely, positively, no doubt in our minds, beat this.

That's all we've got right now. The next 3-4 days will be more appointments, follow-ups and a treatment plan. We will be posting on here what we can. It will be raw; it may be funny some days and hard to read other days. So, hang in there with us, and we will be sure to keep everyone informed. On our first night in the hospital I obnoxiously curled up in the tiny hospital bed with Tom and we chatted for hours and got ourselves a plan to beat this thing. Lots more to come and thank you all for the support!

"I can't wait to beat this," Tom said as he wrapped his arms around me and closed his eyes.

"Me too, babe, me too," I softly replied as we fell asleep.

PART 2
My Preparations

I remember hearing my mom's voice on the other end of the phone. She was supposed to be on her way to pick me up from college. It was the last day of my freshman year, and I was excited to be heading home for the summer. I had made the best friends at college and loved my freshman year, except for the studying part, but I was eager for summer back home in Milwaukee. I had an internship lined up and was also waitressing at night at a new restaurant in my neighborhood. Mom was supposed to pick me up; we were going to spend the night at a hotel before the six-hour drive home from Cincinnati for my busy summer to begin.

"Hi there, little change of plans. Cousin Dan is on his way from Chicago to pick you up later today," my mom said with an emotion-filled voice.

"Wait, what? What's wrong?" I asked.

"Your dad really isn't feeling well, and he needs to go to the hospital. He will be fine; I just need to be here in case we need to make any decisions and he's on pain medicine. Just get yourself packed up; you guys are going to turn around and come right home."

"Are you kidding? Is Dad going to be okay? I haven't even really packed yet because I had my last exam this morning and thought I would have time this afternoon," I said, getting more concerned about my dad's condition.

"Just get your things together and call me when you are on the road," she replied.

I didn't know what was happening, but I called my roommate and filled her in. She hurried back to the dorm to help me pack everything up and say our goodbyes. She called her mom, who had quickly become my mom away from home and had her come say goodbye too. We had become instant best friends from the moment we met, and despite being random roommates never had a single fight our entire first year living together. We were like bread and butter and saying goodbye for the summer added to an already emotional morning.

The word had spread that I would be leaving early, and friends were swinging by to say farewell. My cousin had pulled up to the dorm and came up to help carry things down. I remember showing him our now bare room. I had all my stuff lined up in the hallway. We chatted for a few moments and then figured we better pack up the car. I walked out of my dorm room to see all of my friends each grabbing a box and taking it down to the car for us. I literally carried nothing but my purse, a tote and my dorm key. In less than five minutes we had the entire car packed, and I was giving hugs all around. I remember feeling so supported in this moment despite being completely confused about what the situation was at home. It was the longest car ride of my life.

We pulled into Chicago late that evening and crashed at my cousin's house. I was getting up first thing in the morning and driving the rest of the way to Milwaukee and was up with the sun to hit the road. I drove my cousin's car straight to the hospital – the car completely full of everything I owned. I walked into the ICU and saw my dad lying in the hospital bed.

"Hi, baby," he said, trying to put on a strong face but in quite a bit of pain.

"Hi, Dad!" I happily replied, relieved to have my eyes on him. I reached down to give him a big hug and then went over to my mom to do the same.

They weren't quite sure what was going on, but Dad was in a lot of pain, and they were trying to figure out what had caused it. It hurt him to stand up or lie down, and my mom had been trying to get him to see a doctor for a few days before ultimately coming to the hospital. While I was in the hospital room, the ER doctor recommended seeing a specialist and they would be releasing my dad.

After filling in my parents on my exams, I eventually left the hospital to get things settled at home. I had missed home so much in my first year away at college, and as I drove, I realized that I was going back to a different life than the one I had left. Within days, my dad was undergoing a very dangerous surgery that could alter his abilities for the rest of his life.

I remember waiting in a family cube in the surgery waiting room that each family was assigned. There were a few chairs and a phone in each cube, and we tried to keep ourselves distracted. I remember looking over at my mom and wondering what she must be thinking. Since the moment I had gotten home, she had been so calm, dealing with the facts, calling people that could help us get a plan and never seemed flustered. She explained things simply and even taught my sister and I along the way about what she was doing and why she was doing it. I was nineteen at the time my sister was twenty-one. We were obviously old enough to understand exactly what was happening as it related to the medical side of things, but it's not often in life that your parent has a chance to really break down and explain how insurance works or how to handle doctors and second opinions. My mom was stoic – she always kept everything together. If I knew then that I was getting one of the most important lessons of my life I would have paid even closer attention.

Dad's recovery was a long one. He had to relearn how to walk. The task of getting him in and out of a chair could take half an hour. I was his cheerleader that entire summer. My sister had an internship out of state, so it was my mom and I getting him healthy again. I would work my internship in the morning and then have a break for a few hours before I would work the dinner shift at a restaurant – ironically, the place I met Tom. Caregiving came quite naturally to me, and I wanted to do anything in my power to get my dad better. Most days, I would come home, and we would have lunch together, and then I'd take him on

30

a walk. In those first days, we wouldn't even make it to the corner, but each day we went a little farther. Eventually, we walked around the entire block. It took almost forty-five minutes, but we did it. Most days, we would watch *Cold Case* on TV while I rested after his walk and before my shift.

I remember about ten weeks into his recovery; I had started to doze off on the couch on a cold and rainy afternoon before work. I heard Dad moving around and opened one eye slightly to see what he was doing and if he needed help. He had been getting out of the chair on his own for only a few days, and though hard, he was able to do it. I figured I'd let him try to get up and then see if there were anything I could to do help. I kept my eyes closed, peeking occasionally. I watched him slowly, but surely, get himself out of the chair and grab his walker. It took all I had to not get up to help him. He turned and walked towards the sun room – not where I had expected him to go – and reached for a blanket on the chair. He draped it on the side of his walker and turned back towards the chair. He passed his chair and came over to the couch where he fanned open the blanket and laid it across me. I kept my eyes closed as he did this and listened as I heard him turn around and get himself back into the chair. I tucked my head down into the blanket and tears rolled down my face. For the first time in weeks, I felt like a daughter again. Not one of his caregivers, not a nineteen-year-old who was learning about the harsh realities of life in real time, but just his daughter, who looked cold on the couch as she dozed off between jobs. I never actually fell asleep, and I never told him that I had watched him that day as he tried so hard to take care of me.

I thought about those months of Dad's recovery many times as we were getting ready to meet with doctors for second opinions in the days after Tom's diagnosis. I thought about how Mom had handled everything and tried to stay strong in moments that I wanted to just crumble. She had communicated with family so simply; I knew I had to try to do the same.

Sept. 20 - The Million-Dollar Questions
Tom and I have learned quite a bit in the last week - the most jarring being how quickly life can change. Suddenly, trips that were planned are on hold, priorities shift and we start to embrace the new normal. Among all the messages etc., a few million-dollar questions keep coming up:

*1. **Were there any symptoms**? Did we expect this was coming? No, 100 percent no. On Tuesday, Tom got up early, went for a run, and felt a little weird when he got home. He showered, went to work, was pretty fatigued Tuesday night with a cough, but nothing completely unusual. We figured he maybe was catching a cold or bug. We were up throughout the night Tuesday as the cough worsened and he started feeling worse. In the wee hours of the morning we* *made the decision to head to the ER and the rest is history.*

*2. **What type of cancer is this**? Well, it's rare. Because if you're going to get cancer, you might as well be unique. It has been diagnosed as a germ cell tumor that is currently located in his chest. He is late Stage 3.*

*3. **Has it spread**? Luckily, no. For now, we are dealing with the primary tumor with no additional cancer tumors in his body.*

*4. **What's Next**? Chemo. A long rigorous sequence of chemo and surgery, but one that we hope will completely remove the cancer from his body. We are very optimistic that with the right treatment we will beat this cancer. More to come over the next week as we meet with doctors and get ourselves a plan. Hope this helps!*

Who I Was

Since I was a little girl, I've always had compassion for people. I've always wondered what made other people tick and was always curious about everyone else's story. I remember during my eighth-grade conference, my teacher told my parents that my biggest issue was that kids in class relied on me to solve their problems. In hindsight, I suppose that was true. I didn't necessarily want to save everyone, but as far back as I can remember, I always thought I could help or make a difference. It came very naturally to me. For some reason, I put off a comfortable vibe, and most people open up to me quickly. If there is something I've learned over the years of having this quality, it's that everyone has a story, as I believe Oprah has said many times. There is no truer statement. Good, bad, happy, sad, regardless of the circumstances, everyone has a story, and with every story there is something to learn. Sometimes this quality was a curse; sometimes it was a blessing.

These qualities are a huge part of me – but sometimes they got lost in the hustle of the day to day. I think sometimes, would I get that same RESPECT award I received in grade school for the way I'm acting right now? Am I a person I would want to hang out with? As I've grown up, I've realized that so much of the day-to-day things in life challenge us to stay true to who we are at our core. Not that we intentionally let ourselves wander, but the focus on tasks and activities make it easy to turn life into a checklist rather than a philosophy. I knew that what we were about to experience was going to test every component of my personality.

One of the first times that Tom and I hung out we grabbed lunch after a shift we had worked together. We had quite a deep conversation for a first time hanging out – and I remember his face when I told him about how I try to live my life.

"Do you ever think about how big the world is?" I asked.

"Yeah, it's amazing how small our communities are in relation to the world," he replied.

"Right – so in my mind – there are billions and billions of people in the world. And in the big scheme of things, I'll only get to meet a select few of them. I guess I try to live in a way that if I get to be one of the handfuls of people someone meets in their lifetime that I make it worth it for them."

A little side smirk came across Tom's face as he nodded and looked directly in my eyes. It was that exact moment that I knew he'd be sticking around for a while. He seemed to understand me, and that wasn't an easy task.

A traumatic event like a cancer diagnosis puts everyone under a magnifying glass – sometimes highlighting the best qualities and inevitably shining a light on an area that may need a little refinement. I promised myself I would be true to who I was – but I knew I was about to change and I'll be damned if it wasn't going to be for the better.

Sept. 23 – Late Night Thoughts
In our attempt to keep things positive, and maybe have some good come out of our crappy situation, we were doing some thinking. We like to consider ourselves compassionate and positive people; we like to pay it forward, do nice things for people and/or strangers, and of course over tip nice servers since we both worked in the service world. Last week, as we were driving home from the hospital, Tom said to me, "Do people know how sick I am?" Oofta. Hit me right in the heart, but certainly an interesting perspective.

From the outside looking in, he looks like a normal thirty-year-old guy, and we look like your normal young couple, but dang, that is just the surface. Fast forward to that afternoon when I was picking up the prescriptions and the woman at the counter was irritated that I had a question – my immediate reaction was to want to yell out, "My husband was just diagnosed with cancer and I'm scared and I need help from the pharmacist." But she has no idea….

Now, why do I say all this? Not because I want the world to know our problems, or feel bad for us, or treat us any differently, but because you truly don't know what that stranger next to you is going through. Of course, there are a handful of rude and mean people in the world because they simply are rude or mean people, but if we've learned anything this week, it is to have even more compassion – because you never know what the person next to you is going through.

The Magic 8 Ball

The week following Tom's diagnosis was full of appointments. We were getting second opinions, meeting with his boss, figuring out work and dealing with what felt like a never-ending conversation with our insurance company. It felt strange to be going about our lives knowing how sick Tom was as we hustled through the week. While he still had quite a bit of pain from his cough, other than that, you wouldn't know from looking at him that he was sick.

Our most important appointment of the week was with a specialist at the University of Chicago. We had received this doctor's name from several people and were going to get a second opinion on treatment. We arrived and got caught in the maze of the giant hospital – our local hospital was much calmer and felt much more relaxed than the environment we had walked into. Signs pointed to hundreds of buildings and parking lots. There was a noticeable hustle and energy in the air as we walked into the big atrium of the building we needed to be in – and had somehow managed to find.

We made our way to the doctor's waiting room and dropped off the twenty-four pages of paperwork that addressed every question except for my bra size. We went back, and the doctor eventually came in to see us – Tom immediately nudged me as I smirked upon the doctor's entrance into the room. I had told Tom on the way down that not only was this guy well regarded in his field, he was pretty damn cute too. Tom had oh-so-lovingly rolled his eyes at the time, but I think he knew I was right when the doctor strolled into the room. We chatted and gave him all the copies of scans and reports. He left the room to review them, which was prime opportunity for me to try to get Tom to admit that this guy was good looking. I was trying to keep things light-hearted – even if I had to go to a superficial level.

The doctor came back into the room and discussed what he saw – he recommended a completely different treatment from the one we had heard from our oncologist. In fact, he was recommending a treatment that our oncologist had told us about, but she had given us a litany of reasons that she wouldn't advise that treatment. In that moment I felt like the ball of a pinball machine. We had just been shot up the side and had to navigate our way through obstacles that we hoped would get us to the finish line instead of some unexpected route that maybe didn't lead us where we intended to go. How were we supposed to know what questions to ask? Who was I supposed to trust and where the hell was the Rosetta Stone for medical language? I felt like my mind was going into a tunnel again and my brain was trying to do too much at once, much like when he was diagnosed. When the doctor finished talking, he asked us to go upstairs to see one of his colleagues about the surgery, to supplement his recommendation on treating the cancer. He said the doctor was willing to squeeze us in since he wanted to see Tom. The only advantage to Tom's rare cancer was that doctors wanted to see us; we were seeing the best of the best with very little effort required to get our foot in the door.

We walked upstairs to see the surgeon. His waiting room was also the waiting room for the chemo patients. We checked in and sat in the atrium area where the sunlight was streaming in. We were looking towards the waiting room area and the check-in desk and quietly watched everything happening around us. We briefly talked about what the doctor had told us, but we kept getting distracted with all the movement around us. It seemed like every person around us was either bald or had on a scarf. These were all people in the heart of their cancer fight – this was like looking from the outside into the future and what we were about to experience.

There was a man in a wheelchair that was causing quite a ruckus. His wife had a walker and was trying to get someone to help her because she said that her husband's medications were making him act goofy. He was making comments that made no sense and walking his wheelchair in circles with his feet on the ground. He would randomly erupt with laughter and then start singing "Sweet Caroline." Normally, I would finish the line of the song from "Sweet Caroline" with BOP BOP BOP or would be amused by a character like this, but I was becoming terrified. I felt like we were watching zombies around us, and this man's laughter was making me want to cover my ears and look away. I heard the wife yelling at the receptionist – look at what this chemo is doing to him – I need to talk to a doctor. The longer they were there, the more I started to breathe fast; I kept looking at Tom, and most importantly avoiding eye contact with the man in the wheel chair. My heart broke for this man and his wife, but it was clear that eye contact with someone was what made him react, so I was avoiding it at all costs.

We had been waiting for about thirty minutes with no guarantee of when we would see the doctor and we had another appointment in the afternoon. We had seen the doctor we had come to see – I glanced at Tom who also looked like this crowd was having an impact on him.

"We need to go. I'm sorry; I can't handle this. We can come back and see him when we are closer to the surgery."

He didn't say a word. He got up, grabbed my hand, and we walked towards the elevator. I walked with my head down the entire way. We got on the elevator, and I had my pointer and middle finger on my mouth, playing with my lip. I was trying my hardest not to cry. I was panicky and was terrified that Tom would become that confused man.

"That was more than I could handle – I'm so sorry, I feel like everything just hit me," I said to him.

He took the half step from the other side of the elevator and gave me a hug, my hand still on my face.

"It's okay," he said as he squeezed me. As he pulled away, he tucked my hair behind my ear.

"If you start going crazy – I'm not sure what I'm going to do. I need you to stay with me during this," I said.

As the doors of the elevator opened, he nodded his head. "I will – but if anything happens – you should record me so we can become famous on YouTube."

He started to smirk – not sure if I was in the mood to joke yet. I let out a giggle as I took a deep breath. "You drive me absolutely crazy."

We walked off the elevator, hand in hand, and headed towards the car. I still was walking with my head down as we navigated the crowd. Tom double squeezed my hand, and I looked up at him. He didn't say a word – he just smiled – and that was all I needed.

Later that week we met with our original oncologist. After lots of discussion and research, we knew that we had been lucky enough to have been assigned to one of the best oncologists around. We had met with her the day after all our other appointments and discussed the treatment plan. We had several questions based on things we had heard from other doctors, and she talked through every single question with us and never made us feel dumb. After we all agreed on the direction we were headed, she walked us through each of Tom's three chemo drugs and all of the side effects that we could anticipate. I'm convinced it would have been a shorter conversation had she told us what wouldn't happen as a result of these drugs. These were hard things to hear – how did these drugs become our best option? Hair loss, hearing loss, potential damage to his bladder or liver or heart, confusion, nausea – the list seemed to go on forever.

We left that day feeling like we had a roadmap of sorts. I wouldn't say we felt in control by any stretch of the imagination, but we at least knew we had a plan. Tom is a very data and fact-driven guy, and now he had been told what he needed to do. I never doubted for a minute that he would do it.

Sept. 24 – Let's Do This

We are officially on day nine of our new "normal." I have to say, it's been incredibly weird that some hours have felt like days (typically when we were waiting for results/doctors), and yet, in reality, the last nine days have been a complete whirlwind. We knew when we got the diagnosis that we would have to move quickly, so I went into turbo mode, and we had quite the lineup of follow-up appointments, second opinions, and much more this week. (Translation: A ton of paperwork.) We are fortunate to live near some of the best doctors in the U.S. and were able to go to University of Chicago Hospital & Rush Hospital for second and third opinions this week. We found out some interesting facts along the way, the most mind-blowing being that less than 400 people per year in the U.S. have the type of cancer Tom has. Hence why it was so important to get second opinions and seek out doctors who have seen this type of rare cancer before.

After taking all the information and attempting to process it, we finally have ourselves a plan. Obviously, I use the word plan loosely because so much of this is going to evolve as we go and see how Tom is reacting and how well the tumor is shrinking, but it's a short-term plan nonetheless. So Monday begins what will be quite an adventure for the next several weeks. Tom will be having surgery for his port – we are affectionately referring to this as his Iron Man Surgery. Then, as mentioned, we are moving quickly so chemo starts Tuesday. Tom will be receiving one of the most intense types of chemo treatment possible for a few reasons (1) the type of cancer he has (2) his age (3) we make sure this thing doesn't spread. After our first week of chemo, Tom will have two weeks off, and then we start it all over again. We know this is going to be tough, we know he is going to have to fight hard, but we are ready to get treatment started.

To prepare, we met with our oncologist and went through everything to expect in great detail. After going through all the symptoms of his chemo regimen with us, Tom jokingly replied, "This is like the commercials you see on TV that once you hear all the symptoms/side effects of the drug, you think why the heck would anyone ever take that?" A valid point. But if this gets us to cancer free then we will manage the symptoms and carry on. Despite what has been an emotional week with lots of decisions, we are incredibly grateful for the team of doctors we have and how comfortable they have all made us feel in this process. So now we relax this weekend and prepare for next week…

Medically Limited

I am one of the lucky girls who married one of the most romantic, caring, and loving man a girl could wish for. Three years before this mess, I had a medically busy month with my first ever colonoscopy followed two weeks later by getting my wisdom teeth pulled out. Tom didn't miss a beat, and I remember thinking what a wonderful caretaker he was. He was stern when I tried to avoid listening to the doctor's orders but was never mean. He did things for me that I never said out loud but had thought about asking him to do. He figured them all out and did it anyway. He curled up next to me and was miserable with me, even though I know post wisdom teeth surgery I had the breath of a lion.

I probably thanked him a hundred times in those few weeks, and his reply was always the same. "Don't thank me. I'm your husband, I love taking care of you, but I hate to see you sick." Despite this very minor hiccup of a few weeks, we had been very healthy throughout our relationship; minus a few injuries from poor decisions after a beer or four.

About a year before our wedding, I was pushing Tom to go to the dentist. His fear of dentists and needles had resulted in him not seeing a dentist in almost eight years. With my sweet tooth, I would have already had dentures if I hadn't gone to the dentist in that long. He told me he wasn't a fan of the dentist and especially hated needles. Of course he hated needles; no one enjoys needles. No one wakes up hoping that they are going to get a needle jammed in their gum and drool like a teething child. I gave him a hard time, thinking he was just being a bit dramatic and ultimately found a great dentist for both of us. I told him I'd come with him to his appointment, and surprisingly he didn't argue.

Fast forward to him in the dentist chair and the dentist preparing the needle for the Novocain, and suddenly I felt terrible. First, I had been giving him such a hard time about the needles, which any good wife would do, thinking he wasn't *actually* that afraid of needles and second, I was worried he would never forgive me for bringing him to the dentist. I could see him start to panic; I told him to close his eyes so he didn't see the needle and grabbed his hand so he could squeeze mine when the Novocain went in. In all seriousness, it took everything I had not to laugh. This amazingly tough guy couldn't stomach a needle and a little dental work? If only I knew then what I know now.

On our way to his port surgery, we reminisced about his first dental experience as I tried to keep his mind off the surgery. It was sunny; his teeth looked great thanks to me, and this procedure seemed like the beginning of something that we wanted so desperately to end.

Sept. 28 - Iron Man Surgery

What. A. Day. Our day began bright and early at the hospital for Tom's Iron Man (port) surgery, and despite some nerves – he has never "gone under" before – we were ready to get this thing in and get treatment going. After a brief delay, he was wheeled down to the radiology surgical area and we met with the doctor who showed us the port and walked us through the procedure.

The port is in Tom's upper right chest and is a double-line port – he's got the Cadillac of ports – so that he can use the port to both receive chemo and also take out blood for the various testing required throughout this process. Ultimately, this fancy port eliminates the need for him to get pricked repeatedly and damage his veins. Small victories.

The actual port procedure was only about thirty minutes; the longer part was getting him in twilight and comfortable before and after the procedure. He was wheeled back to his pre-surgical room and had a little breakfast and boom – we were on our way home. I love an efficient operation.

He relaxed this afternoon, got some rest and tomorrow we begin chemo. Chemo sort of feels like this dimly lit road that we know we have to walk down but don't quite know the way. We know all the side effects that COULD happen; we know it's likely not going to be pleasant, but until we do it, we won't know what to expect. Here's hoping this is as pleasant as possible!

Highlights of today include:
1.   A nurse who didn't feel bad for ripping out Tom's arm hair. As she pulled off the IV tape she said "This is payback for the fact that men get to stand to pee."
2.   I'm getting comfortable in our new home away from home at the hospital and creating efficient cup holders with medical equipment.
3.   For the first time in almost two weeks, Tom didn't feel nauseous for a brief time! To make the most of this appetite before chemo starting tomorrow I got him whatever he was craving (and crossed my fingers he didn't request our favorite pasta dish from our trip to Venice, Italy). Lucky for me he was just craving Outback!
4.   While picking up a prescription for Tom, I got pulled over. I can summarize by saying I should have been a lawyer. I was lucky enough to get myself out of a big 'ol ticket.

We will update everyone on chemo soon– thanks for all the love and prayers!

40

Dazed and Confused

The automatic doors slid open as we approached the ER the next morning. We had to go to the ER to get admitted to the hospital for Tom's chemo, and he wasn't coming alone; he was bringing his wife as a roommate. Every single moment of this day was a piece of the puzzle of this unknown chemo world. We already knew we would feel better once we got done with the first cycle since we would know what to expect.

We checked in and waited as they processed our arrival and got a transport wheelchair. An older gentleman came over and asked Tom to get in the wheelchair. He would be taking us up to our room on the oncology floor. I was hoping that we would see some of the familiar faces from our first visit so that Tom would feel comfortable. We went through the maze of halls, turning left and right, getting on elevators and ultimately ended up in our room. 241. One room down from our original stay – we were moving on up!

The room was the mirror image of our first room. I put our stuff down, and Tom grabbed the gown on the bed and began to change. I looked at our surroundings, and my chest started to feel heavy. It felt like we were walking into a jail cell. Tom wasn't feeling great from his port surgery the day before, and we were about to have five days of unknown adventures in this tiny little space. Right as I started to get panicky, Nancy appeared at the door.

We hadn't seen her since our diagnosis stay, and she was eager to hear about how the last week and a half had transpired. We filled her in as she was getting a bunch of needles, gauze and tape ready to use Tom's port for the first time. She was on one side of the bed, closest to Tom's port, and I was on the other holding his hand. She took off the bandages from yesterday's procedure, and it was quite the scene, lots of bruising and swelling and two little bumps where the nurse would put the needle. She patiently walked us through everything she was doing and then prepared Tom for the first of the two needle insertions. I decided to sit on the side of his bed. I hoped he thought it was to be closer to him; actually I was getting a little queasy. The first needle went in as Tom squeezed my hand hard: one down, one to go. The second one followed quickly after, and the part I knew he was really dreading was officially over. In hindsight, it was the worst activity of the day.

Nancy started to explain what would be happening; we would do premeds and fluids, followed by three bags of chemo, each lasting about an hour. With the second bag, Tom would be put on an IV of drugs to protect his bladder that would drip for the entire time we were at the hospital and was the official time clock for our ability to leave the hospital. Each bag lasted twenty-four hours and coincided with the second bag of chemo on day one, so we knew the approximate timing for our Sunday departure. Everything was new; everything that was happening was something we never experienced before, so I felt helpless not knowing what to do or ask as his advocate.

My job was generous enough to let me work remotely from the hospital during Tom's chemo so I could be there for him and help with all of the comings and goings of doctors and decisions. And, of course, bring some humor to the room. Fortunately, I work in change management and communications so working from a hospital was possible. It wasn't going to be easy, but I was determined to make it work. I set up my laptop and was working throughout the day as we progressed through our first day of chemo. Mid-morning, our first bag of chemo arrived. Nancy had on a special gown, special gloves, and was handling the bag very carefully. I remember looking at her, taking all these precautions, following very strict protocols and thinking, that's going _in_ Tom's body. The basic concept of chemo is that making someone very sick will make them better – but that was still a struggle to comprehend. The seriousness of these chemo drugs didn't help with my ability to understand cancer.

The first day of chemo was a blur; it felt like it went very fast, and we were waiting for him to suddenly feel terrible. Our nurses told us he wouldn't feel great but not to expect some sort of epic shift. As the afternoon wore on, we continued to dominate with our answers on _Price is Right_ and _Family Feud_ and I was wrapping up work for the day and preparing for Tom's parents to arrive with dinner. We had arranged for dinner at the hospital each night – which at first I felt terrible about – but came to terms with because it was such a great motivator for Tom. He powered through chemo each day and then got to have some company and good food to celebrate in the evening. It ended up being something that we looked forward to every day and helped propel us through six long hospital days.

As I shut my computer, I asked Tom how he was doing.

"Better than I anticipated so far, but I have a feeling that won't last much longer."

"I know, babe, but to feel better than expected for one of these days is awesome and hopefully a good sign for the week to come."

"I know. How are you doing? It's like we are in jail together."

It didn't feel like jail to me at all; in fact, I was sort of enjoying this random time we were having together – him rolling his eyes or trying to make me laugh while on a conference call, the hug he gave me every time I got up to unplug his IV machine so he could wheel it to the bathroom. It was only the first day, but we had already started a few traditions.

"It's not like jail, babe, though I will say I'd much rather be having dinner on the beach in Aruba again."

Tom and I had gone to Aruba for our honeymoon, which was also his first international trip. He was as excited as the eight-year-old in front of us to get a stamp on his passport as we went through customs, and we were so excited to have a few days in paradise. Our resort had a restaurant that they built each night on the beach and when you checked in at the host stand you took off your shoes. We had decided that dinner there would be our splurge for our honeymoon and booked it for our second-to-last night. The sun was setting as they seated us and we curled our toes into the sand under our table just a few feet away from where the waves were crashing on the shore. This was a dining experience unlike anything we had experienced. The food was unbelievable, and the wine was fantastic. Our meal was almost two and a half hours long, and it felt like we were in a movie. As it got darker, they lit candles all around the restaurant, and live jazz music was playing back near the bar. A soft breeze was coming off the ocean; there was the smell of salt in the air, and the weather was perfect. I never wanted that meal to end – I almost got a second dessert so dinner wouldn't have to end. I could have sat there all night.

As I looked at Tom lying in his hospital bed, I couldn't help but wonder if I would have done anything differently if I had a crystal ball and knew what was to come. I wouldn't have. I lived in that moment; I can still smell the air when I think about it, still taste the food and still remember the headache from the wine the next morning. Those moments and memories all had somehow prepared us for everything we were about to deal with. Today, what put a smile on our face was being able to talk about how amazing that meal was, how lucky we were to have been there, and to discuss where we could go on a trip when this was all over.

Sept. 29 - One Down, Nineteen to Go
Well....so far, so good. Actually no; so far, so great! We've conquered Day One, with nineteen more days of chemo to go (stretched across the next twelve weeks, but nonetheless, we will be counting down the number of days of chemo!). We checked into the hospital this morning, and Tom received his first blast of chemo. During chemo he is on a constant drip of fluids and preventative treatments in addition to chemo treatments throughout the day.

The port proved to be a great decision on our part, as it has made this much easier on Tom, and it's clear that as we have these sessions in the upcoming months that it will make things quicker and more efficient too. We sort of were waiting for the symptoms to rear their ugly heads all day, but for the most part his body responded quite well. Now, we recognize that this is only day one, and often symptoms don't appear until someone has had the treatment multiple days.... but we are just so grateful that he is feeling better than we expected.

43

Set the bar low and you'll always be satisfied – right? I'm sure there is a motivational poster out there somewhere with those exact words on it. We are incredibly grateful for the amazing staff of nurses here who have been so accommodating, educational and helpful. They are truly walking angels on earth! Here's to hoping that Day Two is even better than Day One...and that Tom doesn't beat me twice in UNO again tomorrow night.

July 10

It's my favorite day of the year, July 10th, my birthday. Since I was a kid, I have absolutely *loved* my birthday. I remember distinctly when it happened too. I was turning five years old and that entire day everything just kept coming up Honore. Cake, balloons, friends, family, presents, you name it; it was all wrapped into one day. To top it off I got a Little Mermaid lunchbox for kindergarten, a bike, and a tire swing. What more does a five-year-old need?

I never grew out of it. I have countdowns to my birthday every year and am slightly embarrassed by the number of people that call me on January 10th, my half birthday, or that call me on July 9th, my birthday eve. I recognize it's a bit crazy, but as I've gotten older, it became less about me and more about the concept of a birthday as a whole. What is it about a birthday that makes the day feel different? Even on calmer birthdays, the day does feel special, it feels different, and it feels like you own that day. You make sure to look nice, maybe splurge on something you wouldn't otherwise splurge on that day. More than that, it's about the celebration of what a birthday signifies.

As I got older, and the realities of life became more obvious, I realized that it wasn't about just my birthday; it was on behalf of everyone who didn't get their birthdays that year. My entire life, as expected, there was loss. Grandparents, family, and friends – the inevitable happens and people are suddenly no longer with us. I don't take for granted one single day that I get another day and I especially don't take for granted that I get another birthday each year. It's a privilege.

Unfortunately for Tom, it's a privilege that requires a lot of effort on his part, because he always tries to make my birthday extra special. When I met Tom, he wasn't big on birthdays. I think part of this was due to his early December birthday – I think all December birthdays get cheated a bit. However, to him it was just another day. It took several years, and perhaps some over-the- top celebrations, but eventually I got him more excited about his birthday. I remember on his 27th birthday, he wanted to do something more extravagant and sensed my hesitation about how much it would cost. I don't even remember what exactly it was, though as I reasoned with him, he pulled out the zinger, "But it's my birthday; we need to celebrate." Damn! I had created a monster, and I wasn't even mad about it, I was proud!

On my twenty-first birthday, I had a blowout. I was home in Milwaukee and my parents were throwing me a party with friends and family coming in from all over. We had a big party in the back yard, which eventually evolved to keg stands and ultimately resulted in all the "young ones" heading out to the bar. We had a blast. All my closest friends were partying with me, and Tom kept a careful eye on me all night.

Drink after drink we bounced around the bars, and I managed to get a free three-foot blow-up Jägermeister shark that I named Sergio. I had been a bit overserved by the bartender and took a moment to step outside the bar and get some fresh air. Tom followed me, and we strolled down the block to the Wasted Weiner, a small hut-like place to get a hot dog late at night. Maybe it was the booze, but that was the best damn hot dog I ever had. I managed to sit on the curb as Tom paid and proceeded to sit on the edge of the curb next to me. I was eating my hot dog, with a twenty-first birthday crown on my head. I'm sure I was the picture of beauty, but Tom still gave me a kiss or two despite my face being covered in ketchup as I drunkenly rambled. I think he had had one drink that night. He had fully intended on taking care of me that night so I could have the best time. Tom was a few years older than me, and I met him when he was already twenty-one, so I never was able to repay the favor.

Hours later as all of my girlfriends and I filed back into my parents' house, Tom helped Sergio the shark and me into the house and helped me get settled. My friends and I had taken over the house for the weekend so we had people sleeping on every couch and in every bed. I had offered to sleep on the couch on the enclosed front porch and Tom got me situated as I repeatedly told him I loved him. I laid my head down and dozed off, as I had partied hard. I remember waking up for just a moment shortly after I had dozed off as Tom was sliding a garbage can near my head.

"There is a garbage can here if you need it, babe, I love you," he said as he kissed me on the forehead.

"I love you too – July 10th is the best day ever," I drunkenly replied.

Sept. 30 - Two Down, Eighteen to Go

Well, we are cautiously optimistic again this evening as we have finished Day Two. Today was certainly a bit tougher as it was a second day of very intense treatment and it continues to wear down his body – however, all in all, still a good day. Two down, hopefully only eighteen more to go. Tom received the same chemo cocktail today as he did yesterday. It is made up of three different drugs. We decided that if this chemo was an actual cocktail and had a taste, it would either be a gross rail gin or one of those terrible shots with Tabasco sauce in it. (Tom then proceeded to have flashbacks to his twenty-first birthday – oh, to be in our early twenties again...) You'd be amazed what you end up talking about when you're distracting someone from chemo.

We were reminiscing this evening how this all started just two weeks ago today. It's amazing that in fourteen days we were able to figure out that Tom had a rare cancer, meet with a slew of doctors, get a treatment plan, have surgery and already be two days into chemo. I truly believe the speed with which we did this (and needed to do this) is part of the reason we are going to beat this thing. In the past two weeks amongst all the chaos, we have learned to celebrate the little victories, be grateful for all that we do have, and are trying to do things that make us feel "normal." For example, our evening stroll around the hospital – it's like our evening walks in our neighborhood except with much cleaner sidewalks and less questionable yard decorations.

Here's hoping Day Three of chemo is another decent day and starts October off on a great note!

You Must Be a Parking Ticket – Because You're Fine!

It had become like nails on a chalkboard: "No, I'm fine." Tom is one of the sweetest men you'll ever meet, and never wants to inconvenience people or make waves; he usually takes the path of least resistance. He's the first to apologize in a fight, even if I owe the apology, because he doesn't like when there is tension. It's not guilt, but he puts pressure on himself to not make things complicated for others. It's an amazing quality, except during cancer.

You have to be taken care of when you're as sick as he was, and it was a constant struggle. Originally, despite wanting to be, I wasn't sure if it made sense for me to be at the hospital full time. Would he rest if I were there? Would he rather have some time alone? But I quickly realized that I needed to be there. I only left for one hour during each of the six-day chemo stints to run home and take a shower halfway through the week. I wouldn't have left at all if I hadn't felt so bad about smelling so terrible.

Tom needed that advocate. He needed someone to question what shot he was getting, to mention that we just had someone else in here for a different shot, to help him get up and down from the bed, get his IV pole plugged in and out each time, and listen to what the doctors were saying. It was hard enough to comprehend everything happening without being sick, and as the chemo took hold over the course of the week, it was hard for him to focus. He was in and out of sleep and often confused.

My role was a bit of a puppeteer. I had to deal with our entire life outside of the hospital while being an advocate for Tom and working full-time out of my little corner of the hospital room.

I looked over to Tom and could tell he wasn't feeling well.

"Are you okay? What's wrong?" I asked.

"Just not feeling too well, lots of pain in my chest and with the port."

"Okay, let me call the nurse and have her bring you some pain medicine."

As I was reaching for the phone in our room to call our nurse, she happened to walk in to check on Tom and asked how he was feeling.

"I'm fine," he replied.

"You literally just told me that you weren't feeling well and that you wanted pain medicine," I said, puzzled.

"It's fine, it's fine. I know there is a lot going on," he replied.

I wasn't stupid. He didn't want to inconvenience the nurse.

"Can you please bring him some pain medicine? He isn't feeling well and just mentioned that he would be willing to take some more pain medicine," I told our nurse as I looked at Tom.

"If you don't mind, that would be great," Tom said to the nurse.

"No problem at all; that's what we are here for," she replied.

As she walked out of the room, I looked at Tom, who looked away because he knew what I was about to say.

"I am balancing a lot right now. You need to tell me how you feel and let them help us. The last thing I want you to do is feel miserable when we have all the tools here to help prevent that. I know you don't want to inconvenience people, but it's not an inconvenience. They want to help you too. We are great patients; we only call when we really need something, and I'm here constantly so they don't have to help you with the little things like getting up and down. I know it's not your favorite thing, but I need you to help me help you."

Tom looked over at me and put the cutest damn look on his face. "But that's why I married you; we complement each other so well. You do the confronting in our marriage, remember? I hate asking people for stuff."

"You also married me because I'm a straight shooter. Get over it," I replied with a smirk on my face.

We laughed as he acknowledged it was something he would be forced to work on, now that we were in this situation. As we went to bed that night, three chemo sessions in, I was thinking about what he had said. We did complement each other. We had enough in common, but more importantly, enough differences to keep us on our toes. After nine years, we still had a curiosity about the other that kept us intrigued. Where I was an outgoing, grab life and go kind of gal, he relaxed me. Where he tended to sit back and let life come to him, I taught him to reach. His beliefs were different from mine, and with that came new perspectives and a reminder to be open to other viewpoints. He is the planner; I'm spontaneous. He's compulsive, and I'm more calculated. As I sat there in the dark that night, Tom dozing off to sleep, I thought about what had happened earlier that day and all the circumstances where he as the yin to my yang. I resigned to the fact that we would be adding a new characteristic to our list, at least for a little while. He was the patient, and I was the caregiver.

Oct. 1 - Three Down, Seventeen To Go
Another day is in the books, and these days are getting tougher. As you can imagine, the back-to-back days of chemo is catching up with Tom. There is more fatigue since his body never has chance to bounce back, but that, of course, is what kills the cancer as it continues to quickly try and grow.

We've gotten a little stir crazy but are happy to be over halfway through this first treatment regimen! Since we don't have a ton to update, we'd just like to thank everyone for the texts, comments, emails, cards, etc. It really keeps us going through all of this and keeps us motivated. We are so lucky to have such wonderful friends and family. We are exhausted...time for some sleep so we can crush Day Four of chemo.

The Suffering

There is no worse feeling than that of helplessness while watching suffering. This is true at the broad level – the injustices and pain in the world – all the way down to a person you love suffering. I don't know how others have managed. I'm certainly not the first to go through this but having to sit alongside the person you love while they are suffering so much is heart-wrenching. I cried every night on my hospital couch after Tom went to sleep. I wasn't crying because I was mad about our situation or going stir crazy; I cried for him. I know the ups and downs of my life were tough for the past three weeks, and my body wasn't the one going through chemo on top of it all. The throwing up, the confusion, the nausea, the emptiness – it made me sick to my stomach for him as the week went on.

The only way I could ever get myself composed and redirect my thoughts was to think about all the non-suffering times we had had. Until this point, we had been very lucky. Other than when the Packers would continually whip on the Bears, or he had to go to something he didn't want to go to, we really had a great life. As I tried to think about happy things, my mind kept thinking about a suffering of a different sort and it bought a smile to my face. Tom and I met working in a restaurant. Tom had stayed in Milwaukee for the summer after his junior year of college, and I was home from my freshman year of college. Oddly enough, we had both applied for serving jobs at the same two restaurants, both been offered both jobs and both picked the same restaurant to work at. It was a new restaurant opening at the end of May. We were going to have a few weeks of training before the grand opening, and I had hoped the grand opening would make for a summer of quick money.

About midway through the summer, the corporate crew came waltzing into the restaurant one day to see how things were going and do some quality checks. I walked in for my shift; Tom was already working and warned me about the corporate team. They were standing by the kitchen door with stopwatches. They had jammed down our throats in training that once a party was seated, they should have drinks on the table within two minutes. They would start the clock when a table was seated and watched to see how long it took you to get to the table, take the drink order, and get it back to the table. It was ridiculous, and Tom was having none of it. He waited until one minute and fifty-seven seconds to bring the drinks to the table, not because he wasn't ready or on top of it, but because this was the kind of stuff he hated. The assumption of incompetence that these corporate folks had rolled in with infuriated Tom, and I'm surprised he made it through that shift. That type of stuff was a suffering of sorts, I suppose, and for whatever reason it had popped into my head and calmed me down in one of my darker moments.

What was hardest to watch, beyond the physical suffering, was the mental toll this was starting to have on Tom. I was trying my damnedest to keep him upbeat and positive, and for the most part I was able to, but I knew he was suffering both physically and mentally. I had tried to refocus him on little traditions so his mind was kept busy and he didn't have too much time to dwell.

Every morning, Tom had to use these special antibacterial wipes. They helped prevent infections or bacteria from the hospital. There were six cloths in a pack, one for each leg, one for each arm, and one for this chest and back. They would get heated in the microwave and then he would take this washcloth-type bath. It was our morning ritual. We would squeeze into the tiny bathroom together, Tom still tethered to his IV pole, and I would have the wipes and a fresh gown for him. He would take off his gown, stand in his boxers, I would make an inappropriate comment of some sort, and then I would open and hand him each wipe so he could clean up. We had the whole system down. Once he was done with the wipes, I would snap up the new gown around his IVs and he would have a fresh gown for the day. While this happened each morning, our nurse assistant would change the sheets on Tom's bed and get him fresh blankets. Once we were all done, we would finish our ritual with the most important part, a hug. We would turn towards each other in this tiny bathroom and he would wrap his arms around me, and I would carefully do the same. Sometimes we would stand in the bathroom, hugging, not saying a word for minutes. Those were some of my most favorite moments of the day because for a few moments, we weren't suffering at all.

Oct. 2 - Four Down, Sixteen To Go

It has certainly been an adventure as we started Day Four. Tom woke up feeling weak, very nauseous and in some pain. Not the greatest way to start the day when you've got a whole docket of chemo ahead. I wouldn't say it was an easy day, but he did manage to sleep quite a bit and let his body rest and fight the cancer. I'm SO incredibly proud of him as he forged on and got through the treatment today and even kept me laughing throughout it all.

We were joking today at how goofy it is that we now celebrate the weirdest things like the removal of his heart monitor, less shots, test results, and the ability to take a shower. It really is all about the little things right now! Speaking of the little things, tomorrow is the last day of chemo in our first session and we are VERY excited to finish this first round up and start our two weeks "off"...though rumor has it those will be very tough weeks and likely much worse than what we've experienced thus far. But...we will worry about that when we get there. One day at a time.

Point Freak

I had cashed them all in, over 150,000 hotel points to go on a thirteen-day European adventure. We were going to spend a week in Italy, and just shy of a week in Ireland. I had spent months planning this trip, figuring out all the attractions, setting up tours, and most importantly, researching the best food and wine. It was a trip of a lifetime, and it went perfectly. Not a single flight or train was ever delayed; every tour guide was amazing; every recommendation was better than the next, and I managed not to kill us as the driver of our rental car in Ireland.

I loved every city we went to for very different reasons, but Venice, Italy, stole my heart. It's out of a storybook. It doesn't seem possible that a place like that exists in the world and it oozed with culture and romance. Tom and I had arrived late at night and were roaming the streets of Venice, looking for our hotel in the dark. We'd occasionally pass a bar or restaurant with some action, but for the most part, we were two American tourists wandering around the most confusing city in the world. I'm sure we should have been more scared; we looked like we were the beginning of a Dateline special, but there was something about this situation that was strangely romantic too.

The next few days we explored Venice. We had a recommendation from our hotel owner for a restaurant on the other side of the town. He had called ahead for us and made a dinner reservation and attempted to give us directions. Directions in Venice are sarcastic in some sense; there is no rhyme or reason to the way the roads and bridges turn. We gave ourselves plenty of time to find our way and headed out for dinner. We had both dressed up and were eager for an Italian feast.

As we headed to the restaurant, we saw clouds rolling in and a storm headed in our direction. We figured we would beat it, and kept twisting and turning through the streets of Venice. As we were walking, the rain started and Tom grabbed my hand and dashed for a little restaurant ahead with an empty patio. Tom wrapped his arms around me as we huddled under a table umbrella. It was like a movie, this sudden storm arriving on our way to our fancy dinner when we are both dressed up. The bustling streets were completely empty. We couldn't see a person in this whole courtyard area, and it was strangely quiet and peaceful. It rained hard for about ten minutes and then gradually started to lighten up so we decided to keep on trying to find the restaurant. As we turned the last corner, the sun was shining again. I was in heaven. It smelled like a summer rain in this beautiful country and Tom and I were lost in their world.

We were seated at a table for two in the middle of a rectangular room. We could have touched both tables on either side of us without having to extend our arms very far – it was cozy to say the least. We ordered a liter of the house red and attempted to figure out the menu. By process of elimination, a little bit of help from people around us, and the owner, we managed to order an appetizer as we poured ourselves a glass of wine.

In Italy, the restaurants make their own wines, which are served by the liter in pitchers. The wine is amazing and has a lighter body to it. As a result, it went down smooth and fast as we enjoyed wine and chatted. Tom ordered another liter of wine for us right before our food came out.

"I can't remember if a liter is more than a bottle," Tom remarked as the server walked away.

"I have no clue, but it must be close based on how many glasses we've had," I replied.

An older American couple overheard us from a few tables over and started to snicker. Tom looked over and the woman replied, "A liter is more than a bottle of wine; you two are doing just fine though."

We all laughed as we realized our miscalculation, and they started telling us about their travels and how they've come to this restaurant every time they've come to Venice. Our meal lasted over three hours; we talked with other travelers in the restaurant, had our own conversations and enjoyed the most wonderful food and wine. The whole night had been out of a storybook. When we finally got up, we had to find our way back through the maze of Venice and the two liters of wine did not help. Our navigation back to the hotel took us twice as long, but night had fallen in Venice and all the lights from the boats on the canal and the bridges lit up the city. It was magical, and we enjoyed our time getting lost the whole way back.

We were crossing through St. Mark's Square to get to our hotel and stopped to admire the square at night – it was lit up and musicians were performing "Nessum Dorma" under one of the canopies. We stood there in awe, Tom's arms around me, swaying to the music, as we watched the musicians play the iconic notes. The wine had me swaying and reflective. Tom said something romantic, though I couldn't for the life of me tell you what it was. I just remember looking back and unromantically replying, "I love it here. I love you, and I really love all my hotel points."

Traveling had always been an escape, and I loved traveling with Tom. We are the perfect balance of planner and spontaneity, with a curiosity that finds us the most interesting places. I have always felt that no matter how well you know someone if you go on a trip with them you will find out something new or interesting that you never knew before. In addition, you create all the memories, and these memories aren't just for happy times to look back on. Suddenly these memories, the meal in Venice, our slow dance in St. Mark's Square, every moment of that trip became an escape from the days we spent in the hospital room.

Oct. 3 - Five Down, Fifteen to Go

Day Five of chemo is complete! For those that are following along, that means our first session of treatment is all wrapped up. Unfortunately, there are some post-chemo drug treatments that require us to stay another night, so that has required some creative ways to pass the time. For example – there are twenty-seven ceiling tiles in our hospital room. Cutting-edge stuff, right?

Tom has been sleeping quite a bit which means his body is busy beating this cancer. He also had a bit of a rough afternoon/evening, but while he was awake this afternoon we decided to come up with the Best/Worst list for a five-night stay at a hospital and figured we should share. In theme with our five-night stay, we've done the top five for each – in no particular order:

The Good....

1. *There is a frequent buyer card for the cafeteria! I'm not trying to show off, but I've almost got a full card punched.*

2. *Visitors – lots of love and non-hospital food deliveries have stopped by when Tom has felt up for it, which helps pass the time.*

3. *The staff – doctors, nurses, technicians, transport, housekeeping, social workers, cafeteria staff and volunteers. Everyone has been SO wonderful – and we've meet a few characters along the way too. Though we must say a special shout out to the nurses that are second to none and have been AMAZING.*

4. *Lullaby – At our hospital, when a baby is born, they play a ten-second clip of a sweet lullaby over the intercom across the whole hospital. A sweet reminder that good things happen in hospitals too, and better days lie ahead for us.*

5. *Love – perhaps a strange one but a very real one. Have you ever watched people at an airport right after the security checkpoint when they are hugging the person they came to see? It's usually quite a joyful place to people watch! Same here – despite lots of sadness in a hospital there is an incredible amount of love and care happening around us at all times – in a weird way it's a very special place to be.*

The Bad...

1. *We are not earning hotel points for our stay here – those that know me know I'm incredibly proud of my hotel/airline points and ability to cash them in for awesome trips.*

2. *Vampires. Lots of people come in and out during the night and often draw blood.*

3. *Beep Torture – Tom has been on at least two IVs at all times and sometimes up to four when he's having chemo. If the bag is complete, or there is air in the line, or if it just wants to remind you that it's there, it beeps. And beeps. And beeps. Until one of our amazing nurses comes in and stops the madness.*

4. *"Average Size" – Most medical facilities, clothing, etc. is made for your average-size person. This means they are about 5ft. 7inches. That's a little challenging for my 6ft+ tall husband. Just picture that scene in the movie Elf where he is showering in the little elf shower and the shower spout is in the middle of his stomach.*

5. *TV Channels – yes, this one seems ridiculous, but when you are married to an obsessed Cubs fan, this certainly makes a difference when the limited channels mean he can't watch all of the Cubs games while they are in the hunt for the post season. The good news is we will be home for the big game on Wednesday.*

Safety Net

Tom and I had purchased our first home almost a year before he was diagnosed. We had looked at so many houses and were trying to find the right balance of what we needed and wanted in our price range. For as outgoing as I am, I am truly a homebody at heart, so the feel of the house was important to me. It drove Tom crazy. At one point we saw an amazing house, but I told him it just didn't feel right. I thought he was going to fall over; he was so taken aback by my brutal honesty about the feel of the house.

We found the perfect starter home for us. I'll admit that a large closet in the basement that I wanted to turn into a small wine cellar was what really sold me. Right after we closed, we went straight to the new house; Tom and I were so excited to step into the house as the official homeowners. We pulled into the garage, and Tom started to mess around with something in the trunk. I didn't think much of it and started to grab the cleaning supplies. A few moments later, I heard him yell from the front yard.

"Babe, come here," he yelled.

"What's up?" I asked as I took the few steps from the garage to get to the front yard.

"Happy House Day!" he yelled as he started to chuckle.

Hanging in the rusty flagpole holder was a flag he had ordered. It read "A House Divided" and had the Bears logo on one half, and the Packers logo on the other half. He was thrilled with his purchase and eager to see my reaction. I laughed out loud as I walked over to him and gave him a kiss.

"That's pretty good," I said. I wrapped my arms around his waist as he put his arm around me. It was the perfect start to our new house. This house was going to "ooze" us, and I was excited to make it a cozy place to be.

You buy a house, but you make it a home, and I was eager to do just that. With the new homeowner's budget, we slowly but surely started putting our own personal touches on the house. Months after moving in, it was still one of my favorite places to be, hanging with Tom in the house. Now, it was our ground zero, it was where we were making some terrible memories, and suddenly home didn't feel safe. When we arrived home from his first chemo, I didn't want to be at the house. The hospital was where I felt safe. What if something happened and I didn't know what to do? What if I didn't act fast enough? While being home felt like the greatest milestone, I was a bit scared to be there.

We were exhausted when we got home after that first week. During the week of Tom's chemo, I was up all night with him; at one point on his first night, he got up to go to the bathroom and when he came out of the bathroom to go back to bed I was standing by his bed waiting to help him get his IV plugged in and get him settled back in. For every treatment cycle I got up almost every single time throughout the six days to get him unplugged and resituated; it became one of our rituals. Once I plugged him back in, we would always hug, or vertical cuddle as we joked, for a moment. Some nights I was still sleeping while I did it and the hug was more to hold each other up.

On the first night of his first week, at two in the morning, I was helping him get back into bed. I gave him the usual hug, but he started to cry. I held him so tight. I knew he was exhausted. Knowing he only had one day down was overwhelming to him.

"I don't know if I can do this," he said as I felt his tears hit my shoulder.

"You can do this, and I'm not leaving your side. We will do it together," I replied as he squeezed me even tighter.

"How am I supposed to do this nineteen more times?" he asked, "I just want to be home."

"One at a time and we'll be home soon," I replied.

I got him situated back in bed and he fell right back asleep.

I thought about that exchange as I stood in our house feeling lost. I had turned our office into Medical Central with everything I needed. I wanted everything in that room so that I could close the door and keep the rest of our house looking like the house that we had grown to love so much. I didn't want medications all over the kitchen counter or in the bathroom.

Tom was getting medications every few hours, and we didn't have the nurses or the medical system at the hospital to keep track of everything he was taking and the timing. It was all on me. I was happy to do it, but still scared due to my lack of medical training. To top it off, I was running on little sleep and I was terrified that in my drowsy state I might grab the wrong medication or the wrong number of pills. I set my alarm throughout the night to wake up and give him his medicine and would often be too wound up to fall back to sleep. I would triple check the bottle, the number of pills, the time and then mark it all on my tracking sheet. If I tracked food the way I was tracking these medicines I would have lost twenty pounds in a week.

We were exhausted, we were spent, we were overwhelmed, but we were home, and that's something many people fighting cancer wish they could say.

Oct. 4 – Home Sweet Home

It's well past midnight and I need to be up again in an hour to give Tom some more medicine, so tonight's post won't be long – but it's an important one! WE. ARE. HOME. Delightful! I will say, today was incredibly tough, but we managed to get home. Tom unfortunately started feeling the effects of the chemo overnight last night and into this morning. Nausea, vomiting, fatigue, and general weakness reared their ugly heads. Tom essentially slept until we were discharged in the afternoon. We had to wait for the final post-chemo meds to finish dripping, which felt like DAYS when we were so close to getting home after almost a week at the hospital. It probably felt extra-long for him too since the Bears game was on for the last few hours in the hospital. (Sorry – I couldn't help myself, even if they did win.)

As expected, the symptoms have continued at home, and Tom has slept most of the day. He is on an incredible number of pills to proactively help manage some of these symptoms. The number of drugs along with how often he needs to take them resulted me drawing up a chart so I can keep track of it all. I certainly don't want him feeling crummy because we missed a dose – not on my watch! We are expecting a rough few days with limited action on his part, and then hopefully he turns the corner and can feel more "normal" towards the end of this week and next week before we head back for round two.

Speaking of heading home – quite literally we were able to walk out/get pushed in a wheelchair (I'll let you guess which was Tom) of the hospital today. Our hospital neighbor one door down from us in the oncology wing was saying her final goodbyes this afternoon as we were leaving. Her children, grandchildren, and siblings were all bedside and talking in the hallway about their favorite memories. We are thankful and recognize that we are in the position where we come in, get treated and go home with the intent of beating this cancer. Others are not as lucky as we are – may that sweet woman rest in peace. Sorry, a bit of a late-night tangent, but an important one nonetheless. I digress...

So while we were very excited to get through the first treatment – especially since we now know what to expect – we are still very curious to see how these next two weeks go between treatments. We will feel much better when we know what to expect within the whole chemo cycle and can manage accordingly. So today was a baby step – but I'll be damned if we aren't going to celebrate it – this is a marathon, not a sprint, and we are still moving in the right direction. More to come...

I Watched Too Many Medical Dramas

It was the day after we had gotten home from his first round of chemo. We had only been home that first exhausting night and were in a complete fog. Nothing seemed real. It felt like we were sort of floating and going through the motions of what people were telling us to do. The worst part was that we had to go see our port surgeon's nurse first thing Monday morning. Despite us having just been in the hospital for the six days following his port placement surgery, we had to go in to have the nurse practitioner check it out and make sure that everything was okay. We were less than thrilled but had to be at the hospital anyway for Tom's first "booster" shot, which occurred every Monday following his chemo to help prevent infections.

Now, you've likely seen the booster shot commercials, where two sisters up on the coast of Maine are eating a table full of seafood that was just set out in front of them. The sun is out, the waves are beautifully crashing into the coastal cliffs, and life couldn't be any better. I call bull on that. When we saw the commercial for the shot, we both laughed out loud. It's one of those commercials that I'm sure we had seen one hundred times before, but until the product means something to you it doesn't process. We always wondered under what conditions this woman required a Nuelasta shot because she certainly didn't look like a post-chemo patient.

We drove to the hospital and I was so thankful that we had such a great hospital so close to home. For Tom to be moving around one day after five straight days of chemo was tough enough and being in the car elevated the nausea and fatigue. He was not feeling great but was trying to keep a smile on his face. We went in to the hospital, patiently waited our turn, and then were ushered back to a small room for the nurse practitioner to see us. I could tell Tom was not feeling well, and I wished we didn't have to be in this place at all. The nurse happily entered the room with a big smile on her face and asked us how we were doing. She remarked at how sad it was to see someone so young here – a chorus that had become all too familiar.

Tom had taken his shirt off so she could see the port. She pushed around a little bit and said everything looked fine while asking him a few questions about how he was feeling. The appointment lasted less than three minutes. She stood up to leave, and Tom stood up to put his shirt and hoodie over his head. He immediately sat back down.

I looked at him. "Are you okay?"

"I don't think so," he replied.

"You look really pale all of a sudden," the nurse said. She walked over closer to him and I sunk back into the chair.

I reached out to grab his hand as he started to convulse.

"CODE BLUE, CODE BLUE, WE HAVE A CODE BLUE," the nurse screamed as she ran out of the room.

I had learned after our first stay in the hospital that Code Blue meant they needed immediate help and that a patient's life was at risk. I turned my head to see where the nurse was going as she darted out of the room.

"Where are you going?! What am I supposed to do!?" I screamed as I turned back to Tom. His head was tilted back against the wall as he continued to convulse. I looked him in the eyes, but he wasn't there. It looked as if he was looking my way, but there was no one in his eyes.

"Tom, Tom, don't do this to me. Stay with me. Tom!" I yelled as I screamed his name and squeezed his hand. He slumped into my arm and ultimately fell down my shoulder and was convulsing in my lap. When he hit my lap, I just screamed as I cried out. "Somebody help me, please!"

The nurse couldn't have been gone longer than twenty seconds, but it felt like minutes. I didn't know how to help Tom. One of my arms was now pinned down by his body, and the other was trying to squeeze his hand. Suddenly our nurse was back and eight other nurses and doctors came rushing in. They got Tom upright again and tried to ask him questions. He wasn't giving them anything, even though his eyes were wide open. A bed was wheeled into the room as a nurse grabbed me and told me I had to leave the room. She and one other nurse literally had to pull me out of the room because I wasn't about to leave his side. She took me around the corner and had me sit in a chair in the hallway.

I lost it. I screamed into a Kleenex and bawled like never before. I was convinced that those were the last moments I would ever have with my husband. There was a woman sitting a few chairs down from me and she just stared. A nurse knelt on the floor next to me and tried to calm me down. It was a wasted effort; I wasn't going to be calm again until I knew what was going on with Tom. I kept seeing more doctors and nurses come in and out of the room and not hearing his voice.

It couldn't have been more than five minutes when the nurse on the floor rubbed my back to get my attention. I think she had been talking to me, but I had just been staring at the floor and crying. I looked over to her and saw the doctor who had rushed into Tom's room walking towards us with his head down. I had seen enough episodes of ER to know that couldn't be a good sign. He whipped his head up as he told me that Tom was asking for me.

"What?" I said looking at him and then down at the nurse.

"He's asking for you – he's okay. I think he just passed out from seeing his incision, all the medicine he is on, and the port getting poked."

"Was it a seizure?" I asked, convinced that was what I had just seen.

"It certainly looked like one," the nurse interjected as she guided me back into the room.

I looked over at her as I tried to take a few deep breaths and calm down. "You know, the doctor really shouldn't walk down the hall with his head down. I've watched too much TV to not make assumptions." She laughed out loud as she guided me into the room.

Tom was on a hospital bed that hardly fit the space because they had crammed it into the small room. The bed was tilted so that his feet were above his head. I sucked in as I wiggled around a small space between the bed and the consultation table so I could get to him.

He looked up at me with a puzzled look on his face. "Why are you crying? What's the matter?"

He had no recollection of what had just happened. He remembered sitting back down in the chair and then waking up to a bunch of nurses and doctors around him in a hospital bed.

I looked up at the doctor who was standing on the other side of the bed and saw him smirk at me.

"Seriously, if you had any idea what just happened I would be so mad at you for asking me what's wrong!" I replied with some laughter in my voice as I looked at him and the doctor.

Tom was dripping sweat and clearly confused. They made him stay tipped down for ten more minutes. We still had four nurses and a doctor around the bed watching him. He started to entertain his crowd, and I just felt paralyzed. I couldn't believe what just happened and thought it must have to do with all the medications he was on. I wanted to get him off all of the drugs, but he didn't have many other options.

After a few discussions with the other doctors about whether he should admit Tom to the ER to keep an eye on him, the doctor assured me he was doing much better and we would be able to go home. Again, home was the goal but suddenly also a scary place to be.

"If something like that happens again at home, what should I do?" I asked the nurse.

She wasn't stupid and could sense my nervousness at leaving the hospital. "I really think it was an isolated incident, but I'd call your oncologist when you get home and see if she wants to adjust any of his medications. If something happens at home, call 911 immediately."

"Uh oh, I might be in trouble then. She loses her phone in the house all the time, even when it's in her hand," I heard Tom quip as the other nurse did a final vitals check.

"Isn't he charming?" I said to the nurse as I smiled. "I'll keep my phone close, and thank you for the help. Please thank the other nurses too. I'm sure that's not how you all planned to start your Monday morning."

We drove home and I hardly said a word. Tom had his eyes closed but was awake during the drive.

"You okay?" he asked.

"Yeah, don't ever scare me like that again. I need you here; I need you to beat this," I said, rather selfishly.

"I know, babe; I'm not going anywhere. I think I just got queasy when she poked the port and I feel so weak right now."

"I'll call the doctor when we get home," I replied, wanting him to quietly relax and not worry about anything.

"Okay. In hindsight, knowing what happened now, it was kind of funny to see your face when I asked why you were crying," Tom said with his eyes still closed but a smile creeping across his face.

"Yup. Hilarious," I replied as I shook my head and sighed. What an adventure this had become.

Oct. 5 – Oy Vey

Let the bounce back begin. The five days of chemo is incredibly intense, but it's just scratching the surface. The first few days after chemo are even tougher because his body adjusts to not having the chemo treatments and deals with the effects of all the drugs. I won't sugarcoat it at all – today was the toughest day so far (for both of us) – right up there with the original diagnosis day.

Tom and I had to be at the hospital this morning so the surgical doctor could check his port (typical protocol about a week after the surgery) and to get a shot from the oncologist. Essentially this shot helps his immune system rebound (he has no immune system after chemo because his red/white blood cells are so low) as quickly as possible. This shot is great to help prevent major infections, but it comes with a price because it creates the feelings and symptoms of a flu for a few days following. We ended up being at the hospital a bit longer than we had anticipated because Tom was having a tough time and had a scary episode. Thank goodness we were at the hospital as they were able to quickly help us in a very scary situation. Despite an unexpectedly eventful morning, we got home mid-morning and Tom was able to sleep and recover.

Here's hoping we turn the corner tomorrow and have more of a "normal" week before the next round of chemo. One other important tidbit we learned today? I'm a terrible wheelchair driver! Until next time...

Mind Over Matter

We never officially had a conversation, but it was something that didn't need to be said. We weren't planning to go into this fight with a negative mindset or assuming the worst. We always acknowledged what the worst could be – but only to help prepare ourselves for all the different scenarios that could transpire. From day one, we took a positive approach to his diagnosis and truly believed that laughter was the best medicine. Tom had said at one point during the first days following his diagnosis that he was going to try to have as much fun as possible while having cancer. At first, I was a little taken aback by his comment; it almost seemed to be a mockery of our pain to make light of such a serious situation, but I knew what he meant. He made a decision to not take any one day too seriously, focus on the good things instead of the challenging things, and try to keep everyone around him laughing.

There were days when he was struggling, sick, and miserable, but he always managed to put on a strong face when visitors would stop by. He didn't want anyone to worry about him, and more than anything, he wanted to be positive and appreciative for all the people around us. I was so thankful that Tom could be true to how he was feeling with me, but it sometimes was exhausting. While he could grin through a visit or pretend to feel better than he was, I was left to try to echo those sentiments too. There were times in the hospital or at home when minutes before visitors arrived we were crying, or one of us was having a difficult day, but we didn't want to take others down with us, so we would make a generic comment like "It's one of those days" or "I'm exhausted" to try and keep everyone comfortable.

Despite it all, though, we knew we had it good. We knew we were doing better than most would in our situation, and we also knew that we were the only people who could control these emotions. It was on us to stay positive. It was on us to remember how lucky we were to have the doctors we had, and it was on us to not get frustrated with the little things. It was truly how we spun as many of our situations as possible.

Every possible complaint had a complementary angle that made us grateful, and I tried to find them in as many of our situations as possible. The doctor was forty minutes behind became and appreciation that we were patients of such an amazing doctor. The medical bills which are confusing and expensive became thank goodness we have insurance. The struggle to balance everything became how lucky I was to have so many things that need balancing. Wanting our old life back became I can't wait to see what our new life will bring.

This wasn't easy, but we needed it to get through these days. I tried my hardest to not cry too much in front of Tom, though I often did. Instead, I tried to cry in the shower or bath. It actually became quite therapeutic – there was something about the tears literally going down the drain that made it seem like they could be gone forever.

Things that used to cause bad days had become so insignificant in our new life. The little things didn't matter nearly as much as they used to, and I wasn't quite sure why. It wasn't that the value of those things changed; it was what they meant to us or how we prioritized them that changed. I had a heightened compassion for everyone around me, too – when someone cut me off I wondered if they were on their way to see a loved one who was sick, or were in a rush for some other serious reason. When a woman was frustrated in the aisle at the pharmacy, I tried to help her in case she was new to caretaking and felt overwhelmed. I had always had compassion, but our situation had turned it up high. It was that compassion and that positive and somewhat humorous view of our situation that saved us. We didn't always do it perfectly, and some days we had to try extra hard to be positive, but damn did we try.

Oct. 7 – How are You Doing?
How Are You Doing? It's the question that we've been getting a lot lately – but a difficult one to answer. Personally, I think we are doing quite well considering how fast our lives have changed, how many quick decisions we have had to make, and how scary this whole experience has been. We are staying as positive as possible, trying to find humor in this chaos and feeling incredibly supported by our friends, family and work.

However, I also don't want to misrepresent our reality – we would take our old lives back in a second. The hardest part of this whole experience has been how quickly we had to figure out – and adapt – to our new "normal." I have alarms set all throughout the night to get up and give Tom his medicine, "good" has a whole new meaning, and we are at the mercy of not being able to plan anything because we won't know how he feels – but what gets us through this is knowing this will only be temporary. There have been moments in all of this, like yesterday, where I stopped to breathe for a moment and really questioned if this is all real life. Sadly, it is; but I know months from now, we will look back at this few months of our life and laugh about how crazy it all was. (This conversation will likely happen with a glass of red wine in my hand.)

I'm glad to report that Tom has turned the corner on the forty-eight/seventy-two hours post-chemo and is feeling MUCH better. We knew those first three days post chemo would be the toughest in these three-week cycles (along with the chemo days), and with the help of some medication adjustments we managed to get through these rough days without too much pandemonium! Now if all goes as the doctors say...he will start to feel better and better each day just in time to get his next round of chemo. We still have to be very careful since his immune system is quite compromised even if he feels better – but we are encouraged by his progress!

My grandmother was a journalist and recently I read some of her writing – in one of her articles she wrote that without a few bad days, you would never be able to recognize the good days. So despite some bad days, it will only help us appreciate the good ones ahead – and we know we've got plenty of those to come. So to answer the question, considering our situation, we are all good.

Let Me Show You How It's Done

Two weeks before Tom was diagnosed, we had a comical foreshadowing of our life. It was 7 am on a Friday morning and Tom and I were going to the fertility doctor for blood work for both of us and a quick scan for me. I knew Tom was a bit nervous about the blood work, and until that point he hadn't ever needed it. I knew he wasn't a fan of needles based on our adventure with the dentist, but had never witnessed him dealing with blood until this point. Ours were the first appointments of the day and I got us checked in with the receptionist. I asked her if we were doing our blood work at the same time and, if not, could I go back with Tom. The receptionist looked at me a bit puzzled as I whispered, "He doesn't do so well with needles." She laughed and nodded, probably thinking I was a crazy wife.

We got called back and were escorted to the blood draw room. We sat next to each other, our chairs separated by a trash can. The woman was making small talk with us and we were laughing, warning her that he didn't do well with blood. As she was prepping Tom, she had him grab one of the stress balls to start squeezing and get his blood moving. Tom reached over and grabbed the stress ball that looked like a house, passing up the one that was a cartoon sperm that was smiling. One of the sperm donor banks had a brilliant marking plan by creating a smiling sperm stress ball.

I looked at Tom, disappointedly, and told him that wasn't the one I would have picked. He rolled his eyes at me as the nurse turned her back to us to get the vials ready. I mouthed to him that I was going to try to take one of them when no one was looking – I'm no criminal, but for some reason I needed to get my hands on this sperm stress ball. If nothing else, for a little humor around the house as we continued to deal with the fertility rollercoaster.

The nurse was about to put the needle in Tom's arm and gave me the look.

"Hey, look at me," I said as I grabbed his hand.

"I'll be okay," he replied, trying to play it tough.

"I know, I just want to hold your hand and stare into your eyes," I said with a smile on my face.

The nurse put the needle in his arm and began the blood draw. At that moment, another nurse walked in to grab something.

"Oh boy, he looks pretty pale," she remarked as she looked over at us. I looked back at Tom and his head was now against the wall. He was pale and his lips were white.

"Uh oh, here we go," I said to the nurse as I looked up at her.

Tom looked over at me and seemed a bit drowsy. The nurse pulled out the needle as Tom began to sweat. His shirt was actually wet as he reached up for the orange juice that the nurse was handing him. As I was about to reach down, Tom beat me to the punch, grabbed the trash can, and began throwing up. I looked up at the nurse who was now having an amazing start to her Friday and had no words to say to her.

"Are you feeling lightheaded, Tom, should we lie you down?" she asked. I was rubbing his back and squeezing his hand. Our blood nurse, the other nurse and I were all just trying to figure out how to help him.

"I'll be okay," Tom replied as he continued throwing up. He was obviously feeling quite optimistic.

He gradually stopped throwing up, drank a little water and started to eat some crackers.

"I'm so sorry," he said to the nurse with embarrassment in his voice.

"Don't apologize, it's okay," she kindly replied, trying to put Tom at ease. We chatted as Tom's color and energy started to come back.

"Can I steal your wife for a moment?" the other nurse asked as she walked into the room.

"Go right ahead, I'll be right here if she needs me," Tom joked as I got up.

I walked down the hall and into the exam room. The nurse and I were joking a bit about Tom's reaction and she said she hoped for me that Tom didn't always react like that to blood. She commented on how sweet he was, and how men have a lower pain tolerance than women, or at least that's what we choose to believe. I was in and out of the scan in about ten minutes and headed back to the blood draw room for my own blood draw. As I was coming down the hall, I heard the nurse laughing with Tom and turned the corner to see him smiling as he excitedly told me he was feeling much better.

"Can I switch chairs with you?" I asked, since it was now my turn for a blood draw. Tom got up and got into the chair I had been in. I sat down.

"Are you sure you want to stay in here?" the blood nurse asked Tom, trying to avoid another vomiting issue.

"Oh no, I'll be fine. I'm good with other people; I just don't like needles or my blood being taken," he replied, with a matter-of-fact tone.

"Well, there you go, now we know," I said to the nurse with a laugh.

As the nurse prepped my arm, I made an immediate grab for the smiling sperm stress ball and looked over to Tom.

"Ready to watch the pros do it?" I teased.

"Oh shut up, I can't help if I have a reaction!" he said, laughing.

The nurse took four vials of blood, two more than they had to take from Tom, and stuck a Band-Aid on in a matter of seconds.

"Wait, is that how it's really supposed to go?" Tom asked the nurse, trying to hold back a laugh.

"That's the more common experience, yes," she replied. "You two are funny."

It foreshadowed the situation we would be dealing with just days later. In the midst of Tom throwing up, me trying to steal a semen stress ball, and the undertone of our fertility nightmare, we had managed to somehow make it fun, and made memories in the process. Later that day, I called to get the results of some of the preliminary tests, and the receptionist, upon hearing my name, asked how Tom was feeling. I couldn't help but laugh; we now had a reputation. She asked to schedule a follow up appointment, which was precisely when I realized I had forgotten to steal the damn sperm stress ball.

Oct. 8 – Phobias

Well, in addition to cancer, my dear husband has a little thing known as trypanophobia/ hemophobia. That would be a reaction to needles/blood draw. I used to joke and give him a hard time about it, because I honestly thought he was just being a little dramatic, but I will publicly take that back. It's not that he doesn't like them, or gets scared; it's that he really has a physical reaction when he needs blood taken, which usually results in him either passing out, vomiting, or going pale (almost my Irish level of pale) and sweating. As you can imagine, between chemo and blood work this has created a whole separate challenge. The good thing is he does have the port in, so they can get blood from that and not have to take it from his arm every time, but even so, he sees that needle or knows he has to give blood and it's all over.

Tonight, I was doing some research online to see if there were any tips or tricks on how to help combat this issue. No joke, he was getting queasy reading over my shoulder; the very thought can make him have a reaction. Luckily, he doesn't take himself too seriously and makes lots of jokes about it all and usually has the nurses cracking up.

Anyway, he did some blood work today (see above paragraph to take a guess at how that went) and the counts were low, which is expected for a week out of chemo. We will know more tomorrow and next week on his blood work when we meet with the doctors. So maybe he's not great with needles and dealing with blood, but he's totally crushing chemo, and if I had to pick between the two, I pick chemo!

The Golden Ticket

When Tom was diagnosed, there was a brief moment, during his initial diagnosis conversation with our oncologist, that I saw him crack a smile.

"There is a specific drug that has great results for managing symptoms, specifically the nausea, which I may recommend. That is medicinal marijuana," she said with a very serious yet quiet tone.

A brief smirk came across Tom's face as he glanced at me and then glanced back to the doctor.

"It's not yet legal in Illinois, but it can really make a difference," she said, and she briefly paused.

It wasn't medically legal in Illinois for a few more weeks so there wasn't much else she could say to us. Tom had smoked in college, and a bit after college too, and I knew that if there was going to be any silver lining to this situation, this might be it. A few days before his next round of chemo we were approaching November 1 and wanted to get all the paperwork to apply for his medical marijuana card. Sadly, it's harder to get a medical marijuana card in the state than it is to get a firearm – talk about the systems being backwards. We had gotten all the paperwork filled out, a background check and fingerprinting done, and had everything ready for the doctor to sign.

The good girl in me, the girl that had attended Catholic school for sixteen years and always associated drugs with evil, was having a hard time wrapping my head around it all. I had a puff or two in college myself, but still had felt an overwhelming guilt, or believed that it was some kind of gateway drug. Through college and after, my view on marijuana had evolved since I had seen so many people be quite successful while still enjoying the relaxation it provided. It wasn't such a scary monster to me anymore, but still wasn't something I chose to do.

When we were in Colorado the year before, I had no problem walking into the recreational shops with Tom and seeing what they were all about. It was interesting to me, and the business girl in me was fascinated about how fast this industry had to get itself together with all its rules and regulations. I had always thought the medicinal side of legalization was just a way to soften the legalization of the drug. But now, all I wanted was for Tom to feel better and experience less nausea and chemo symptoms. It had been so hard to watch him go through this first round of chemo and I was willing to try anything in the world to make it better. So I got on board and made sure it was on the list of things to talk with the doctor about in a few days when we checked back in for the next round of chemo.

"Alright, everything's ready to go for Dr. Sobol to sign. I even put a stamp on the envelope for her so you'll have no delay in getting your marijuana card," I said.

"It's not a marijuana card," he said seriously.

"It's not? Then what is it?" I asked, walking right into his trap.

"It's my Golden Ticket," he replied with a smirk on his face.

Oct. 10 – Good Momentum

We've turned the corner! Hell, we've turned the corner and are almost on the next block. I'm SO proud of my husband who has made it through the first round of chemo and the initial post-chemo days, which were incredibly tough. However, now he is feeling much better – the Cubs wild card came probably had something to do with that too. In fact, yesterday, there was a chance that we were going to need to go back to the doctor to get some fluids and supplements depending on his blood results from Thursday, and they called and said everything was looking great so far and there was no need. Woo hoo! With the initial post-chemo days complete, he is on way fewer medications, sleeping through the night (hallelujah!) and his appetite is rebounding a bit.

In a weird way, it almost plays with our minds more that he's feeling good because (1) good has a whole different meaning in his current condition (2) we still have to be careful of lots of people/crowds because he still has super low counts and (3) we still have this cloud of knowing we've got to do this all over again in nine days. However, in our quest to be positive we are encouraged by how well he's doing and being able to figure out what the ups and downs of these chemo cycles will be – and the fact that it looks like we will have a good stretch of "ups" within these chemo cycles is wonderful.

Today felt sort of normal as I ran some errands to pick up some stuff we needed (including my own self-prescribed medicine – wine!). All in all – we are preparing for what we hope is a calm week – more to come...

Reality TV

If I had to grade myself on my ability to relax, I wouldn't necessarily give myself high scores. I'm always going and my brain just simply won't turn off. Tom often has to bring me back to reality when I come up with all these great ideas, like writing a book, or starting a company, or coming up with an invention. I just see the world a bit differently and seem to think about it differently. It's comically tragic. When it comes to TV, and we had to watch quite a bit of TV, I struggle to focus. I am usually doing something else, like writing or medical bills or playing on my phone. I wish I was kidding, but it's a real struggle for me.

The only times I can focus on the TV are for sporting events, especially my Packers. Who wants to take a chance at missing a shot of Clay Matthews or Aaron Rodgers? Not me. As a bit of a reality TV junkie, I truly see sports as the ultimate reality TV. It happens in real time, the story lines can't be producer-fed, and its raw emotion. It's simply the best, and part of the reason I have always enjoyed sports so much. I played sports growing but my fondest memories include watching sports with my dad. I could sit with my dad on a Sunday in his big chair and watch the game, asking him a thousand pesky questions and enjoying the action of the games. I knew I would always marry a guy who liked sports, but didn't necessarily think I would marry someone who was the exact rival of all my teams. And yet, we were a perfect match.

Oct. 12 – A House Divided

So for those that know us well, you know Tom and I love our sports teams. In fact, prior to our wedding, Tom randomly sent me an email at work with the subject line "Sports Prenuptial Agreement" that requested all children from our marriage be Bears/Cubs/Bulls/Blackhawks fans. I wish I was kidding about that, but I'm not. For the record, I laughed out loud and deleted the email. We don't disagree over too much, but we disagree over a few things:
Bears/Packers
Brewers/Cubs
Other less important rivalries like Xavier/Marquette and Bulls/Bucks
...and who is funnier.

I'll let you all be the judge of these (and remind you that the Packers are 5-0), but I must say for the first time in my life I am not rooting against one of his teams. Tom has been a lifelong obsessed Cubs fan – he watches almost all of the games, coaches from the couch and is quite invested in the team. He was very excited for this season and the late season push into the playoffs prior to the cancer diagnosis, but now it's really become a lifeline. As silly as it may seem, having games throughout the week gives him something to get excited

*about and look forward to in a very isolating time when he's required to
minimize his exposure to people.*

*Anyway, the Cubs won tonight – and that certainly helped make Tom's good
week better. The trickiest part about this third week prior to the next round of
treatment is that though he is feeling better (i.e., less nausea, fewer
medications, etc.), his body is still very much fighting this cancer. For example,
we took a walk down the block yesterday and he was SPENT. With his reduced
red and white blood cells, it's challenging for his body to keep up with lots of
activity. So while he feels better, his body's ability to do what he thinks he
should be able to do doesn't necessarily align, which can be frustrating. But he
is at least feeling better...*

*For the record, I'm a big fan of the Cubs manager, Joe Maddon. As a Brewers
fan, I just can't root for the Cubs, but I will certainly root against the Cardinals
since they are a division rival... and of course I will continue to root for my
husband's happiness. More to come...*

A Nightmare

I heard Tom roll out of bed to go to the bathroom at about 5 am. Until recently I had always been a hard sleeper, but ever since Tom was diagnosed, I would wake up at the slightest movement. I heard him close the door, and I dozed in and out as I waited for him to get back to bed. I knew he had been in there a bit longer than usual, and I lifted my head to try and hear if he was throwing up. I didn't hear anything serious, and then moments later heard the door open. He came back to bed, and I could tell something was wrong.

I lifted the blanket up for him and he crawled into bed, facing me and grabbed my entire body as he started to sob.

"It's coming out in chunks, it's literally just falling out if I touch it," he said between sobs.

"I'm so sorry, babe, that has to be scary to wake up to," I said rubbing his back, now wide awake and realizing that there was loose hair all over our pillows.

"I thought there was a chance I wasn't going to lose it since I almost made it through week three. I don't want to look sick."

"I know, but I really do think you are going to be sexy without hair. Do you want to get up and we can cut it now?"

"No, I think I'll go to the barber later today and just have them do it."

"That's a good idea, it will probably be the safest option for you," I said as I tried to make him laugh.

Tom giggled as he tried to regain his composure. This was only the second or third time he had a really good cry, and it broke my heart. Tom is not a guy who cares too much about vanity, but he really felt like now he was going to *look* like a cancer patient. He would often say that in the big scheme of things, it wasn't a big deal, but I think most days he was trying to convince himself.

Later that day Tom got his head shaved at the barber. They had done it as close as possible, but it looked splotchy, and I knew we were going to need to do another round.

"It looks great, babe," I said with a smile, knowing Tom was both eager and nervous to see my reaction.

"This is awful," he replied, trying to not cry.

"I think it will look less like a sick person if we do the close shave. We can do that tomorrow if you want; it can be a date night," I said, trying to keep him positive. "And in the meantime, we will rock these bad boys."

I tossed Tom his Cubs hat and I grabbed a beanie from the basket in the closet. As we put on our hats, he looked over and assured me he would be fine and once again made the best of the situation.

"I really just did this so your dad has some company," referring to my dad's bald head, as a smile came across his face.

Oct. 14 – Hair Today, Gone Tomorrow

Well, today was a very emotional day. The hair loss took a dramatic turn and was literally coming out in chunks this morning. Now, in hindsight, Tom did pull at his hair quite a bit during that dramatic Cubs series win last night, but by this morning it was clear that the hair loss was in full swing.

As many cancer patients will tell you – this is an especially hard day for many reasons. For Tom, it's that no hair makes him "look sick" versus look like himself. He has been incredibly strong throughout this whole journey, and I have such admiration for the fact that he is being so strong, trying to remain positive and attempting to make his life as normal as possible for himself and for the people around him. I don't care how strong you are, losing your hair is tough, and it totally sucks. So, Tom made the decision to shave it today once he woke up and realized it was officially necessary – it's not 100 percent gone – he chose to do a very close shave and will let the rest continue to fall out on its own. Luckily, we are approaching a Midwest winter, which requires hats, and he looked good with the haircut!

So as positive as we are trying to be – this was a tough day. So tonight, we rocked hats – and rocked them pretty well if I may say so myself. Until next time...

Did You Hear That?

We were in Colorado for a visit in April, four months before our never-ending life of no relaxation and intensity began. On our honeymoon, Tom had convinced me to get a couples massage with him, and I was hooked. I had never been to a spa before, but it was relaxing and fun to do as a couple. It had become a tradition of sorts; whenever we took a vacation, we would get a couple's massage. Colorado was no different, and I had scheduled a couple's massage in Boulder, the last stop of our week tour in Colorado.

We got to the spa, checked in, changed, and Tom met me back in the waiting area and tried to figure out how to appropriately sit in a robe. This spa had a beach theme. Everything was a teal blue or white with shutters to make it look like a beach house. It was sweet and quaint, and I was enjoying the ambiance as our masseuses arrived in the waiting area to take us back, one male and one female. Tom was going to get his massage from the woman, and I would get the man. My masseuse was well over six feet tall, and had the stature of a giant. He had paws for hands so I figured I was about to get a pretty amazing massage.

We went back to the room and they left for a moment as Tom and I got on our separate massage tables.

"He's so tall – I feel like his back is going to hurt by the time he's done, considering how low these tables are."

"You're weird," Tom replied as he rolled his eyes and got under his sheet.

I followed suit and proceeded to take off my robe and get under my sheet too. We were both lying on our stomachs and had our heads turned towards each other. If we had both reached out, we could have touched fingertips.

"I'm looking forward to this – I'm glad we waited until the end of vacation to do this; it's a good way to finish our fun week," I said to Tom.

"Me too – are you going to be able to relax and enjoy?" Tom asked, knowing that I have a hard time relaxing.

"Oh, shush," I replied as we heard a soft knock on the door and our masseuses walked back into the room.

We tucked our heads down as they began their massages. Soft music was playing in the dimly lit room and I tried to slip into a state of relaxation. It usually doesn't work. I laid there and tried to justify how thinking about things I needed to do when I got home should count as relaxation because I'll feel better knowing I thought through some things. Instead a whole series of random thoughts came floating in and out of my mind, including how I was right about my masseuse's hands. He was doing a great job and working hard on the kinks in my shoulders and neck.

It was about halfway through my massage, and the masseuse had just finished my neck, back and legs. He asked me to turn over, under the sheet, so he could start the next part of the massage. I knew this was coming because I had just heard Tom's masseuse ask him to do the same thing. He sat down by my head, his knees damn near my ears, and worked on my shoulders and head. A few moments passed, and he leaned down and whispered into my ear.

"Please excuse me for a moment," he said, catching me off guard.

"Sure," I replied, a little confused on where he was going.

I turned my head over to Tom to see if he had heard the exchange but he was in la-la land, looked quite peaceful and didn't move an inch. Less than a minute passed, a strangely short amount of time, and he returned. I kept my eyes closed to avoid eye contact but wondered what on earth he had done while he stepped out of the room.

As he started up again, I started thinking about all the possible things he could have done, and then started breaking down their jobs. I would get so bored massaging one person for an hour. Knowing myself, I was pretty sure I would start tracing words into people's backs with my fingers and see if they could figure out the word, or tapping beats of a song on their backs and see if they would recognize it. Tom and I were awesome at that song-tapping game. My mind continued to wander.

As my masseuse was finishing, he was back up by my shoulders and neck. My eyes were still closed, but I could tell that's where he was. I assumed he was done and was about to open my eyes when he leaned down and whispered into my ear.

"Thank you, Honore," he said, as he put one hand on my shoulder. As he was doing this I heard Tom's masseuse start to wrap up and speak to Tom too.

I opened my eyes and looked up at the masseuse. "No, thank you," I replied with a smile.

He leaned back down near my ear. "You have a beautiful body," he remarked as he stood up and left the room.

I made a confused face as I looked over at Tom.

"Did you just hear what he said?" I asked.

"Huh?" Tom replied as he started to snap back into reality.

"He just leaned down and said I had a beautiful body. Don't you think that's strange? And did you see when he left for a few seconds during the massage?" I said.

"You do have a beautiful body, it's not strange – it's a good strategy for a better tip, and no, I didn't because I was enjoying my massage," Tom said.

"That was just so incredibly awkward," I said to Tom as I started to get up and put my robe on.

We discussed that exchange many times later that day and over a dinner that night, and each time we laughed a little bit harder. These little dates that happened throughout our lives, from a calm Friday night at the house to an awkward exchange with a masseuse always had one thing in common – we always had fun.

Oct. 15 - Date Night – Hair Today, Gone Tomorrow Part 2
I'm sure many people get excited about dinner and a movie, a show or some other event when having a date night with their spouse. Tom and I? Our hot date tonight was the final stages of the hair loss saga – and let me just say, though still emotional, we made the best of it.

As you know, Wednesday started the hair loss adventure. Yesterday, Tom left his hair alone for the most part, and then this morning in the shower a majority of what was left fell out. It was clear it was time to just shave the rest off because the spots were so scattered. So...our date night began on the back patio, with him wearing a garbage bag, and me shaving his head with the clippers. I did what any logical person would do and immediately shaved an "H" in his head. Considering we all know how he handles needles, I would never anticipate a tattoo with my name on it – so I felt like this was an important thing to do. (For the record, I'm kidding and would never want him to get a tattoo.) I got as close as possible with the clippers we had, but we knew there was more left to do after our first round on the patio. I'm sure our neighbors thought we were absolutely crazy, but I doubt that was the first time they thought that due to an incident with a bee and a tennis racket over the summer, so I'm not going to lose any sleep over it.

Later in the evening after some dinner and a movie on the couch – we started part two. The razor blade to his head. Do you want to have a trust exercise for your marriage? Have your spouse cover your head in shave gel and trust them to take a razor to it. Luckily, we had some guidance from a friend who has experience shaving his head... so I quite literally took a deep breath, closed one eye (just kidding), and went for it. Fast-forward twenty minutes... after some laughs and one close call with the tip of his ear and we've officially taken ownership of the hair loss!

I personally feel like he's rocking it but some of my favorite quotes from him while getting adjusted to his new look include:
"I can't take a picture and not look like Lex Luther!"
"I feel like an evil mastermind now – I'm taking over the world!"
"My head is cold."

Tom is feeling very good, which is exactly what should be happening before our next chemo. We met with both oncologists yesterday and they are both very happy with how well he is doing and the results of his blood tests. Our one oncologist was shocked at how well Tom was doing – I'm so incredibly proud of him – he's really trying hard to beat this thing and it's working!

So this weekend we get ready for another round of chemo and try to salvage every moment of him feeling a bit better. Plus, tomorrow starts the next series for the Cubs' quest for the World Series – so if you don't have a team to root for, feel free to support the Cubs (or root against the Mets) so we can keep these games going through treatment! Until next time...

Trust

I figured out the puzzle. I figured out the nagging feeling that perpetuated my hatred of cancer. I lost all trust. I lost trust in a moment; I lost trust in the day; I lost trust in the mood, and I lost trust in statistics. I was forced to lose my trust.

When we woke up on Sunday, Tom said he was feeling the best that he had felt since he was diagnosed. Our doctor told us this would happen, but we didn't trust him. We didn't know how Tom's body would react, or if he would start to feel better, but he did. He had a little more energy, was starting to get his appetite, and was eager to have a few stronger days before our second round of chemo. When we woke up that morning, Tom rolled over in bed and pulled me close to him like he did every morning. I got a kiss on my forehead as I woke up and we gradually began chatting. We laid in bed for almost two hours talking. It was one of the most intense talks we had since he had been diagnosed. We hadn't had a moment to take a deep breath or realize what was happening and really talk about how insane this whole experience had become.

As Tom was talking, I remember looking at him and thinking that for a moment, things felt normal. We were just lying in bed, on a Sunday morning, curled up and chatting – life was good. Then I snapped back into reality as I looked at his bald head and focused on the topic – cancer. I wanted so desperately to go back to that moment where it all seemed normal. I tried to stop dwelling about that and instead was thankful that Tom was having a good day, and that we could enjoy these next few days together and not have such a dark cloud over us.

It wasn't but six hours later that we were checking into the ER where it was determined that Tom had blood clots. I couldn't trust a moment in time anymore.

Tom's pain had progressed throughout the day and when we were back in that ER, I felt sick to my stomach. I knew there was a high possibility that he was going to have blood clots; that was something we had been warned about. On the way to the hospital I was worried that perhaps the pain could be coming from a new tumor in his body, or a more serious complication that would make blood clots seem like a walk in the park.

Tom and I laughed as we were immediately ushered back to a room.

"Apparently telling the receptionist you have cancer and your oncologist thinks you might have blood clots is the jump-the-line card," I said to Tom as we got escorted into a room.

"Hey, at least cancer is good for something," he joked as we turned the corner into his room.

As they wheeled Tom away for his scans I sat in that room by myself, a few doors down from where we had been diagnosed just a month before. I was paralyzed again. I was mad at cancer. I was mad that I couldn't trust the day. I was mad that I had been naive enough to think that I could ever trust a moment prior to this. Life can change quickly, and until it happens to you it's just an abstract notion. My whole life I've heard people say, "Seize the day," "Appreciate every moment," "Life can change in the blink of an eye," "You never know how fast life can change," and all the other fluff people say to make sure you are living life to your potential. As I sat in that room by myself, I hated that I had to acknowledge that all that fluff was true, that it had always been true, and I just was fortunate enough to not have to know it firsthand. The only thing I could trust was that Tom and I were doing everything in our power to beat this and that our hard work would pay off.

Oct. 18 – One Step Forward, Two Steps Back
Well, sadly, I'm writing this post from the hospital (I'm fully aware I should be sleeping right now) after a crazy day. It seems that despite how great things have been going, we've taken a few steps back. We rushed to the ER this afternoon after what we thought was back pain became much more serious over the afternoon. After calling our on-call oncologist and determining we should get him checked out, we confirmed what we hoped wouldn't be the case. Multiple blood clots in the arteries around the lung. Punch. In. The. Gut. I won't lie – this has been tough to swallow. We are VERY thankful we caught the clots before, God forbid, they got to his brain, heart or lung – but this 100 percent absolutely, positively, sucks and took the wind right out of our sails. Tom feels like he got cheated out of two of his "good" days. We didn't want an extended stay at the hospital, and it's frustrating to feel like we are doing everything the doctors tell us to do and yet we still hit roadblocks. He's in a lot of pain but taking it like a champ and continuing to make me so proud.

Adding insult to injury, after I ran home to pack us bags, grab our laptops, etc., I parked and loaded myself up with our cargo – two laptop bags, two overnight bags, my blanket, a pillow and one extra bag of hospital stuff. I got to the entrance of his building, and it was closed because it was after hours and I had to literally walk all the way around the hospital grounds to the emergency entrance and then trek from there all the way back to his room. We are lucky; we have amazing people in our lives; we both have jobs we love; we have each other, etc. – but after the day we've had, we simply reserve the right to hate cancer today. We meet with our great team of doctors in the morning...more to come.

What's The Return Policy?

Tom and I were waiting in line at the courthouse to pick up our marriage certificate. I was oddly excited. It seemed like our wedding was becoming a reality. We found the little room tucked away in the courthouse and walked in to fill out the paperwork. A couple was in front of us, dealing with their own marriage license, minus the love. The woman working at the courthouse was being as patient as possible, but the couple was in the middle of an argument and didn't seem too thrilled to be there in the first place.

As they were fighting the woman handed us our paperwork to fill out. We took it over to the island that was in the middle of the room. We had our backs to the other couple, who were still having a hard time with the paperwork. Tom and I were starting to laugh a bit and look at each other as this exchange became weirder. We had filled everything out we needed and had all the different documentation. As we turned around to get back in line to pay and hand in our paperwork, the other couple was finishing up.

"The total will be $105," the employee said to the couple, eager for them to be on their way.

"A hundred-five for a marriage license?" the soon-to-be groom replied in shock. Neither of them reached for their wallets; they just looked at each other. After a moment, the gentleman reached into his pocket and begrudgingly pulled out his wallet.

"If this doesn't work out, do I get my $105 dollars back?" he asked as he handed over his credit card. The bride just rolled her eyes and didn't say a word as she looked in the other direction. Tom and I could hardly keep it together and couldn't look at each other for fear of laughter.

"No, sir. You are paying for services rendered, not a guarantee," the clerk replied as she grabbed his card. Clearly she had handled this question before and it took everything I had to not applaud her response. Tom squeezed my hand hard, probably knowing I wanted to start a slow clap, and to keep from laughing out loud. They wrapped up and walked out; we stepped up to the counter, and the courthouse worker smiled at us as she shook her head watching them walk out the door.

"Well that was interesting…I think we are all set with our paperwork," I said as I handed it across the counter to her.

"And I'm not worried about a return. She's stuck with me for life," Tom said to her as he leaned over and kissed me.

I kept thinking about purchasing our marriage license when we were "stuck" in the hospital for the extended stay. Because, in a way, we weren't husband and wife right now; I had to let that go the day he was diagnosed. We abruptly had to shift to patient and caregiver, and while he was obviously still my husband, in the day-to-day our dynamic was so different. It wasn't a bad thing, but there were days where I missed the old days, our usual banter, singing in the kitchen, or him dancing down the aisle of a grocery store. More than anything, I missed our freedom. This hospital had really become a jail of sorts. It was our favorite month, October, and we had to watch the colors change and the leaves fall from a hospital bed. I wanted to be stuck with Tom for the rest of my life, just not in a hospital room.

Oct. 20 – Extended Stay – Hospital Adventures
It's been a crazy few days here at the Hospital. I almost posted at 2 am last night, but then realized I should probably attempt to get a little shut-eye before morning. I was still hating cancer pretty hard and figured I should be a little more positive before I post again. Per the name of the post – we've been here since Sunday and sadly did not get to go home prior to chemo. That makes for a seven-night stay this push, and we are already counting down our nights remaining – but the good news is we've got the blood clots under control.

Essentially, Tom was high risk for blood clots because of his chemo treatment. They had warned us of all the symptoms to look for, so I'm glad we were smart enough to put it all together and get to the hospital. Due to his pain, Tom lost track of the fact that we came to the hospital a few hours before the Cubs game, to which he said, "It's a good thing you didn't mention it, because I probably would have avoided coming." Apparently, he is willing to jeopardize his health for the Cubs. He will require shots every twelve hours – for the next three months. So, starting tonight, I got the lowdown on administering the shots and will be moonlighting as Nurse Honore moving forward. Remember our trust exercise with the head shaving? The repeated shots make that look like a piece of cake. I had three nurses watching me/teaching me as I (sort of) confidently stabbed him or should I say poked him with the needle. I'll continue to do the shots while I'm here to make sure I'm good to go at home. However, for now, I've totally got the dramatic doctor/nurse glove-snap thing down.

Today was another busy day, but I'm glad to say that we are done with Day One of our chemo treatment. He rocked it as per usual. We saw our regular oncologist first thing this morning to prepare for the day, and she had great reports from his blood work. We definitely have started to kill this tumor! Unfortunately, it didn't reduce in size greatly (yet), but the blood counts show great progress so that was a great way to start our day after a rough two days here dealing with the clots. As for now, Tom is trying hard to keep his eyes open, despite meds that make him drowsy, to watch the whole Cubs game. More to come tomorrow…

Older And Wiser

I had a professor once say that sometimes life gives you the test before it gives you the lesson. This was usually the case for me anyway because of how my brain worked. I winged it in high school and college. I could listen to lectures, take a few notes and pretty much be set except in economics or math. I always used the approach of common sense and logic to figure out the answers, and I think it's part of the reason I've been successful. I never focused on remembering what the answers were supposed to be, but instead I assessed the question and figured it out. If there were a manual to life, I'd probably leaf through it and then figure out the rest on my own. I'm more of a baptism-by-fire kind of girl.

By the second round of chemo, we had just about everything figured out. We knew the routine; I would work from the hospital; I could pack our bags for the week in the hospital without thinking twice; I blogged to help manage all the love and keep people informed, and I had created relationships with people at the hospital. Logic told me that I couldn't do anything to take Tom's cancer away from him any faster than the path we were on, so once I reconciled that, it was a matter of execution. In fact, it's essentially what I do for a living; taking complex changes and breaking them down into actionable steps people can take to get from Point A to Point B. The only difference here was that I wasn't quite sure where Point B was, when we would get there, and what we would need once we got there. But those were the details, and the details have never been my style.

However, my style evolved. Throughout this entire experience, I wondered how much our ages affected how we handled things. Would I have handled it differently if this had been two years earlier? What about ten years from now? Of course I knew I couldn't spin in the land of "what ifs?" but it puzzled me. We were repeatedly told how unfair it was that it happened to us so young, or how shocking it was to see two young people fighting such a serious battle, and in a way it upset me. It implied that there was a "right" time for this to happen, and that if we were in our eighties this would somehow be less difficult.

What about a child and their parents dealing with a cancer diagnosis? The thought of a child going through what Tom was fighting made me want to hurl my insides out of my body. The parade of older people I saw every day fighting this disease were the matriarchs and patriarchs, potentially leaving large holes in their families or a partner on their own for the first time in years. Was it fair then? They lived their lives right? Bull. I call bull. It implied that these tragedies are less painful at a certain age. They are painful no matter what, to the patient, the caregiver, their family, their friends, and the friends of friends who don't even know them but know their story.

It wasn't about our actual age, but the assumptions that go with being a certain age – where people are at in their lives and how they will handle something. When a gentleman told me he was shocked and taken aback at how young we were, what he really was saying was our current challenge was a lot to take on for people who haven't lived that long. It wasn't our age he was talking about but whether we had the wisdom and ability to comprehend what was happening. Because those older than us are always wiser than us at some level; they've lived that little bit longer, they've learned one more lesson than us, and they've felt pain that the younger generations have not yet felt.

It stretches well beyond a cancer diagnosis, and I realized I had been guilty of this myself. At the age of twenty-eight, I was still fortunate to have healthy parents. When I hear about someone dying and leaving behind children, it's entirely unimaginable to me that a young kid could comprehend and cope with the loss of a parent. This incomprehension doesn't change that they will experience it, though, and who's to say a child wouldn't handle the loss of a parent differently than I would at the age of twenty-eight because of their approach to life and resilience?

In addition to personality, it's about the life experiences that dictate how you will react, and for some, those experiences come earlier in life than others. Right before we came for the second round of chemo, we received a gift in the mail with a card and kind words – *"It breaks our heart that you're experiencing the true test of a marriage so soon."* I didn't disagree, but I wondered if it really was too soon. Because in my mind, the sooner, the better. If this was in the cards for us, then so be it. Let's deal with this now, before kids, before we could realize the difficulty of shifting to patient/caregiver and most importantly before we got too old without yet being wise.

Oct. 21 – Cancer & Cubs

Day Two is in the books! We had a relatively calm day with our second day of treatment of the cycle. This cycle has actually been quite different from our first in one very important way – much less pain. Our first cycle was more challenging because Tom was just coming off his port surgery so he was taking a lot more medication than he is now. Currently, we are just getting chemo prep/chemo drugs during treatment. It may not seem like that big a deal, but it does make him less of a medication zombie and helps reduce his fogginess. He's feeling quite well considering we are already done with day two, but during our first round of treatment day two into day three was the toughest for him and when it really started to "hit" him.

Speaking of hitting him, I got to poke him again tonight with his needle, and he says it was less painful than yesterday. When I did it the first time I was nervous so I went slow – the trick to these shots is to make them quick – so Jack be nimble, Jack be quick, he got that shot fast tonight. Regardless of his (alleged) pain, my glove snaps were perfect this evening.

The hardest part of his day was the end of the Cubs post-season run to the World Series. I have to say it's actually kind of sweet to hear the different rooms cheering and providing some joy to these otherwise quiet halls. As I was walking down to the nurse's station tonight, an older gentleman was here with his loved one and he had chatted with Tom and I earlier in the evening when we were out on our hallway stroll. When he saw me walking to the nurse's station (during the game), he was also in the hall again and commented that he heard Tom clapping and was hoping they could pull off the win for him. We chatted for a bit, and he showed me an actual card in his wallet that anointed him as a lifelong Cubs fan – he got the card in 1954 at his first game. I was impressed, mostly because I can't find a gift card that I know is in my wallet and he readily pulled out a card he's had for over fifty years.

Anyway, he then went on to tell me how much it hurt his heart to see such a young couple fighting such a tough disease and that we had caught him off guard earlier when he first saw us taking our stroll. Yes, we are young. Yes, we don't look like your average couple in the oncology unit. However, I wouldn't wish this on anyone, at any age, including my worst enemy. If anything, we are lucky to be fighting this at a younger age because Tom's body has the ability to fight it and he and I will be stronger than ever when it's all over. This gentleman was not the first to react this way, and I'm sure he won't be the last – but we're going to beat this – and we might as well enjoy people referring to us as young.

Anyway, the best way to summarize our day is the t-shirt that his Aunt Paula and Uncle Rick gifted him today. "Cancer Has Nothing on Me – I'm a Cubs Fan!" No truer words have been said, and cancer's got nothing on us! More to come tomorrow…

I Get By With A Little Help From My Friends

I felt incredible guilt for every one of my friends and family. I don't know what I would do if I were in their situation, and they were grasping for any chance to help us. For me, the greatest help was to talk to my friends and family, and sometimes to talk about our situation. I talked to my sister when she was having a bad day and she remarked, "I know this is nothing to complain about considering what you're dealing with…" and proceeded to tell me about a particularly irritating day. There was nothing wrong with her having a bad day, and her frustrations didn't count less because they weren't as serious as mine.

I've been fiercely loyal for as long as I can remember, and the thought of my friends and family not feeling like they still had a two-way friendship tore me up inside. Yet some days I really just needed to vent, to talk things out so I could process them, but I didn't want it to be about me. I wanted to hear about their crazy coworkers, and their spouses being silly and the milestones of their kids. I wanted them to still have a friend even though my days didn't quite match up to their everyday lives.

The day we got home from Tom's diagnosis hospital stay, I called my best friend Katie on my way to Walgreens to pick up a prescription. She answered the phone and I sobbed. I don't think she understood a word I said for the first two minutes. I just sobbed. It was one of the first times I had cried that hard and she listened. In her shoes, I would have been itching to do something, and I knew she was. I knew she wanted to figure out a way to help, and she did; she listened. I said everything that had been circling in my head for days. Why is this happening to him? I'm scared. I don't know if I can do this. What if we can't have kids? She let me cry it out and reassured me that everything would be okay – but my heart broke for my friends and family.

Katie and I had been random roommates in college – from the first night we were best of friends and have rarely gone a day without talking. We were two peas in a pod and have always supported each other to the max – she was like another sister to me. I have only known her one year longer than she has known Tom, and I knew she, and all my girlfriends, were probably grieving a bit too. I felt bad venting to my friends and family because I knew they were dealing with this all as well.

Tom's parents and family were another group of people that were very much in this same boat. He was their child, their nephew, their brother, their friend – and he was very sick. I found myself wanting to comfort everyone else instead of grieving for myself. Taking care of others was always how I took care of myself. The night Tom was diagnosed, his Aunt Paula and Uncle Rick told their kids what had happened. I texted them both late that night from the hospital.

"How are you two doing?"

His cousin Stephen replied, "Better question. How are YOU doing?"

I knew I didn't have a good answer. I had been carrying such guilt since Tom was diagnosed and wasn't sure how to make it go away. Especially with an extended stay at a hospital and the perception that things were getting worse, our friends and family were being put through the wringer.

What's interesting about that guilt, though, is that is also creates awe. There are very few times when you see your network of love come to life. Sure, people come to your wedding, attend baby showers, send love on your birthday, but it is remarkable to see the network of people you love tap into the network of people that love them to make connections with doctors, make blankets and gifts for us, and send cards.

For every person that we were close to, I would guess at least five people close to them heard about our situation, whether from their parents, siblings or coworkers. Suddenly our network became this large web of people, many of whom we didn't know, who were filling the world with good energy and prayers for us. It was the only thing that helped my guilt subside because we had done the same for someone else too. We've been that network for others and that's why we are ultimately all on this earth, to love, to help each other out and to be forever tangled in these webs of love and support.

Oct. 22 – Three Down...Two to Go

Day Three – DONE! Two more days to go. We are going a little stir crazy in the hospital, but know we are getting closer and closer to our stay being over, which is what is keeping us going. Tom is starting to feel the repeated days of chemo and getting quite fatigued and tired, but he's been rocking it. We were incredibly close to needing a blood transfusion, but his blood counts were just at the cutoff point so we avoided that. Phew! Given how he reacts to blood being drawn from him, I can't even imagine what the reverse would do!

All in all, his counts look good. He's managing to get by with little nausea, but he is sleeping and resting quite a bit. He was a little bummed all day, but we have the Cubs to thank for that, not the chemo.

I'll be honest; we are exhausted. It's been a long week already and we are going to try to catch up a bit, so a brief post tonight, but for good reason as we try to keep ourselves ahead of what will be a long few days after chemo too. Thanks for all the great blog comments, the text messages, emails, calls and cards – it really brightens our day and keeps us going through this all! Until next time...

Your Wishes – Minus the Genie

Tom and I were curled up in his hospital bed late one night – our dinner visitors had just left, and I knew Tom would be asleep shortly. I nuzzled into his arm as I looked up at him. He looked exhausted and had no color in his face. I turned my head back against his chest, looking down to the edge of the bed.

"I can't decide if we are tall or if this bed is short," I said as I rested my feet on the foot of the bed.

"I don't think it matters. Either way it's uncomfortable," he said. "This is my idea of hell."

"Stuck in a room with your wife for seven days, or an uncomfortable bed?" I quipped, looking back up at him.

"The bed part," he replied, "I like being stuck with you."

"Well, you are stuck with me, just remember that. No funny business, you're beating cancer," I replied.

"I'm trying, babe – that's the plan," he replied, with a sense of calm in his voice.

"Can I ask you something? I don't want you to get mad, but it's been on my mind," I inquired, nervous about approaching the topic I knew we had been dancing around for weeks.

"Of course," he replied. I was convinced he knew where this was headed.

"I know you are going to beat this, but just in case something was to ever happen to you, what would you want? I know we talked about this years ago but I can't remember, and it's been bugging me. The last thing I would want if something was to happen to you, not just with cancer, but life in general, would be for me to not remember your wishes."

Tom didn't say anything for a minute; I still had my head on his chest. I turned up to make eye contact with him.

"Cremated for sure," he replied.

"Really?" I replied, though I wasn't shocked.

"Yeah, and then I want my ashes put in an urn that my oldest child has to wear around their neck for the rest of his life," he said, chuckling.

"Oh stop, seriously, what would you want?"

Tom took in a deep breath. "I want to be cremated and then you can spread me in a few places. But I think I would still want a gravestone, too," he said. I could tell he hadn't thought about this too much, or he was pretending to make me feel better.

"Where do you want your ashes spread? It better not be somewhere that might get me arrested," I joked.

"First, you need to get some Cubs bleacher seats and drop some into the ivy," Tom said as a smile came across his face.

"Are you serious?" I asked. "Am I even allowed to do that as a Brewers fan?"

"I mean, it's not ideal, but what are my options?"

I shook my head as I put my head back on his chest. "What else?"

Tom thought about it for a while longer. "McClain State Park."

I took in a shallow breath to try and not cry. McClain State Park was located up in the Upper Peninsula of Michigan – known as the UP – and the location of our July family reunion each year with my dad's family. It's an all-day event of swimming, games, food, and relaxation. Each year we go to the same spot within the park, a bluff that hangs over Lake Superior. The fresh air of the Great Lakes is special; the temperatures are always reasonable and some of my fondest memories of growing up took place there – especially with my dad and grandparents. The sunsets from this location are spectacular; and sunsets and water were the two things that calm me the most.

Last year, when we were in the UP, we had spent the whole day at McClain. Early evening, everyone packed up and headed back to the hotel. We had my parents in our car so we went back to the hotel to drop them off. As we were unpacking our beach things, Tom suggested we make the drive back out to the park and watch the sunset. He knew it was one of my favorite things to do and thought it might be fun. He didn't have to ask me twice. On our way out of town we grabbed Chinese takeout - because you can eat whatever you want on vacation and not gain a pound - and headed back to the park. We sat in a gazebo overlooking the sunset as we ate our dinner. The weather was perfect, and the sky was lighting up in shades of orange and red – it was one of the best sunsets I had seen in years at McClain. Tom had grown to love the UP in the years he had been going there with my family. The fact that McClain had such meaning to him almost made me sob.

"That's sweet," I mumbled, still not able to look up at him. "Anywhere else?"

"Yeah, the little park area where I proposed to you and where we hung out when we first met," he said.

I smiled as I looked up at him. "Doesn't that seem so long ago?"

One of the first times Tom and I hung out we went to the lakefront in Milwaukee. We were sitting on Bradford beach, in the moonlight, and Tom was playing his guitar. We chatted as he strummed on his guitar and talked about music. I played the fiddle for years and thought it was so awesome that he was passionate about playing music too. We sat there for two hours talking; it was when I first realized we might have something special.

Five years later, on my birthday, Tom was walking down that same beach with me, moments away from proposing. It wasn't where he had initially planned to propose but the hot-air balloon ride he had planned was canceled due to weather. Just steps away from where we had hung out that first time, he dropped to his knee and proposed. It was a special spot to us both.

"That's another good one. I can do that one and probably not get arrested," I replied, trying to lighten the mood.

"The rest can go at a gravestone somewhere. I'm not sure where, and I'm not sure what I want on my grave. I'll have to think about that more," he replied. "Whenever it happens though, I want a celebration. I want an Irish wake style celebration. I'm sure people will be sad, but I want people to celebrate," he said.

"Lucky for you – you married an Irish girl," I said as I looked up to him. He was starting to talk with his eyes closed and was dozing off for the night. I got up on my elbow and gave him a kiss on the cheek.

"Get some sleep," I whispered as I got out of his hospital bed. Tom opened his eyes, looked up at me, and smiled. He didn't need to say a word. I reached over and turned off the light and grabbed the remote. I looked over at him in the light of the TV and stared at him sleeping. As I looked at him, I reached for a pen and my notebook. The seriousness of the conversation we had was starting to sink in. I looked down and flipped to a blank page. In the left column I wrote TOM'S WISHES. To the right I wrote:
- Cremated (Irish Wake)
- McClain
- Wrigley Ivy
- Proposal Park
- Gravestone

I looked back up at Tom as he slept and the tears that I had tried to keep welled up in my eyes finally broke free. I looked down at what I had written as a tear dropped right on top of where I had written TOM'S WISHES. I took a deep breath and closed my notebook as I started to quietly put my things away for the night. The only wish I had right now was for this to all be a bad dream.

Oct. 23 – So Close...

Phew! Another day in the books; we are so darn close, yet it feels so far. One more day of chemo and then two more nights here in the hospital. We can do it. As we get further into the week, he tends to get more fatigued, and that continues to be the case this week. I would anticipate tomorrow he will sleep quite a bit as he gets his last treatment, but so far this cycle, we've been very lucky with the nausea. Perhaps we have gotten the mix of anti-nausea medicines figured out for him! So tonight, for your reading pleasure, we came up with a list of things that happen when you spend a full week at the hospital: 1. I get a little crazy in the gift shop. I'll be honest, this is a really good hospital gift shop; they've got some awesome home décor stuff, and it feels like everything is on sale (and not the kind of sale stuff that is so ugly you totally understand why it's on sale). As much as I was tempted by the hospital sweatshirt – because much like a college sweatshirt I will have paid this place enough to wear it with pride – I got some cute décor, and a sentimental piece we will hang up in the house when we get home to always remind us of this experience and how lucky we are.

2. Tom is cynical about commercials. As you can imagine, he's been limited in what he is able to do, so he has watched a more than average amount of TV. The following commercials bother him specifically:

- *Chevy Commercial with Wi-Fi in the Car: He's irritated they don't tell you there is a data plan required AND that almost everyone has internet on their phone. He thinks it's the silliest campaign ever and yells at the TV people when they act so excited – never mind that they are actors.*
- *Domino's Pizza: He feels that the pizza emoticon campaign is misleading because you obviously have to do some setup work before you text Domino's your order. I'm not sure why this one bothers him so much, but it's at the point where I laugh out loud when it comes on.*

3. We make lots of new friends. I'm a pretty social person and have made friends here at the hospital. The checkout ladies in the cafeteria are wonderful and keep an eye to make sure I'm eating well. I've made some friends on our floor that are also here supporting their families, and of course we have gotten close with some of our favorite nurses, technicians and the cleaning staff.

4. Crazy Conversations. Imagine being with your spouse holed up in a room for seven days. Minus our scare earlier in the week, we try to make treatment week as fun as possible. It's kind of cool that we've had some random conversations and learned stuff about each other that we never knew despite being together for nine years. For example, he never knew that as a child I once made the poor decision to swallow a penny (for the record, I thought it was chocolate).

5. Not All Late Night Boredom Activities Are Encouraged. Let's just say drawing funny faces on the masks seems to be frowned upon.

Thank you all for the prayers, good energy and great vibes. We truly feel it all and know we've got so many people rooting for us. THANK YOU! More to come tomorrow…

The Student and The Teacher

We were the Guinea pigs of the oncology floor. Almost every single day we had two nurses administering the chemo. One to teach, and one to administer; the nurses have to practice a certain number of times to become officially certified. The staff was always kind enough to ask if it was okay, and we of course always said yes – if we could help, we were happy to.

However, Tom had mastered his own chemo process. He could tell you what bags went where, what bag lines could be combined, when a filter was needed, and what lines required an alcohol cap. During this round of chemo, one of our nurses was administering chemo for the first time and talking herself through the process. The experienced nurse was standing behind her, listening to her talk through it. I looked up from my work to see Tom nodding or shaking his head. She kept smiling as Tom helped remind her what she had learned during her training session. If he needed to, Tom could have hooked himself up to those bags; he had figured out every piece of the puzzle.

We were repeatedly thanked for our patience, as this process often took longer than normal since there was lots of stop and go in their teaching moments. We had nothing but time, and if anyone deserved an award for patience it was the nurses. Plus, they had a little help getting certified thanks to Teacher Tom guiding them to all the answers.

Oct. 24 – Round Two – Check!

Round Two of Chemo? Check! Phew, what a week, but we've almost made it through. We had a bit of a rough day with some more blood clot pain returning out of nowhere, after four days of no pain, and then Tom getting sick (nausea – one, Tom – zero). But we are done. Tonight is our last night here. Then we can go home. I'm beyond excited for this – as is he!

We've had a tough week, a bit of a roller coaster. We came in feeling pretty down with the blood clots, got some momentum once we started chemo, and then had a rough last few days of hospital fatigue and Tom's symptoms coming back. I truly think just being home will help lift spirits and make life seem "normal," even if he's feeling very sick.

When we leave tomorrow, we are done with two of four treatments, so halfway done with chemo! We know we've got surgery too, but for now we celebrate chemo. I'm exhausted so my apologies for the short post, but more to come...

Writing for the Soul

I've always had a creative brain and enjoyed writing. I attempted some writing ventures before, but never followed through. To be honest, I think it was lack of inspiration. When Tom got sick and I suggested that I would do the blog, he said, "You do that, and I'll do this," pointing to the tumor. It had started as a communication mechanism, and morphed into a lifeline.

There were so many nights I wrote what I really wanted to say, saved the file and then edited it to have less swear words and be a bit more positive. I wasn't being deceitful, just trying to process. A shock of this size was not something that could be reconciled in the mind alone – I needed to think it out, talk it out, and write it out. I never quite knew what I was going to write, but the pages always seemed to fill themselves. There were days when I felt like I was reading someone else's writing. I hadn't realized what I was writing; it just flowed from my fingertips onto the page.

I was hearing that the blog was inspiring; I was hearing people checked the blog each morning; I was hearing that I should write a book. The fact of the matter is while I was writing I heard nothing; all the chaos subsided for a moment. I was coping, I was processing, and for a brief moment, I was at peace.

Oct. .25 – Halfway

HOME. HOME. HOME. Any guesses where we are? HOME. Those were some of the longest seven days of our lives, and we still aren't sure why seven days on vacation goes so fast, yet seven days in a hospital is like a never-ending march...but we did it.

Today was challenging. Tom was getting sick again, and we were so anxious to get out of there, so it felt like a very long morning and early afternoon. Here's the trick with our last day – we know exactly, down to the minute, when we can leave because of the treatment cycle. Luckily for us, the nurses love us, and our nurse was waiting in our room for the IV machine to beep and immediately removed all of his port IVs and got us out of there quickly. We already had gone through all the discharge paperwork and our medicine matrix, so we really just had to wait for that last drop of medicine before we could leave. At one point, Tom was shaking the tubing of his IV to help it move along; of course, the nurse laughed and said that would do absolutely no good.

It's hard to believe we are halfway done with chemo, and by hard to believe, I mean Hallelujah. We have tried to stay positive, and Tom has been doing SO incredibly well. The doctors are surprised at how well his body is handling his treatment but don't get me wrong, we have had some really, really tough days.

93

A "good day" for him is not having to feel like he is going to throw up all day, and being able to walk down the block and not feel like he climbed Mount Everest, but he has been putting mind over matter.

The beautiful thing about going home is that it lifted his spirits. High spirits help as we go into a few of the hardest days of the chemo cycle, so it is comforting to be home in his own bed, in a normal-sized shower, and not be hooked up to IVs. We hate the IV machine so much we took a photo of it turned OFF. Anyway, we came home to a stack of cards – which he loved – they really make him smile and help keep spirits up into the post-chemo days.

A month ago, when this all began, we had started the blog to keep everyone informed, but it's morphing into more than that. First, a side effect of Tom's treatment is a mild amnesia, so it's likely he won't remember most of his treatment details – for which I'm actually thankful. They say he will be able to remember this period of his life, but likely not specific conversations, etc. I thought that seemed odd, but it was clear this week he remembered very little about his first treatment and events of the past month. This blog is a way for him to look back and have some memory of this time, all the love that was around us, and how many people were rooting for him. Second, it's become a little bit of humor and therapy for us to try to think of creative things to post that aren't just about treatment and might bring a smile to people's faces. I'm glad people are enjoying it so we will continue on and perhaps get more creative as we go.

Perks of this stay?
- *We are halfway done with chemo...*
- *I got another full loyalty card in the cafeteria – and an extra punch because the guy dropped my omelet on the floor...*
- *It will make chemo three feel fast because we won't have an extended stay...*
- *Tom watched a segment on tiny houses and tried to convince me that it would be a good idea to sell our house and live in a tiny house attached to one of our cars.*
- *Multiple times we laughed so hard we cried...*
- *We avoided a hospital stay on a special day – we got home the day before our wedding anniversary...*

Sorry for the rather scattered post tonight, but stay tuned for a special anniversary post tomorrow....

Mrs. Independent

I always knew I was the marrying type, but never had a specific physical type in mind, other than tall - because I'm tall. What mattered were personality traits. Sure, an element of attraction needs to be in every relationship, and Tom and I have plenty, but I could never point at some picture and say: that's what I want my husband to look like. Instead I had relationship criteria – he has to make me laugh; we have to have fun; we needed similar goals and ideals, and he had to be a family man. To me those were the most important qualities I could ask for in a life partner.

We were engaged in July and planned to get married the following October – fifteen months later. I never quite got into the wedding planning thing. I enjoyed it, but there was a bit of drama within my own family, and my sister was getting married in September of the year we were engaged. By the time my wedding rolled around, my family was tired of wedding fuss. We made it fun, but I was trying to prepare for a marriage, not a wedding. Some days I got lost in the wedding piece more than the marriage piece, but the marriage was where I tried to keep my focus.

I remember bits and pieces of our wedding day – some for better reasons than others – but to be surrounded by all these people we loved was a special experience. We made that day our own, but as I look back there are so many things I would change. When the evening wrapped up, we headed back to the hotel. We got to the room and there were rose petals on the floor, champagne, and chocolate-covered strawberries. We talked about the insane day, who we had talked to, and that we felt like we hardly saw each other because were busy mingling with 200-plus guests. It was already the wee hours of the morning and I was starving.

"Are you hungry?" I asked Tom.

"Starving," he replied.

"Where can we get food right now?" I asked him, hoping he had a solution because I was too tired to figure one out.

"I still have the Jimmy Johns number in my phone, and they are open late because of the campus," he replied. Tom had attended Marquette University and during poker nights with his buddies they had all become regulars.

"That sounds epic," I replied.

A few minutes later, Tom said, "Done!" and the food was on its way. In no time our food arrived at our hotel door. We sat, legs crossed, on either side on our big king bed, eating our Jimmy Johns and drinking champagne.

"This is amazing," I said to him as I wolfed down the sandwich.

"Happy Wedding!" Tom joked as he leaned his sandwich towards mine. I grabbed my champagne glass and we first clinked of our champagne glasses, and second bumped our sandwiches together.

That was our first official bed picnic – three years later I'd consistently be sitting cross-legged on my husband's hospital bed eating meals. Our vows were being tested, and this cancer diagnosis wasn't a quiz; it was the final exam straight out of the gate. On that day, we celebrated a wedding, but that same day we started our marriage, the part that lasts well beyond those hours. Who would have thought late night Jimmy Johns on the bed would prepare me so well for what was to come.

Oct. 26 – Three Year Anniversary – To the Edge And Back
Three years ago today we made vows to each other on our wedding day – it's hard to believe how fast the time has gone – and it's amazing to think how little a clue we had for what lay ahead. This diagnosis has taken us to the edge of our vows and back and has truly put all those words to the test.

We said, "I (Honore or Tom) take you (Honore or Tom) to have and to hold, from this day forward, for better or for worse, for richer or for poorer, in sickness and in health, to love and cherish, until death do you part."

I've got some thoughts on this. It goes more like this for us right now:
"I, Honore, take you, Tom...
to have and to hold close so I don't fall off the edge of the tiny hospital bed...
from whatever the hell day it is, because I lost track of days in the hospital, forward....
for better, and there will be better, or for worse, but let's hope not much worse...
for richer, when I finally win a lottery scratch card, or for poorer...
in cancer and in health, which we will never take for granted...
to love, more than I ever thought possible, and cherish you through a brief brush with death, because we are going to beat this thing..."

Seems more realistic, don't you think? All kidding aside, we know we will be stronger for it all when this is over and we have our lives back.

As you can imagine, we had a bit of a low-key day. Our big anniversary date consisted of us getting up early and going to the doctor to get his booster shot, which really exhausted him. It's amazing what these first few days post-treatment do to him. It is no exaggeration when I say he is out of breath if he walks around the house for longer than a minute. He is completely wiped out. Once we got home, he dozed while I worked all day from home.

Despite everything going on in our lives, when Tom was having his "good week" before chemo he figured out a way to get to Hallmark without me knowing and had an anniversary card for me. It was the sweetest thing he could have done, better than any gift in the world. I made him his favorite dish for dinner tonight and we caught up on some stuff on the DVR. He was feeling pretty down today that his situation made for a rather mild anniversary, and I'd be lying if I said there weren't some tears from both of us, but I think it was a perfect anniversary considering our situation. More to come...

Forty Days And Forty Nights

I went to Catholic school for sixteen years. My parents made sacrifices to make sure I attended a fabulous Catholic grade school and high school, and I made the decision to go to a Catholic university. You'd think I would know the bible backwards and forwards, but my faith had shifted over the years.

One thing always stayed true, I always gave something up for lent. Lent is the forty-day period in the Christian Liturgical Calendar between Ash Wednesday and Easter when you are encouraged to give something up (a sacrifice) or try a new positive habit like not swearing or volunteering. I always tested myself at Lent, and always took on a challenge. My whole life, it has been hard to stay challenged. I tend to pick things up quickly, do well at my jobs, and easily get comfortable in most situations. The greatest challenge for me? Giving up sweets – cookies, cake, candy, ice cream – it was a feat, but one that I did every year and I never once cheated. That may seem like a small feat, but I don't have *a* sweet tooth, I have a whole mouth full of sweet teeth.

All we had left for chemo was a "Lent" – forty days. For some reason, this was very comforting to me. Every year during Lent there was a point when I wanted to give up and give in. This usually involved Shamrock Shakes at McDonalds. Yet inevitably, I would power through and would be surprised how fast the time had gone when I reached Easter. I knew we had much further to go after chemo, with surgery and potentially more chemo, but knowing there were only forty days until the end of chemo made it seem digestible. It felt like we had made some progress, that we might be at the end of this nightmare sooner than we thought.

Thinking about Lent brought to mind my religion and my faith. I had sort of blocked it out of my mind during the initial diagnosis. I believe in a higher power, for me that is God, and I believe in many things about the Catholic faith.

Some people, after a diagnosis like Tom's, put all their faith in God and prayer; they trust that things will work out. Others question the existence of God, and wonder why God would let such terrible things happen. They get lost in the "Why". Most days, I didn't know which I believed either. I believed in the power of prayer, energy and positive thoughts, but I'd be lying if I said there wasn't a part of me that ventured down the path of "Why," which started to have a cloud of anger and frustration surrounding it. I was too mentally and physically exhausted to put much thought into solving these centuries' old questions about faith and religion, but I knew deep down that we weren't fighting this alone. Regardless of what you call it across a variety of different religions, I felt the energy of our family and friends and knew that we weren't fighting this alone; on earth or elsewhere.

Oct. 28 – Turning The Corner

Well, we've made it through the few days post chemo. What a difference seventy-two hours can make in our life. Tom is feeling much better, and the nausea is starting to subside, but the extreme fatigue/exhaustion still lingers. Unfortunately, there isn't a magical pill that can help boost his energy or prevent exhaustion, so that is more of a gradual climb back to his "normal." Plus, if there were a pill that worked that type of magic, I would have started taking it six weeks ago!

Today marks forty days until the last day of chemo – not that we are counting. His diagnosis was forty-three days ago. I'm not even sure how to describe the past forty-three days, but if I had to summarize it, I would say one word –blur. The last day of chemo will be a huge milestone for us and then we will have the final hurdle of surgery – so let the countdown begin – forty days until the end of chemo! Some days, I'm not even sure how we have kept it together so far, but I'm hopeful that the next forty days are quick and calm, without any major disruptions!

In other news, Tom thought it would be funny to fake a reaction to one of his shots that I give him at home. I gave him the shot and he looked at me with a panicked look, dropped his head back and started shaking his arms. Worst. Joke. Ever. However, I know he's starting to feel better when he starts to joke around again. Such a double-edged sword...but I don't think he'll do that again because I threatened to take him back to the hospital...and he says my father-in-law is to blame for teaching him those kinds of jokes. Until next time...

The Waiting Game

There was no place I hated more than the oncologist's waiting room. We were there every week for a shot, blood work or an appointment. I'll remember the smell for the rest of my life, and not in a good way like the smell of a grandparent's house, or summer rain. We were so caught up in our day-to-day struggles that it had all become normal to us – except when we went to the oncologist's office.

Our new day-to-day was challenging, but we controlled it. We chose to be positive, we chose laughter as medicine, and we chose how to handle bumps in the road. In the waiting room, we were surrounded by all types of people, in many cases people who didn't choose the same road as us, or never had a choice. There were family members having a hard time smiling through heart-wrenching situations; there were familiar faces that we saw every week – and that looked weaker each time – and there were people holding puke bags in case they got sick.

I always wondered what everyone was there for that day. Were they coming in for routine blood work? Were they finding out if they had beat cancer? How sick were they feeling? Were they finding out that they were out of treatment options? There was such a spectrum of possibilities with these people in the waiting room, and the sad part was that it was usually packed. Sometimes it was standing room only, and it was a tragedy to see how many lives cancer was touching – to think that this was just one oncology office in the world was overwhelming.

And yet, at some level, this place was comforting. It was a tribe. I could look around and get a nod from a caregiver who was having as hard a time sitting in that waiting room as I was. Tom could look around and see others who had lost their hair. I remember Tom and I overhearing a gentleman scheduling his appointment. He didn't have to come back for six months for a checkup. Tom looked over and said he couldn't wait for the day when he could just have a checkup.

In our life, which had become a bubble, this place reminded us that there are many other people also living in their cancer bubble, that things could be worse, and most importantly, that things would get better.

Oct. 29 – Blood & Gore

Well, unfortunately Tom got more into the Halloween spirit than I had hoped. After blood work today, it was determined he needs a blood transfusion tomorrow due to his red/white counts, so we will be spending our Friday at the hospital for his transfusion. We should be in and out of the hospital tomorrow (thank goodness we don't have another sleepover), and in theory it should be a relatively simple process, so fingers crossed all goes well. The great thing about a transfusion is that he should be feeling much better afterwards since the new blood will boost his red/white blood cell counts way up. Hopefully, it's a small bump in the road and this will be the only time we have to do this throughout his treatment.

He's not looking forward to this, as you can imagine, but we were talking tonight and what's most challenging for us right now is the constant unknown. It's incredibly hard to not be able to trust any moment in time. This morning we woke up thinking he just has to get his blood checked, and then has the weekend to rest, and now we have a blood transfusion tomorrow. Certainly, this happens in life no matter what, but the constant waiting for test results, checking progress, etc. can be draining and make it hard to not doubt good days since his health can change so fast. So tomorrow is a whole new adventure...more to come...

Full Circle

Tom and I were sitting in the infusion room and getting everything ready. This wasn't quite the day we had planned, and as per usual, I was doing work as the infusion was happening. About an hour into the infusion, both of our phones buzzed.

"Who could this be?" Tom asked as he reached for his phone.

"Greg," I replied, opening the message.

"What?! The baby is here?!" Tom excitedly proclaimed.

A sweet newborn baby boy's photo was looking back at me with the caption "Oh, Hi there."

I quickly replied, "Greg!!!!!!"

And Tom followed with "What?!?!? Oh my god!!!"

Tom and I looked up at each other and we both had a huge smile on our faces. We had been anxious to meet this little guy and were so excited for Greg and his wife May to have this little bundle of joy in their lives.

I quickly texted to get more information. "Name? Everyone well?" I laughed out loud as I saw Tom's text that just said "Baby!!!"

This was a big deal for Tom. He knew that Greg was going to be a top-tier father and was eager to be the first person to buy beer for his son, likely at an age well before twenty-one. We both were eager to see more photos and most importantly see the baby, which is when the mood began to shift.

We had to make sure it was safe for Tom and the new baby to be around each other. We certainly didn't want to cause an issue for the baby and couldn't risk Tom getting sick either. Yet in any other circumstance, we would have met the baby within the first few days or weeks. It was a reminder that cancer was having an impact on our day-to-day life in so many ways, and on this day it was a tough pill to swallow. I looked over at Tom, who was texting with Greg, and thought about what an interesting turn their lives had taken. Greg was welcoming a new life into the world, and we were fighting to keep Tom alive. Every day that we were in the hospital we wished that we could be headed to a labor and delivery floor, but our plans had been derailed. We tried our best to remain focused on the joy of this newborn, and we did for the most part.

"I can't believe Greg is a dad – I feel like they just told us they were pregnant," Tom said as he looked over at me.

"They are going to be great parents, and now we might just have to have a little girl first so she falls in love with their little guy," I said, thinking about what a fun wedding that could be.

"That would be insane," Tom said with a smile on his face, but I could see in his eyes he wanted to badly to feel the joy Greg was feeling.

"We will get there soon enough," I replied, acknowledging what I knew he was thinking but only half believing what I was saying.

I wasn't sure what I meant by soon, but Tom was here fighting for his life, for us, and the future we wanted. As I looked over at him, literally hooked up to a life-line of blood, I smiled. His drive and fight had become my lifeline.

Oct. 30 – An A+ Day

I have one major regret for today, and I don't typically have regrets. There was a moment of today that I wish I had Tom's reaction in a photo or video – but unfortunately, my story telling will have to do…

Tom woke up feeling decent this morning but a little apprehensive about the blood transfusion. Now, we knew this would be a relatively simple process, but Tom was overthinking it and wondering how it would all work, which got him a little uneasy. Mid-morning, we headed to the infusion center – an unexplored floor in our favorite hospital. We can now check that floor off the list! Anyway, we got registered, and then sat in the waiting room and waited for our infusion nurse. Now, remember, tomorrow is Halloween. The receptionists were not dressed up at all so it wasn't even occurring to us that someone in costume would come and get us…

We hear "Thomas" and both get up and turn toward the nurse and she is dressed as the greatest thing ever. A cheese head. GO PACK GO! If you've been reading along, you know I'm a Packers fan, which creates the big rivalry with Tom and his Bears. Of all our rivalries, that is the one we are most serious about. I have a love for the Packers, have a celebrity crush on Aaron Rodgers, and would probably bid an unhealthy amount on eBay for a lock of Clay Matthews' hair. I literally burst out laughing and yelled, "Go Pack Go" and as Tom laughed and replied, "I honestly didn't think today could get worse." This is where I WISH I had gotten this exchange on camera – his face was priceless.

In the big scheme of things, he got the best nurse for many reasons, but especially because the other costumes we saw were more complex. The nurse dressed as Mickey Mouse (including giant Mickey hands) would have been challenging, and who trusts a mouse with four fingers but not opposable thumbs anyway? I'm actually quite shocked none of the infusion nurses were dressed as vampires, seems like a logical costume choice for their careers… Anyway, we got settled in our infusion room, which was actually quite nice. It's a private room with a big TV, an infusion chair, and even a chair with a desk for me to get some work done. They prepped Tom for the blood and walked us through the potential reactions someone can have to an infusion and what they would be looking for. Luckily, he had no reaction! In fact, once we got it started (it's quite the process), it was a pretty simple few hours. He just had to be hooked up and gradually receive the blood. Interestingly, the blood is cold when it is delivered, which makes the patient cold when they start the infusion. They had warm blankets, and he was all cozy in his infusion chair throughout the process. For the record, the blanket warmer device looks exactly like a wine fridge. Coincidence? I think not.

As we finished up, our nurse said despite how much fun she had with us, she hoped she wouldn't have to see us again. We agree! Tom did great and hopefully this is the only transfusion he will need – but it did make him feel much better and put a little pep in his step. Hopefully with this extra blood, his blood levels will continue to rise and he will be better prepared for our next bout of chemo. We hope everyone has a great Halloween, more to come...

Drop the Beat

I was going to pick up some of Tom's prescriptions and it was pouring rain outside. I was exhausted, as the weeks had been catching up to me, and gave Tom a kiss as I ran out the door. I was gone less than ten minutes. When I returned home and pulled into the garage, I had to walk by Tom's car to get to the door and noticed there were wet tire tracks and that Tom's car was wet. I was puzzled as I walked into the house; Tom wasn't supposed to be driving and I didn't know where he would have gone since I was taking care of everything.

"Did you go somewhere?" I asked as I walked in the door. I was already on the verge of being angry.

"No," Tom replied, forgetting that I had missed my calling as a detective.

"You must have gone somewhere; the car is wet."

"It was nothing."

"It must have been something – did you need something else? I was just out and could have grabbed it."

"No, I'm fine."

"I'm so confused – where did you go in the ten minutes that I was gone?"

I could tell Tom didn't want to tell me. I figured I would drop it for now and give him a few minutes to calm his thoughts. I turned to start walking up the stairs, when I heard him take a deep breath.

"I drove around the block with the windows down and the music up. I just needed to feel the air and the rain for a minute."

"Well, that makes a little more sense," I replied as I kept moving up the stairs.

I wasn't mad, but I got to the top of the steps and felt my eyes welling up with tears. My heart broke for him. He had been in cancer jail for almost a month, and he just wanted to feel free for a moment. I knew that music was special to Tom and was confident that a five-minute joy ride was better than any medication he could have been prescribed.

"I love you," I heard from downstairs.

"I love you more. Was it a good song at least?" I asked, to make sure he knew I wasn't mad so he wouldn't come upstairs and see the tears rolling down my face.

"Of course, would you expect anything less?"

I walked down the hall and went into our bedroom, lying down on the bed for a second. I took a deep breath and for a moment, out of character for me, basked in the silence.

Nov. 1 – Music Makes The World Go Round
Tom and I love music. He's an awesome guitar player, and I've played the violin/fiddle since I was four years old. We often play together. Sometimes I

hold a tune and sing, but we are always jamming out to something. Maybe if hell freezes over, I'll post a video of one of our jam sessions. I assume this is normal, but if he or I start a sentence and it happens to be part of some lyric, 98 percent of the time a lyric battle breaks out. For example, Tom feels bad asking for help, so I said to him today, "I need you to tell me what you want." Tom's reply? "I'll tell you what I want what I really really want, I wanna, I wanna, I wanna, I wanna, I wanna to really really really want to ziggazig ha." Old school 90s Spice Girls. Music to my ears, and of course, a terrifying flashback to a poor talent show performance.

In addition, I tend to make up lyrics that apply to what's happening around us when I've got the radio on in the car. Lately, lyrics have changed to me hating cancer, singing about his bald head or whatever else works with the lyrics. Anyway, my tendency to be a closet songwriter inspired our cancer-themed playlist below. Anything in parentheses is a slight addition to the current song title to make it relevant...

To me physical art decorates space; music decorates time. This certainly isn't an ideal time in our lives, but one that will be full of many memories regardless of the situation. For us, music is a therapy of sorts, both playing it and listening to it. We are cautiously optimistic that he will continue to feel better and get stronger each day before our next round of chemo – it makes such a difference to start chemo strong versus coming off surgery or with blood clots. So enjoy our goofy list below and let the countdown continue. Thirty-six days until chemo is over...

Hit Me (With Chemo) Baby One More Time – Britney Spears
(I'm) Toxic – Britney Spears
(Chemo is a) Wrecking Ball – Miley Cyrus
I Say A Little Prayer – Aretha Franklin
(Cancer) I (Don't) Want You Back – The Jackson 5
With a Little Help From My Friends – The Beatles
(Hey Chemo) We Are Never Ever Getting Back Together – Taylor Swift
Stayin' Alive – The Bee Gees
Pour Some (Antibacterial Hand Soap) on Me – Def Leppard
Stand By Me – The Temptations
Do You Think (My Bald Head) Is Sexy – Rod Stewart

Plans, Milestones, and Goals, Oh My!

It took me until my mid-twenties to have the epiphany about planning. If there is one piece of advice I would give to anyone in high school, college or their twenties, it would be to have a goal but not a plan. It may seem contradictory, but I believe a detailed plan is the culprit of disappointment.

I was never one to say things like "I want to be married by twenty-five," or "I want to have my first kid by twenty-eight," or "I want to be a manager before I'm thirty." It never made sense to me because the goal was too specific and created a life that wouldn't include spontaneity, trusting my gut, or taking a chance. If I wanted to have a kid by twenty-eight, and hadn't met the right guy, or it wasn't in the cards for us, there would be disappointment. Instead, my goals were more generic. For example, one of my simplest goals: I want to have a family. That goal of a family might not be until I'm older, might not happen the way we thought it would, but there are many things I can do to create the family I envision without leading myself down a path of disappointment.

For my career, my goal is to have challenging work that interests me and serves a purpose for the world. The number of jobs that could fulfill that goal is almost infinite, which is exactly what I hope for. The people in my life who have a degree in one area and found themselves on a completely different path are almost the majority, and it's the most wonderful thing.

I got to a point in the cancer diagnosis that the thought of our situation not being part of our life seemed strange. Sure, milestones have changed, timelines have been extended and short-term goals have shifted, but it would all still fit into the plan.

Nov. 3 – Feeling Good!

I am thrilled to say that Tom is feeling great and getting stronger each day as we get closer to our next round of chemo. As I was looking at the blog today, I saw that on the archives section we now have three months listed. WHAT?! I will say this, for some reason November was a breath of fresh air. There is something about knowing that we are in November that means major milestone #1 - finishing chemo – is near, since that should be the first week of December. (Thirty-three days!) It also helps that we've got the holidays coming up to give us other dates to anchor to and get excited about, but regardless, I can't believe this madness started eight-plus weeks ago.

Now we begin the rather daunting task of starting to get all of our ducks in a row for the surgery that he will need (major milestone #2). We were told that we would start this process after his second round of chemo, because there isn't a whole lot they can do until they start to see the numbers drop and can anticipate what will need to be done via surgery. There was a 1 percent chance that he wouldn't need surgery, but that has already been ruled out. Never mind that he dominated the odds of getting this cancer but can't catch a break on that 1 percent. ;-) So now we just hope that it gets small enough that it doesn't have to be a major procedure and instead can be done in a less intrusive way with a short recovery time. We do know that surgery won't be until late December or early January because they won't do surgery until his body has had time to bounce back from his last round of chemo. Realistically, since that will be his fourth round, it will take little time for all his levels to get up to an acceptable range that the surgeon deems safe for surgery. But for now, we start meeting with the doctors and getting ourselves educated on this last little adventure of getting rid of cancer. We meet with his doctors on Thursday and will get blood work done again – hopefully no transfusion needed, and hopefully good news from his doctors on progress.

For the record... the remaining major milestones after #1 and #2 are:
#3 CANCER FREE
#4 a YouTube worthy happy dance
...and last but not least...
#5 a strong drink.

More updates to come on Thursday when we know more!

The Big Red Nose

We were standing in a large industrial kitchen as I gave Tom the rundown of what we would be baking. Tom and I had taken the day off to go to the Ronald McDonald House and make cookies for the kids. It was seven months before he was diagnosed. If only we knew how close to our future we were when we were standing in that kitchen. To help make the house feel like a home, volunteers come in and cook meals or bake cookies. Tom and I spent a few hours making cookies, chatting with some of the families, and seeing the excited look on the faces of the kids when they realized it was a cookie day at the House.

We made several dozen, and then the coordinator offered to take us on a tour. She showed us the rooms, the various programs that they offer and the roof-top garden. The space was beautiful, fun, large and bright, but I couldn't shake the feeling at the pit of my stomach. As I saw families during our tour, my heart would sink into my stomach. How could such a little kid be handling so much? How could these kids even understand what was happening inside their bodies?

The coordinator took us around a corner and showed us the chapel – it was a beautiful, small space that had some stained glass décor. In the corner was a white light that wasn't lit. It was the shape of a tube with a textured glass.

"If we lose a child, we will turn on that light on in the chapel," she said as she pointed to the unlit light. "We try to not bring up a lost child around here, so it's a subtle way for us to acknowledge it, but not upset the kids."

It was hard to hear, and if that had been lit, it would have probably stung even more. Cancer touching a child then seemed impossible, but now, having had such a close-up view of cancer, chemo, and the pain, confusion and nausea that come with it, I was rocked to my core thinking back to that day. It pains me as a wife to see Tom go through this; the thought of a mother and father dealing with it for their child seems like torture.

We remained as positive as possible during cancer, but there were days when it just felt like too much, like we were fighting a never-ending battle. And on those days, we would think back to those kids at the Ronald McDonald house and be reminded of all the others who have had this fight. Without bad days, you would never know a good day, so we took them one by one, and bad days were okay – we were only human.

Nov. 7 – We Don't Like Cancer

I don't like cancer. I don't like it one bit. Admittedly we had a sort of downer day with cancer. We certainly are continuing to be positive, and won't let one bad day dictate the rest, but we have our moments of frustration. We are wearing down a bit, and the constant appointments, confirmations, insurance calls, blood draws, and wondering what's next can get exhausting. I remember the day of Tom's diagnosis, our nurse said to us both, "Right now you are at the bottom of Mount Everest." She was so right, and once treatment started we sort of started to feel like we knew how to tackle this and make progress. We are approaching the mid-point of chemo, and the beginning seems like it was a long time ago and the ambiguity of when cancer will be over seems unrealistic, so we feel sort of lost in the middle. But...the middle is better than back at the beginning, so we are grateful...

We had a discussion with our doctor about the upcoming surgery and we will get lots more information about that next week while we are in the hospital. Tom is eager for his last few "good" days of the chemo cycle and is ready to knock out week three. I must say this second cycle has been significantly better than the first and is really helping us get through tough days like today.

In my attempt to remain positive I'll finish tonight's update with a funny story. I've been having a hard time sleeping. In addition to that, when I'm stressed it usually takes a toll on my body, and often my back/shoulders. So this morning, I woke up and my neck/shoulders were totally locked up and painful. Now, I think it was a mix of stress/sleeping but nonetheless not very pleasant. I had been trying to rub my own shoulders all morning (that's a beautiful mental picture for you) and stretch my neck/shoulders with no success. This afternoon we were waiting in one of the chemo chairs/stations for Tom's blood work and results. The chemo chairs are all lined up out in the open, so there are lots of people/and friends and family around. Tom saw me wince in a bit of pain when I turned my head and offered to rub my shoulders for a second. Since we had nothing else to do while we waited and I was sitting right next to him I said alright....it took me all of five seconds to burst out laughing and tell him never mind as I realized that to all of these people it looked like this poor cancer patient was giving a shoulder massage to the healthy one! It gave us a good chuckle, and the folks around us got a kick out of it too once we explained ourselves. Shame on Tom for being such a nice guy! More to come...

The Next Generation of Trouble

Tom and I got the all clear to go see Greg's baby and we were excited to see the little guy and have a moment of normalcy. We walked in to meet the most beautiful baby. Greg and May were beaming, and we heard all about the labor and how they were transitioning to life as parents. We visited for a little over an hour and then said our goodbyes. My mom always told me to never overstay your welcome when visiting someone who is just home from having a baby. As we were leaving, we took a picture of Greg, Tom and the baby. It was the first photo of the next generation of this friendship. I got teary taking the photo. Tom first met Greg when he was that size, and here they were thirty years later with Greg's child.

We headed home and the car was quiet for the first few blocks.

"He's a real cutie and it looks like they are doing well," I said to Tom to break the ice.

"Yeah, I'm so happy for Greg. He's going to be the best dad in the world," Tom replied, with a crack in his voice.

I looked over as his eyes welled with tears and reached over to squeeze his hand.

"What's making you upset?" I asked.

"It's mostly happy tears; I'm so glad I got to see him and the baby. It's just a lot all at once with everything going on and the week we've had," he replied as he wiped the tears away from his face.

"I know, babe, it's totally understandable. And don't worry, we will have a baby soon so he has someone to get in trouble with in fifteen years," I replied. Tom squeezed my hand and took a few deep breaths. I knew he needed a few minutes so I drove and occasionally squeezed his hand. As we got to our exit, Tom looked over at me.

"You okay?" I asked, making sure that the silence wasn't the wrong decision for the ride home.

"Yeah – I'm okay. I'm going to have so many stories to tell that little guy about his dad. It's going to be great," he said as a half-smile came across his face.

Nov. 8 - Let's Get Ready to Rumble

I'm quite glad that I haven't had many updates lately! We are doing well and trucking along as we get prepared for chemo this week. We start session three and then we will only have ONE LEFT! This time last treatment we were already in the hospital with blood clots, so the fact that we are home is a victory itself.

Tom has continued to feel better, still not his normal healthy self, but feeling stronger. It's a bit of a trick on the psyche to know that starting Tuesday we get snapped back to square one and start the climb to feeling better again, but I do think knowing this is the third round, so close to the last one, will help make this next three-week chemo cycle seem manageable. We will also start to work out the details of surgery, which will help us feel more in control.

This past week has been a bit of a roller coaster, but we continue to try to be positive and keep ourselves in the best frame of mind possible; it really does make a difference. We appreciate all the cards and messages – it really keeps us going! More updates to come this week!

The Arrival

I was exhausted. I could hardly keep it together and Tom was having an especially hard time sleeping. I decided it was best to switch our mattress with the other mattress in the guest room. I wanted to get it done before we left for chemo so that when we came home everything was set.

The complication was that I was on my own. This was far too much for Tom to help with; even the simplest of tasks were a strain because he was so weak. For weeks, I had been doing everything. Every dish, meal, grocery run, laundry, appointment scheduling, insurance calls, bills, caretaking and working full time. I did it happily, but for some reason the day I needed to move the mattress, the reality of what I was juggling came raining down on me.

I stripped the bed and tried to start wiggling the mattress up so I could drag it. The ceiling fan, nightstands, and TV quickly became obstacles. Not only did I need to change the mattress; I also needed to switch the mattress cover that we had put on to protect the mattress from chemo sweats. I was on empty. I dropped the mattress and sat on the floor and cried. I knew I could do this, but I wasn't sure I had it in me that day. However, I was still going to find a way to get it done.

I reached up to the nightstand and grabbed my cell phone. I hated to do it, but I texted my sister-in-law Christina, who lived in my neighborhood, and asked her if she could swing by. I'm sure she thought I was ridiculous, but having two sets of hands to slide this cover on and off and swap the mattresses was going to prevent a complete meltdown. She came in and helped me, probably wondering why on earth I couldn't figure out a way to do this on my own, but she helped without question. When we finished, we were chatting and Tom came upstairs from his nap to say hello. As we walked her out, Tom reached into the mailbox. I was still talking with Christina and we heard a gasp as Tom started ripping open an envelope.

"It's here! My golden ticket!" Tom proclaimed.

I didn't even have to look over. I looked at Christina as I explained what was happening. "His medical marijuana card has arrived."

"Ah! I'm so glad I was here to see the excitement!" she proclaimed.

After a lot of laughter and a few munchie jokes, she was off. The mattresses were swapped which made me feel so much better, but what I was most proud of was that I had asked for help. It wasn't easy, but I knew I wasn't going to be able to make it to the end of this fight unless I started asking for the help I needed.

Nov. 9 – Chemo Eve

It's Chemo Eve! So this is really our first Chemo Eve. Our first round, we were coming out of the surgery and focused on his quick recovery. The second one never really happened because we got checked in for blood clots before chemo and were dealing with all of that. This round is really the first time we've had a calm night before chemo where we were able to prepare. So this evening we were discussing Chemo Eve and laughing at ways that Chemo Eve is different from Christmas Eve....

1. Tom isn't excited to wake up since he knows his only gift is the gift of nausea and chemo side effects.
2. We don't leave cookies out – we eat them so they don't go bad while we are away. (Seriously, one of the MVP of Tom's treatments is the button on the top of my pants – it's hanging on for dear life)
3. Instead of a Christmas tree, we wake up and go to the IV tree/pole.
4. There are no last minute sales for medical bills.
5. There isn't a constant loop of Christmas songs/carols (but there is a constant holler of me singing songs I've made up about cancer).

We pick Christmas Eve over Chemo Eve! Tomorrow we continue our quest to kick cancer's butt and head to the hospital bright and early. We are hoping for a calm week, with no major issues so we can knock out these six days and be one step closer to our last round of chemo. Twenty-seven days until chemo is done... Thanks for all the prayers, positive vibes, and energy as we head into this round. We truly feel all the love! More to come this week...

Insanity

A wise man once said the definition of insanity is doing the same thing over and over and expecting a different result. In a similar way, chemo created a bit of insanity because you were repeating the same activities over and over, knowing the negative impacts, but not knowing what the final result would be.

The morning of Tom's third chemo, I was walking around and closing up the house for our six-day hospital stay. Usually Tom would stay in bed until right before we left as I packed the car and got things ready. Except this chemo round was different. As I turned the corner from the kitchen, Tom was on the couch with his head in his hands.

"Are you okay?" I asked. Tom didn't reply for a few seconds.

"How am I supposed to do this again? I don't know how much more of this I can take," he said with sadness.

"I know, babe, I know," I said as I sat down next to him and rubbed his back. "You can do this; I know it's hard to think about the next six days ahead of us, but we can do this." I wished I could take the weight of the chemo off his shoulders, but the only thing I could do was be there with him.

He looked up at me as he wiped a few tears away from his eyes. "I don't know how I would do this without you."

"Well then, it's a good thing I'm going to be with you for the next six days," I replied. "Now let's go knock out number three. We can do this."

I stood up and put my hand out to help him up. He got up, took a deep breath and gave me a hug. No words were needed. We headed to the hospital, and I could tell this was really wearing Tom down mentally. As we got out of the car, I grabbed our bags and headed in. Tom reached down to grab my hand as the automatic doors opened and we walked into the hospital.

"You've got this," I said as I looked at him.

He leaned over and kissed me as he replied, "I know…thank you."

Nov. 10 - Eleven Down – Nine To Go

We've hit single digits for our remaining chemo treatments! Only nine more to go! Woo hoo! Today was an interesting day, but a good day. Tom woke up feeling a little blah (I can't blame him at all) and overwhelmed by the thought of starting another round of treatment. He basically woke up at 4am and never fell back asleep because he couldn't turn off his mind. Anyway, we got up, and got checked in here at the hospital to get things moving.

It's like a mini-reunion when we come in for treatment. We truly have gotten close with many of our nurses and they all get excited, say hi, fill us in on the past few weeks of their lives, and of course see how Tom is doing. As we were doing all the catching up, we got escorted to our room and our nurses reserved us the BIG room! I know, I know. Small thrills, but it's the closest thing to a hotel upgrade here and quite exciting. Our room is a corner suite so it just has a little more room to breathe between all the furniture/computer/IV/medical equipment, etc. It probably seems trivial, but it makes a difference, especially for me since I'm working all day out of the hospital. It helps to have a little more room and a cart for my office setup. Plus, he got a bed for tall people, which they publicize to the world outside of our room as "Hercules." So basically, Tom is Hercules. Which presents a problem for me since Hercules' love interest in the Disney movie always had questionable eye shadow choices. Anyway, back to my point, the location of this room has less traffic, so it's much quieter too. And, for some reason, it's the proud home of eight ladybugs. (I'll figure that out before we leave.)

Treatment went well today and our doctor came in with great news about Tom's blood work. He is definitely killing this cancer and making incredible progress in doing so. The levels show that his body is rapidly attacking the bad cancer cells and those reports came before we even started treatment today, so we are hopeful this round can have a great impact too. With that said, treatments are getting tougher and tougher for Tom as his body has gotten weaker and having a harder time fighting back. For example, in previous cycles, the first day of treatment hasn't hit him too hard. Certainly he feels nausea, etc., but for the most part he doesn't feel miserable. However, tonight at around 9 pm he really hit a wall and said that he was feeling closer to how he feels on Day Three than on Night One. I'm hopeful that is partly because he was up so early and is just tired – but we may have a long week ahead. Either way, we will power through.

All the love, prayers and good thoughts you can send our way would be appreciated – more to come tomorrow...

My Private Accommodations

When Tom started his chemo at the hospital, I was no longer allowed to use his bathroom for my own safety. I would walk to the end of the hall to use the family waiting room bathroom or walk downstairs and use the bathroom by the gift shop. It was strange at first, but then began to feel normal. By his third round of chemo, the hospital was a place where I felt comfortable. In addition to our doctors and nurses, I knew the cafeteria staff, the cleaning staff, the gift shop people, and not just because I purchased a lot there. There was a sense of comfort – it became the smells and sounds of safety. It became a welcoming place because my brain associated it with progress. I no longer measured time by a single day; I measured it by where we were in a three-week chemo cycle. A new chemo cycle meant progress.

The comfort scared me. For our accommodations for the third round of chemo, we had a larger room but a smaller bathroom. I remember laughing so hard with Tom one morning as he tried to wiggle into the bathroom. I helped him in, and when he came out we were still laughing. It felt like we were in our living room. If you took out the chemo pole, IVs and hospital gown, this could be a laughter-filled exchange at our house.

At some level, this was comforting. If we had to be in the hospital for almost a week, knowing familiar faces and rituals was calming. It showed me that we were dealing with cancer the way we wanted to deal with it, and that we weren't letting it take away who we were. But the other part of me didn't want to make any memories here. I wanted to come in and come out. I didn't want the hospital to be normal; I didn't want it to be comforting. I felt that if I let it get normal, cancer had some right to stick around. The only comfort I wanted was a guarantee that the cancer would be gone and that we would get our lives back.

Nov. 11 – Twelve Down, Eight to Go

We continue to make progress through our treatment cycle – what a week! I'm currently sitting in the hospital and Tom is fast asleep and we are under "Code Black" in the hospital. There is some pretty gnarly weather outside, so Code Black means they run around and make sure windows are closed and covered and that everyone is safe. It's sort of sad that we know what all the codes stand for and could probably help if needed – I know all of the safety protocols for the different codes including weather, fire and child abduction. Perhaps I'll nominate myself for Hall Captain.

I know yesterday I raved about our fancy room, but we did find one flaw (I'm not counting the ladybugs as flaws because they are good luck). The bathroom is about a third of the size of our other bathroom in the smaller rooms – go figure. Now, typically that wouldn't matter, but when Tom uses the bathroom he has to take his giant IV pole with him since he is constantly hooked up to the IV drugs. No joke, we were in tears laughing today at his attempts to turn the IV pole gradually to get into the bathroom, which then requires a whole adjustment once inside just to shut the door since the door opens into the bathroom. I don't know why it makes me laugh so hard every time, but it's just hilarious. Due to the amount of fluids he receives in addition to the chemo fluids, it's no exaggeration that he is back and forth to the bathroom at least once an hour. During the nighttime when he gets up to use the bathroom, I typically wake up and help him get his IV machine unplugged from the wall and get him back into bed. It drives Tom crazy that he repeatedly wakes me up since he wants me to sleep – I don't care one bit – so he always tries to sneak by without me waking up which he has done successfully only once in the past two months. With our new bathroom arrangement there is ZERO chance of him sneaking to the bathroom when he's pounding the IV pole into the doorframe and swearing.

Tom took chemo like a champ today and is continuing to feel worn down, but I'm in complete awe. He has been trying so hard to not "be sick" when people are around and sometimes even when he is just with me. There have been points where I've looked at him and said, "It's okay to be sick!" He wants to be the cheery, happy-go-lucky guy that he is. I know he doesn't always feel great, yet he worries about everyone around him, not wanting them to worry. I'm in complete amazement that on many days he makes this chemo treatment look "easy" and continues to crack jokes, thank every nurse, doctor, or employee that walks in the room and be so positive. It's truly an amazing gift to those around him and it is helping everyone cope through this fight. I knew he was a strong guy – but he has shown me strength at a whole other level these past two months. I'm so incredibly proud of him. More to come tomorrow...

Guilt & Anxiety – My New Best Friends

There were days when the guilt and anxiety that came with our life was all-consuming. It would keep me up at night; I would fixate on it, and it would continue to build. Being a good Catholic, I am all too familiar with guilt, but this was different. Every time I opened a card or a care package, I was overwhelmed by the love but then immediately consumed with the guilt. I would wonder if they felt like they had to do whatever they had done for us; I would immediately send a text to acknowledge it; I would write it down so I could make sure I sent a thank you note. Sometimes it got so bad that for me it took away the joy of the many kind gestures. I didn't want friends and family to feel helpless, and whenever we received something, I would think about that person and what they must be feeling.

It was even worse for people who were close by. My sisters-in-law would stop by with lunch or Starbucks and I felt terrible that they went out of their way or that they wouldn't accept my cash. Often people would ask if they could bring us something and I would decline, not because I didn't want whatever they offered, but because I felt guilt. The days that I conceded were usually because I needed a visitor versus needed any particular thing. As Tom's treatments progressed, he napped more and the hospital room became lonelier. Visitors during these days or our nighttime dinners were what kept me sane.

The guilt and anxiety I had about people dealing with our situation made me so sad. I knew that people were heartbroken for us; it's why I tried to keep everyone so informed and feeling like they were part of this fight. One person gets diagnosed with the actual cancer, but an army of friends and family also get the diagnosis. They may not have the day-to-day fight, appointments, pain, agony and sadness, or have to look death in the face, but they have the love and empathy that creates a whole journey for them too. We never forgot that; it's why we handled things the way we did and why the guilt and anxiety was so real. I believe that most of these feelings were just gratitude boiling over – we were so appreciative, thankful and in awe of our support that it didn't feel like we would ever be able to repay those that made such an effort to make our hell a little bit more bearable.

Nov. 12 – Thirteen Down, Seven To Go
Well, the bad chemo symptoms have reared their ugly heads earlier than usual. Tom is having a tough time with this round of treatment and feeling the effects much earlier than usual. This makes these last few days especially tough since he thought he had a few more days with less of the intense symptoms. He was trying to avoid extra medicine today but ultimately needed some of the stronger anti-nausea medicines. As we were figuring out the medicines with the nurses, he was trying to describe how he feels, but couldn't. He and I were talking and

he said it's just an indescribable feeling; it's partly an intense amount of focus so as to not think about the nausea; it's an overwhelming sense of fatigue, and then the achiness of the flu. However, he says that doesn't even describe how it all feels. Ugh. Regardless, we are hoping that these early symptoms don't prolong his bad days on the other end of the chemo cycle too – but that will remain to be seen.

Our day was a bit of a comedy of errors. We made it through chemo but unfortunately – as mentioned above – our day matched the crappy weather outside. To top it off, my dad and sister drove down from Wisconsin to have dinner at the hospital with us and got in a car accident on the way. No major injuries, but just not the greatest feeling when we have people coming to spend time with us, and then they get in an accident. Yuck. We know we have to have some bad days – if nothing else – to know the good days. So we chalk today up to that and hope for a better tomorrow. More to come…

Who Am I?

At the core, we all know who we are. We know our strengths and weaknesses – though some are more in touch with that than others. Our situation changed me, even if only temporarily. I wasn't always confident in how I handled things, and some days I just wanted to talk about anything but cancer.

As a caregiver, a wife, a daughter, a sister, a friend – there were days that I just needed to be who I needed to be that day to make it through, even if it seemed out of character for me. Some days I couldn't help but cry hard; other days I couldn't access my emotions. I was who I needed to be that day to survive. It sounds extreme, but it was subtle – I was both aware of it and not aware, and I don't know if anyone else noticed. Yet who I was at the core and who Tom was at the core were exactly what was helping us survive. It seemed backwards that some days I had to abandon that all just to survive.

When I looked at Tom, on some level I felt like I never knew him until he got cancer. I never saw his greatest qualities in action so overtly. It was a beautiful gift to see his personality come alive in so many different ways. I loved him more than I ever thought possible.

Nov. 13 – Fourteen Down – Six To Go
Honore: Tell me four things you're thinking about right now, what should I write about tonight?
Tom: I'm sleepy…. I'm sleepy…. I want to go home…and I'm sleepy.

Most of his answer was with his eyes closed too. So, that pretty much sums up where Tom is at! We had another tough day of chemo, but he powered through and stayed on the strong anti-nausea medicines all day. We are SOOOOO close to Round Three of chemo being complete – we just need to do one more treatment tomorrow and then we have one more night at the hospital and are on our way to Round Four! I am hopeful that his early symptoms don't make Sunday – Tuesday worse than they already are, but the doctor led me to believe that likely won't be the case. She also thinks another blood transfusion will be in our future. Yuck. Tom needed some supplements today because some of his counts were low, but hopefully that will help perk him up for our last few nights here.

Tom wants to be anywhere but in this hospital – I couldn't agree more – but a few days in the hospital leads to millions more outside of the hospital so we continue on. It's been a hell of a week and we're exhausted, so a brief post tonight. More to come tomorrow…

Loneliness

"Stop looking in all the rooms!" Tom said to me as we were on our nightly walk around the hospital.

"I'm just glancing. I hate seeing people with no one to keep them company," I told Tom, rationalizing my nosiness.

"Not everyone is in our situation, babe," Tom said as he squeezed my hand and pulled me closer to him, making me look at him versus in the hospital rooms.

"I know; it just makes me sad that some of these people lie here all day without a single visitor – especially in this unit!" I said as we were about halfway down the geriatric unit hall.

"Right, but everyone gets old and not everyone is here for only six days," he said. Sometimes his rational nature and practical analysis drove me crazy.

"You know, it's taking all I have to not go make friends with all these people," I said to Tom as I begrudgingly moved down the hall with him and his IV pole.

"I know, babe – but then you wouldn't be with me, and you're the only reason I make it through some of these days."

"Oh, that's not true," I replied. "I just think it's a wonderful reminder of how lucky we are to have so many people that want to visit you and help us."

I wanted to help everyone. I wanted to fix everyone. I knew we had more love and support than most – and if I could, I would have spread it across our entire hospital.

Nov. 14 – Chemo #3 – Done

Round Three is COMPLETE!!! WOO HOO! This was a tough treatment for Tom, but he powered through and we are one step closer to our last chemo treatment. We know we've got a crappy three days (at least) ahead of us, but then he will start to feel better and improve each day from there. I'm very happy that his "good" week lines up with Thanksgiving so we can enjoy a good Thanksgiving meal and great company. Then we check in for our LAST ROUND OF CHEMO and leave the hospital on his birthday. How's that for a happy birthday?

We've got a busy week ahead with additional blood work, and an appointment we are excited for – the first surgical consultation. It's a little early to have a completely clear picture of what the surgery will be, but just getting an idea of it will help put us both at ease. Like everything through this process, the hardest part has been the unknown. Tom is very nervous to be put under and wants to know what the recovery time will be, so hopefully we will at least get some general answers. I'm not expecting too much concrete information since

122

we don't yet know how small the tumor has gotten, but even if we know best case/worst case scenario for recovery times, etc., it will help our planning.

As we were talking to the nurse tonight, she mentioned how lucky we are that people stop by to see us and bring us non-hospital food. She said there are people that are here for days or weeks who never have one visitor and they have to call a cab for them when they are discharged. Can you imagine? I actually almost cried just hearing her tell some of the stories. Unfortunately, because of HIPAA laws, she couldn't tell me if that's the case for anyone here now, because I promise you I would have taken the wheel break off of their beds, pushed the bed into our Hercules room and had them hang out with us. (Plus, perhaps Tom could beat them at UNO since he's been having trouble beating me!) It's so heartbreaking, and another great reminder of how lucky we are to have such an amazing support system. I don't know how we would do this without all the messages and love that everyone has been sending our way. We truly appreciate it all. I feel like a broken record, but I don't care and I will continue to say it, we are incredibly lucky and thankful. More to come tomorrow from HOME!

Mac & Cheese

"Do we have mac and cheese? I am craving some mac and cheese," Tom said as he slowly and exhaustedly walked upstairs into the kitchen.

"Are you serious?" I asked, shocked that he had an appetite for anything.

"A hundred percent," he said with a bit of a smile emerging on his face.

That's the moment I put it all together – last week we had gotten Tom his medical marijuana. The technicians sat with him to determine the best type of strand for his symptoms, and Tom had a vaporizer that he was using to administer the THC. With a vaporizer there was no smoke – which was critical for Tom because we couldn't have smoke in the lungs before the surgery.

Tom had never wanted food the day we got home from chemo. He usually had to force himself to eat just to have something in his stomach with all the medications. If nothing else – this is where medical marijuana is a game changer – every one of Tom's medications helped with nausea, but none of them gave him an appetite. Food and nutrients are critical in how we feel, and that's what marijuana provided him. It was remarkable. It was getting harder for him to bounce back from each chemo, but the marijuana was making it seem so much more manageable.

"If you want mac and cheese then I'm making you some mac and cheese," I said as I reached out to hug Tom. "How do you feel?"

"Pretty awful, but the THC from the marijuana definitely helped settle some of the nausea and made me hungry. I wish I had used it sooner," he replied, holding his head up on my shoulder in our hug.

"Go lie down, I'll bring you the mac and cheese," I said as I pulled away.

"Do I need to stock up on munchies for you now?" I asked with a smile on my face.

"Ha. Ha. Ha," he sarcastically replied as he headed downstairs to the couch.

If you had told me three months earlier that I would have no problem with my husband vaporizing marijuana in the basement – and making him mac and cheese to satisfy the munchies – I would have laughed. Tom would be thrilled to hear me say words I don't say often – I was wrong. It should be legal for medical use – I will go as far to say that it played a critical part in us staying so strong through the fight. It helped Tom deal with the all the symptoms from chemo, the anxiety about the upcoming surgery and helped calm him – which in turn made things a bit easier for me. It also became a replacement for some of the stronger prescription nausea medications, which made him less of a medication zombie and afforded me the opportunity to fight this with my husband, not a heavily medicated version of my husband. When he was heavily medicated, he wouldn't laugh and it seemed like he wasn't in his own body –

when he was using marijuana instead of those stronger meds, I had my husband.

It was the best money we spent through this entire fight – and the most effective medication – yet we didn't get to bill one cent of the costs through our insurance company. It didn't matter – I would have paid double for what it did during his post-chemo weeks. It was truly a game changer. I'm grateful that we had the medical marijuana card – and so was Haribo Candy – that stock has to be through the roof from the number of gummy bears Tom consumed.

Nov. 15 – Home.

HOME HOME HOME HOME HOME HOME HOME. WE. ARE. HOME. Not only are we home, but we managed to get out by 1 pm today which was a treat since we usually are there until about 4 pm. Yes, I know, we have cheap thrills these days.

Tom is feeling rough, as we expected, but managed to eat some food today and that makes a world of difference. With all the medicines he is on having some food in his belly helps so he doesn't get a stomach-ache, or worse, throw up, since so much of his medicine is in pill form. It's hard for his body to process everything without some food. Add to that the complete exhaustion that comes with these post-chemo days and it's not too pleasant for him. As per usual though, he's taken everything with a smile and is trying to stay positive. As we were leaving the hospital today, our nurses/technicians were all stopping to give us hugs goodbye. They were sad to see us go, and all said they are looking forward to our return in a few weeks. I can't say the feeling is mutual about coming back – though I do enjoy their company!

Tomorrow we go in for his post-chemo shot bright and early and meet with a surgeon to get an idea of what this surgery will entail. I'm hoping somehow we can incorporate a post-surgery super power into this procedure. More to come...

Down & Out

Tom took a deep breath as we walked towards the elevator. I squeezed his hand and looked over to him.

"Are you okay?" I asked.

"I'll be fine, just a lot to process," he said, clearly lying to himself. "What about you?"

"That was really intense – I knew this surgery was going to be a big deal but I couldn't process everything we just heard," I replied as I pushed the elevator button.

I wished this appointment had been any other day. We were one day home from his third round of chemo, and the physical impact had taken its toll. Tom had finally lost most of his other facial hair, so the lack of eyebrows and general paleness made it glaringly obvious that he was dealing with something serious. He looked even paler after hearing about the surgery.

The doctor was a wonderful guy – and the first doctor we had ever seen who didn't sit in the doctor chair with wheels but instead sat next to me in the stationary chairs. I immediately felt like he and I could have a beer together – he just was a comfortable guy. He talked about the surgery like someone giving directions. It was casual and confident – a great encouragement that surgery was what he did every day – he knew what he needed to do.

The downside of this appointment was that there was still so much in flux. He didn't want to commit to anything until after the fourth round of chemo when he had a full understanding of how much the tumor had shrunk, if at all. As a result, we ended up with a lot of "if" paths – some more scary than others. If the tumor didn't shrink away from the heart, then he wanted to do the surgery at a different hospital where he could have a cardiac bypass team on call in case something happened to his heart. If the tumor did shrink away from his heart, then we had three other "ifs" that could transpire – all of those potentially involving Tom losing part of his lung.

While we felt like we were gaining some understanding of our circumstances, we also felt like it had become more complicated. The seriousness of this surgery and the reality check of potential outcomes – both positive and negative – were front and center. The scariest part of it all, though, the true slap in the face of that day, was walking to that elevator, tears coming down our faces and realizing that, while we were headed towards the fourth round of chemo, this fight had hardly yet begun.

Nov. 16 – Who Moved Our Finish Line?
We've had quite the day. After getting home last night we had a bit of an up and down night, but for the most part Tom is feeling okay. It's about the same as the last round of treatment – it's just a rough few days. We got up this

morning and headed to the cancer clinic to get his post-chemo shot. We decided today that we should get a plaque in the waiting room with the tagline that says, "Tom & Honore – Bringing down the average age of the cancer waiting room since 2015."

In all seriousness, then our day took a turn. We briefly met with a potential surgeon for Tom, and though we knew this surgery would be quite the endeavor, it was even more than we had bargained for. Granted, it's only the first opinion, but we do know that this is going to be one hell of a final obstacle to get him cancer free. The doctor was great – and incredibly calming, which was needed for us both. There may have been some swear words and elevator cry/tears post appointment, but per our own rules, we have given ourselves a little time to react, process, and now we carry on with a plan. We will meet with some other doctors for additional opinions and will fill everyone in more once we have more of a definitive plan of what surgery will entail – but it will likely be the beginning of January.

Coming off yesterday and into today, I felt like we had turned that final corner and could see our finish line. Today, we feel like someone picked up the finish line and put it back out of sight. Brutal. So today became one of those tougher cancer days, but tomorrow is another day, and one day closer to that new finish line – wherever the hell it may be. More to come…

I Was Sitting In A Sink

Two months is an interesting amount of time. In the big picture, it's short, but sometimes time seems to drag on to eternity. Why is it that days spent on vacation seem to fly by but the week leading up to vacation doesn't? Is it because we focus so much on what's going to happen? How come the hour at church sometimes feels like a whole morning? Is it because our thoughts wander? Why do the first few months of a relationship seem to always fly by? Is it because you're getting to know someone? It's all the way our brain works, focuses and fixates.

Right after Tom and I started officially dating, I was hanging out with him at his job – where he also had his bowling league. It was an awesome group of people casually hanging out, with Tom and I in our honeymoon stage of getting to know each other and having fun.

"You can roll my next ball for me if you want," he said as he pulled himself up to sit on top of the bowling ball case.

"You've never seen me bowl before – how do you know I'm good?" I asked as I leaned into his legs dangling down.

"I don't – let's see what you've got."

I don't remember how the rest of this conversation went, but I do remember Tom blurting out that he loved me. Luckily, he said it right as it was my turn to bowl. I made a shocked face and then immediately turned to bowl. I remember thinking he was either crazy or just had gotten caught up in the moment. We never really mentioned it after that moment until we *actually* said I love you.

A few weeks later, I headed back to college for my sophomore year; Tom was headed into his senior year. We had been hanging out for most of July and started dating officially at the beginning of August. We were planning to attempt long distance dating from Milwaukee to Cincinnati – a solid six hours away on a good day. This was pretty out of character for both of us, but we figured we'd give it a shot with the caveat that we would see how things went and that we wouldn't abandon our college lives to see each other all the time.

It never seemed strange. I would almost recommend starting relationships this way. Having to rely on daily conversations instead of interactions helped me learn things about Tom that, otherwise, I might not have known for years. For us, it worked. My fierce independence liked a long-distance relationship.

At the end of September, Tom made his first visit to Cincinnati. It had been just over five weeks since we had seen each other, but we had been talking and texting all the time. I didn't feel like we were in a long-distance relationship because I felt like I was always learning about him. The distance wasn't causing a delay in the progression of the relationship which had been my only concern. I was so excited for him to come to Xavier and meet all my friends. He arrived late on a Friday night and I went darting out of the dorm and jumped into his arms.

I introduced him to everyone, and we all grabbed some food before heading out to a party for the night. We were so happy to be together and he was having a blast putting names to faces and having some drinks. Later that night we found our way back to the dorm, perhaps a little inebriated on crappy college beer. I went straight for the mini fridge to get some cheese to go with my Triscuit crackers – my go-to late night beer-drinking snack. Like any college dorm, space was lacking, so I jumped up on the bathroom sink, located in our room, and proceeded to fall into it. I sat in the sink, looked up, and offered Tom a cheese and cracker.

"I love you so much," he said as he walked towards me.

I wasn't sure at that point if he was talking about the cheese and cracker or me. I could see it play out both ways. As he got closer, he reached out to grab my face and kiss me – so I knew he was likely not talking about the cheese.

"I love you too!" I enthusiastically replied, giving him a brief kiss because I wanted to eat the cheese and cracker I had just prepared in my hand.

I did love him, and it had only taken two months from when we started hanging out, but it felt right. I remember thinking that maybe this was too fast, or too soon, but how can you put time limits on love. It was real – and as I sat in that sink eating my cheese and crackers, I could tell by the look in his eyes that he meant it weeks earlier when he blurted it out in that bowling alley too.

Nov. 17 – Two Months & One Day

Tom feels, and I quote, "Better than Monday." He got a lot of color back today, and though still quite fatigued, he's starting to feel better. Yesterday was an interesting milestone for us – but one I didn't mention since we were processing the surgery news. Monday was exactly two months from Tom's original diagnosis. There are very few words to describe the past two months of our life. How can some hours/days seem so incredibly slow, but the two months as a whole feel like a complete blur? It's as if we are in a weird time vortex. I'm still working full-time, so it's almost as if I picked up another full-time job, which is why I think life has gone by so quickly. For Tom, I think it's been a mix of being on all the medications, a blur of appointments and a focus on getting through each day that has made time seem to rush. Late last night I read the blog from start to finish – there are posts that I didn't even remember until I read them again. It's amazing how our brains work!

All in all, we've managed the past two months the best we could. We've had some of the best days together and some of the absolute hardest days together. Two months from now will be mid-January, and Tom should be on the road to recovery from surgery and – dare I say – cancer free. So as tough as the past two months have been, we know the next two months will yield much brighter days with happy milestones including the holidays with our families (including a Bears/Packers game on Thanksgiving), the end of chemo, surgery, a cancer-free diagnosis and more. On that note, nineteen days until chemo is done. More to come...

Babies' Intuition

My sister, Mame, had her first baby the January before Tom was diagnosed. We were already an aunt and uncle to three nieces and one nephew on Tom's side. Tom's oldest nieces were the daughters of my sister-in-law, Staci, and had been around quite a bit when he had moved back home after college. They loved to jump on Uncle Thomas' bed, and he adored the girls. My other sister-in-law, Christina, gave birth to the first nephew just two months before our wedding and gave birth to our third niece just short of two years later. He adored them too – Tom's an animated guy and loves kids, so they often are drawn to him.

Yet he would be the first to tell you he was terrified of babies; he didn't want to "break" them, as he would say. He confused beautiful newborns with Humpty Dumpty. When Mame went into labor, we headed to Milwaukee and were there to meet the little guy, Rookie, just hours after he was born. Tom was hesitant to hold the baby, but did, and I was still in shock that my sister had just become a mom. We were in Milwaukee a lot those first few months to help and spend time with the baby. As he got older and more alert, it was more fun to FaceTime with him, and he knew who we were when he would see us in person.

When Tom was diagnosed, Rookie was nine months old. I firmly believe that babies have a special intuition. Perhaps the timing lined up with when he was starting to be more alert and mobile, but he loved his "Tom Tom." I was old news to him – but I like to think that's because I look so much like his mom. He was running all over the place, but when he would come to visit when Tom was sick, he was calm.

They came down the weekend before Thanksgiving. I had purchased a big Elmo balloon for him to play with while he was at our house. As we were visiting, we heard the strongest belly laugh from the little guy who was perched on his Uncle Tom Tom's arm. Tom was making a dramatic noise to the balloon bumping into his head. Tom needed that laughter more than any other medicine in the world that day; Tom laughed as hard as my nephew did when he whacked his head on the balloon. I leaned down and took a video as I held back tears. It wasn't anything crazy, but watching those two play was a special moment. It was the power of visitors and the innocence of a baby not knowing what an impact he was having on Tom.

The cancer had been a distraction, but the fun days with the little ones reminded us of the gap in our lives. We had wanted a baby for a long time before he was diagnosed. For months before his cancer, we had regular heartbreak, hoping every month that it would be different.

It is hard to describe the struggle with fertility. It's heartbreaking every time you find out that it didn't happen. Yet this false climb of hope continues;

you fool yourself into thinking this next month must be the month, trying to think of all the positives. One month I was so upset, I convinced myself it was okay because the baby wouldn't come in the middle of flu season.

Baby showers are even harder to sit through, though it's not because you aren't happy for the person who's pregnant. It's because it reminds you of the hole in your heart that you so badly want to fill. One day while shopping for a baby shower, I had a full-on panic attack in the middle of Buy Buy Baby. And, of course, the constant reminders of people's pregnancies on social media made those platforms something I had to stay away from for my own sanity. Even worse were stories in the news about abused or beaten children. It becomes personal; it becomes a mockery in a way, that someone would torture a child as you sit in your own torture of wanting to have and love a child so badly.

Despite our family being on a delay, the lullaby at the hospital made us smile, we would talk about baby names or how we wanted to raise our kids to remind ourselves that it hadn't gone away. There was one thing we both agreed on to our core – we wanted to raise happy and healthy kids.

Nov. 19 – The Climb Back Up
Tom is feeling much better! Tuesday night he started to turn the corner and yesterday was feeling much better. Today was even better than yesterday and so begins his climb back to feeling "good" for a few brief days before he gets hit with chemo again – for the last time!

Tom had blood work today, and though his numbers were cutting it SUPER close, he did not need a blood transfusion. I wouldn't be surprised, given his numbers, if he will need one next week, but for now he's thrilled. We've got some visitors coming to see us this weekend because he's feeling better, which will be great and keep spirits high – this whole diagnosis/treatment can be incredibly isolating – especially when we have the added issue of flu season approaching. Then we've got Thanksgiving next week for which I will probably have a sentimental holiday post. Consider yourselves warned.

So…fingers crossed we keep our momentum going and can get him as strong as possible before this next round. The stronger he is going in, the quicker he can bounce back and get extra strong for surgery…More to come…

The Bucket List

The list just kept on growing – Tom would randomly think of something, usually prompted by TV, or we would be imagining all the things we'd rather doing than treatment, and he would add a new item to the Post-Cancer Bucket List. I knew he deserved it all but had to remind him that we wouldn't magically have a large beating-cancer budget. As expected, many of the things on the list weren't things at all – they were experiences. Traveling, enjoying restaurants we had always wanted to try but couldn't justify, starting a family, and one he snuck on there without asking me first, getting a dog.

The only "material" things were a new mattress – which we really needed – and his new golf clubs. As fall approached, Tom had looked over at me one night out of the blue and said he was glad he got sick in winter, because missing golf would have been horrible. Our two material objects were not just material. The mattress was more than just a comfortable place to sleep at night; it was a reminder that we got to be home and not in a hospital on an uncomfortable bed or an old rickety couch. The clubs were his freedom – out on the course, with people he cared about and enjoying life.

The bucket list was strangely important to us, and I'm not sure why. Often, a bucket list itemizes things people want to do before they die or "kick the bucket," yet our bucket list never meant that. Everything on our list was going to happen once he beat cancer, not things he wanted to do in case he didn't beat it. The bucket list was a series of ways we were going to celebrate, and on the especially tough days, it was a reminder that better days would come. Tom named his list "Things I want to do without cancer," and sometimes his list just made me laugh. I like to think some of it was the power of good TV ads and his medication. We added more to it, but it started with:

Go skiing
Take Honore to a concert
Go to a beach
Go to Wrigley
Golf…. a lot
Run a 5K
Eat a lot of crab legs
Couples massage
Take a trip
Eat sushi
Cubs Bleacher Game
Shoot Clay Pigeons
Get a new mattress
Go to Vegas
Get a dog

Day at the horse racing track

New golf clubs

It wasn't extravagant; it wasn't extreme – assuming we didn't win millions in Vegas – but it was our little escape and reminder that we would get our lives back one day.

Nov. 22 – Two Weeks Until Chemo is Done

Happy Thanksgiving Week to all! Tom is feeling well but still has some fatigue. We were so happy to have a variety of visitors stop by this weekend, which is great to break up the monotony for him, but it's amazing how that can also wear him out. But as he says – I'd rather be a little tired and get to see people and have some company. We are happy that he should continue to feel better and stronger this week and start to get more of an appetite – just in time for Thanksgiving!

Two weeks from today we will be coming home from our last round of chemo. Fourteen days to go! We are so excited! Certainly, it's not the end of the fight, but a huge milestone that we are going to continue to work towards and of course celebrate. This week should be relatively calm. We meet with our team of doctors on Wednesday because of the holiday schedule and are hoping that he won't need a blood transfusion, especially because the clinic is closed on Thursday and Friday. So we head into this week with a positive and thankful mindset...More to come...

Master Planner

I hate planning – it's one of my least favorite things to do unless it involves travel. I like to have a general idea of what I'm doing, but I hate to get too involved or obsess over details. Plans don't allow for the spontaneous things in life, and sometimes those are the most fun.

The planning required to coordinate our lives was exhausting; first, because there were so many moving parts, and second, because I hated doing it. Not only was I planning every appointment and component of our life, I was also doing the daily planning of my work. It was all consuming, but it made me more efficient than ever.

The irony was that I couldn't plan much at all. The day always started one way but almost certainly would end another. It was a plan-filled life of uncertainty, you would think my perfect combo, but it was exhausting; it was untrustworthy, and it was our life.

Nov. 24 – Phone Calls and Paperwork and Hold Music –
Oh My!

I feel like cancer is one giant event-planning activity – without an open bar. The number of phone calls, coordination, paperwork and sign-offs required is mind boggling. Sadly, I know the numbers of most of our doctors, can hum along to the hold music, and have sarcastic answers for some odd new patient questions. As we ramp back up for our last round of chemo, I will be in mega-coordination mode, as we will have several appointments that will be needed post-chemo, including scans, blood work, lung testing, second and third opinions on surgery, surgical prep meetings, a potential blood transfusion, etc. We need all this done as soon as possible so we can get surgery lined up for the beginning of January. Add to that the doctors' holiday schedules and running against the insurance clock, and it's going to be a whirlwind.

We've got to move fast so that the cells don't continue to multiply, so that we can get the tumor out and not need more chemo after surgery. In our perfect scenario, this last round of chemo kills all the cancer, Tom has a few weeks to bounce back, and then we do surgery in early January to get the mass out. We meet with our oncologist tomorrow and will get a better idea of what we can expect in the way of tests between the last round of chemo and surgery. So we are planning to enjoy this long holiday weekend and try to get some rest before what will be a crazy week of chemo and post-chemo activities that will require a lot more activity than Tom is used to in his recovery weeks. More to come...

Caregiver Back Burner

"I'm going to go in the hall and reschedule my appointment," I said to Tom from the corner of the waiting room.

"Please don't; I feel terrible – take the car, and I can call someone and have them pick me up," Tom replied, with guilt in his voice.

"It's really not a big deal; I'll reschedule it. I would never leave you here alone. This appointment isn't urgent," I calmly replied.

I had a late afternoon checkup with my doctor, which I had mistakenly thought I would have plenty of time to get to. I stepped out into the hall and called the office. They were very understanding of the situation and could reschedule me for a few weeks later. It wasn't a big deal – but I knew it was to Tom.

Through the entire fight, he was always worried about me taking care of myself too. I had so much on my plate, wasn't sleeping, and wearing out physically. Tom felt terrible about how much I was doing and dealing with, about all the medical bills, and the delay on starting a family. It was a challenge for him to watch me take care of things.

Every Sunday, we put out our garbage for pickup early Monday morning. I lost track of how many weeks I would gather everything up, drag it out to the curb and walk in the house to him holding back tears or giving me a defeated expression. Tom prided himself on taking care of me. He was so damn sweet – and I hated that he felt guilty about his situation.

"It was no big deal at all – they moved me out a few weeks and I can still get in before the end of the year," I told Tom as I walked back into the room.

"I hate this. I don't want you to stop taking care of yourself," he said.

"This is just a checkup, babe. If I were worried about something serious, we would figure it out. Seriously, not a big deal at all," I tried to reassure him.

He knew to drop it at that point. The appointment had already been moved, and I hoped my words had convinced him that everything was fine. I understood where he was coming from, though – I was struggling with my own feelings of guilt when people helped us, and I had to imagine it was multiplied by a hundred for him. We sat in the waiting room eager to get out of the oncology office as soon as possible. I looked over at Tom and smiled. "Channel all that guilt toward the amount of food we are going to eat at Thanksgiving."

Nov. 25 – A Three-Hour Tour

Well. Usually I avoid holiday crowds, meaning I don't do the shopping during peak times, etc. However, I didn't realize that going to the cancer clinic the day before they are closed for two days was such a mess too. Add that to the list of things to avoid in the future – along with cancer in general.

So our appointment was a bit of a nightmare this afternoon. Here's a tip for everyone – ALWAYS get the earliest appointment available with any sort of specialist; otherwise, they get behind. Usually I get the earliest appointment, but given the holidays, this was the only appointment they had. After we were sitting in the waiting room for thirty minutes, I went to the counter and made sure there wasn't an issue – nope, the doctor was just running approximately fifty minutes behind. Oofta. We finally saw our doctor an hour and twenty minutes after our appointment time. Now, we certainly are patient people and understand that emergencies happen (in fact, Tom has been the emergency before, so we are especially forgiving), but today was challenging. It's tough to be in the waiting room for that long because it's depressing. The place is usually busy but it was just jam-packed today. It's heart breaking to see some of these folks come in – and for us, especially hard to be the youngest and feel like everyone is staring at us.

Anyway, once we saw our doctor (who acknowledged the wait and apologized, unlike many other doctors), we did blood work. Unfortunately, Tom will be having another blood transfusion on Friday. His levels are low and they are trying to bring them back up before we start our next round of treatment. So, at this point we were circling the wagons at about two-ish hours, and then we find out we need the blood transfusion – which we assumed would be the same as last time. Nope – we had to go to a different part of the hospital to once again do a blood draw (third of the day), so they could match the blood. This made zero sense to me since we know his blood type, but they needed to do it again for a bunch of medical reasons that certainly sounded legit – but was still irritating. So by the time everything was said and done, I was singing my Gilligan's Island *version of our Three-Hour (Doctor) Tour on the way out the door. Long day – especially for Tom who had to suffer with my made-up lyrics.*

The transfusion is less scary this time since we knew what to expect but certainly not what we were hoping to deal with on Friday. The good news was we got all the orders we needed for his post-chemo, pre-surgery testing. So while we were doing all this hustle and bustle of waiting for the additional blood work, I was multi-tasking and making a bunch of the appointments. It was a bit of a puzzle to coordinate when the different doctors were available based on our time crunch – in fact, I called one office a few times to shift things around to accommodate other schedules – but I think we've got most of it figured out. Phew! Tomorrow is Thanksgiving, and I've been attempting to write a Thanksgiving post. We will see if I can pull together the emotions to get up a post tomorrow – to say we are thankful this year is an understatement. More to come…

What Is Thanks?

Thanksgiving is one of my favorite holidays. No pressure of gifts and a day focused around food, napping and family. What more do you need? That morning was strange. While Tom was feeling better, he was still getting so worn down from the chemo. It felt like a holiday – but not one like any other. I thought about years prior and how I would always say the same thing when it was my turn to tell the table what I was thankful for – usually my family, friends, job, health and something that was relevant at that time in my life – very "all encompassing" types of things.

This year was one of the first in my life where I really felt the absence of one of these main staples. I was always thankful for health, but never from the perspective of it being in such jeopardy for someone I love so much. I was always thankful for my job, but this year I had a whole new appreciation for our employers, what they were doing for us, and that they provided health insurance. My family was always at the top of my list, but seeing them all rally around us was something I couldn't even wrap my head around.

Yet as I was in bed that morning watching the Macy's parade with Tom, I didn't know what exactly thankfulness was. Was thankfulness an acknowledgment – or was true thankfulness doing something that demonstrates thankfulness? I suddenly felt panicky about Thanksgiving dinner – it almost seemed like a mockery to sit at that table later that day and say I was thankful for a myriad of things. I was so much more than thankful; these things were not just components of our life that we appreciated – they were lifelines. Our family, our incomes, our insurance, our friends, our doctors – they deserved their own holiday of thanks and gratitude.

I knew it was going to be an emotional day, and to top it off we were receiving so many texts from friends and family saying how thankful they were for us. One in particular had us in tears on the way to Tom's parents' house. People thanked us for being so open about our fight on the blog, for demonstrating courage and being such a drastic reminder of how precious life was. It was that text on the way to Thanksgiving that gave me my "aha" moment. The greatest thank you for so many people was to feel like they were part of our fight – it was a comfort to those who felt helpless. If our hell made people more aware and more thankful of all they had on Thanksgiving, then our fight was a little bit easier. It gave us additional purpose. We weren't beating this just for us; we were beating it for everyone who was part of his cheering squad. Successfully beating cancer was the greatest thanks we could give to the never-ending list of people we owed gratitude.

Nov. 26 – Warning: Sentimental Post

We had a wonderful Thanksgiving that included an attempt to sleep in – I made it until 7 am! We had a lazy morning and were able to relax. Tom and I alternate holidays and this year was our Thanksgiving with his family and Christmas with my family, which worked out well with our current situation. We were able to go over to his mom's house for Thanksgiving – and as usual – my in-laws hosted an awesome Thanksgiving with lots of yummy food.

Like most families, we go around the table and say what we are thankful for. The very thought of describing what I'm thankful for had me choked up. Luckily, crafty Aunt Paula incorporated a pack of tissues into the place cards – she's so damn clever! Needless to say, the tissues were used!

Well. What are we thankful for this year? I blubbered a few things at the table today as I tried not to cry, but in all honesty, I could write a list that would take days to read. In our attempt to really think about it, we pulled together some things we are especially thankful for this year, in no particular order, and of course not all inclusive. But a few sentiments for this Thanksgiving:

Our Nurses/Doctors/Technicians/Hospital, Office & Clinic Staff: The patience of these folks is remarkable. These are people who have truly found their calling. It has been incredibly powerful, and a privilege, to be around that type of energy for the past two and a half months. A handful of these people have become like family during this, and we are forever grateful.

Our Family: You never know the power of your family as a unit until you are in a time of crisis. Our families have been our strength on rough days, smiling faces and shoulders to cry on. Whether it is in person, a care package, a message, FaceTime or any other means of communication, it has been remarkable. Love and gratitude don't even begin to describe this feeling.

Our Friends & Support Network: We have had support at every turn, from every imaginable person. The outpouring of love has, at times, overwhelmed us to the point of tears because we felt we could never repay what we have received. From people helping us with referrals, meals, cards, etc., we are forever in your debt.

Our Marriage: When we got married three years ago, I never thought we would be spending days on end holed up together in a hospital room, or our house, with me as the primary caretaker. I am so thankful that we have the marriage and partnership that we do. Tom has not let more than a few hours go by without thanking me, and we've actually had quite a bit of fun despite our situation. We are stronger for it, and for that, I can't be anything but thankful.

Humor: We truly believe laughter is the best medicine, and I believe that mindset has helped us get this far. Some days I think our humor made this seem easy – though, trust me, it's quite the opposite. I also think you get back what you give, and having a positive mindset made it easy for our doctors and nurses to communicate with us in the same way.

Science & Medicine: Tom has said it repeatedly, but thank goodness he got cancer in 2015. I have been blown away by the power of the human body and all that it can do/tolerate in addition to the medical capabilities that support it all. We are not foolish to think cancer-free means this will all be over; in the years following his "all clear," there will continue to be many scans and tests so we can avoid a situation like this again – and we plan to have many thankful days of clear scans ahead.

Our Employers/Bosses: We both work for incredible companies that have shown us such grace during a dark time of our lives. Tom's company has been absolutely amazing and supportive while he has been away – they are constant cheerleaders for him, making sure we have everything we need. My company has been equally phenomenal and has provided me with flexibility and support that has rendered me speechless at times. I've continued to work full-time throughout this entire endeavor, but working for an organization like mine that knows the importance of family is an incredible gift.

Rough Patches of Life: Let me be clear – I wish that Tom didn't have cancer. However, this diagnosis has given us more than it has taken. Many people say, "Seize the day" or "Live life to the fullest," but rarely do people live that way. We are forever changed. At the age of twenty-eight and thirty, in a matter of hours, our lives were ripped from us, and months of intense, scary and life-limiting events followed. We will never be the same – and I know we will live differently for it. I wish it weren't at the expense of Tom having to go through this – but we are forever grateful for our new perspective on our lives.

Our hearts are so incredibly full – we wish you all the happiest Thanksgiving…

Ho Ho No?

"Let's just not set up Christmas," Tom said.

"No way – you have lost your mind," I replied, shocked at his suggestion. "Do I need to call your mom? You'll give her a heart attack."

Tom's mom loved Christmas. If there was a word bigger than "loved," that would apply too. Since the day I met her, I knew how much she loved Christmas, and her house at the holidays was always one of my favorite places. It had such a warm and comfortable feeling, glistening with lights and decorations. I knew if I told her that Tom didn't want to decorate, she would have been on my doorstep to help me - and yell at her son.

"Let's not do that. I feel bad that I can't help; it takes so much time and we are going to have a crazy December and January," he replied, trying to sell his terrible idea to me.

"That's precisely why we need to decorate! First, it's festive and second, I'm not letting cancer take away the feeling of Christmas for us," I said, getting unexpectedly choked up. "How about I don't set up everything but at least some decorations and the tree?" I was trying to compromise but had zero intention of backing down.

"Can I help?" he asked, already throwing in the towel.

"If I need help with something, I'll let you know. Go downstairs and relax."

Tom begrudgingly shook his head. He knew this wasn't an argument he was going to win. I followed him downstairs to start pulling out decorations. I loved decorating with Tom the day after Thanksgiving and had some specific requirements which included hot chocolate and watching *Elf*. While I was sad that this wouldn't be our usual festive Christmas bonding, I knew he would be happy when it was up, and that made me happy.

I started dragging everything upstairs. I was going to limit myself to the big Christmas tree, some garlands around the house and a few other small things. We had a lot more, but this felt like the right amount considering our circumstances. It took several hours, but I got everything up and was putting some finishing touches on the tree. Tom and I had a lot of opposing team ornaments and since I was solely responsible for the tree this year, most of the Bears/Cubs/Hawks ornaments suspiciously ended up on the back of the tree. I left some of Tom's more sentimental ornaments out and called him upstairs to help me with the finishing touches. He came up and remarked how nice everything looked. As *Elf* was wrapping up, he and I put the final decorations on the tree and called it done.

Later that evening, we were watching a movie, and I had dimmed the lights but turned on the tree. Everything was glistening and looked so festive. Tom leaned over and kissed me on the side of my head.

"Thanks for decorating, babe. I really appreciate it and am glad you did it. It means a lot," he said.

"Of course! I'll be damned if we don't keep things as normal as possible. Plus, your mom would have killed us both if we didn't decorate for Christmas," I replied.

"It looks really nice," he commented looking over at the tree.

"I think so too. It looks the best it has in years – but I'm betting that's because all my sports teams' ornaments are front and center."

Nov. 28 – Blood Friday Is More Fun Than Black Friday
We hope everyone had a wonderful Thanksgiving! We had an eventful few days – including a blood transfusion yesterday at the hospital. It went very well and, most importantly, relatively quickly! Three and a half hours for the whole check-in, prep and transfusion. In blood transfusion time (sort of like dog years), that's pretty good! However, he still was feeling pretty fatigued and exhausted in the afternoon, so he rested up since we've got another week of chemo ahead.

Today we relaxed and started to get ourselves ready for our LAST round of chemo. This included putting up some Christmas decorations. Now, originally, Tom didn't want to put up any decorations because of how crazy December will be and the upcoming surgery, but I think it's important to keep life as "normal" as possible. Plus – he loves Christmas – and for as much as he has been stuck in the house, I think he should have some good Christmas juju around him. We compromised, and I didn't put up all of the decorations – just the tree and some garlands – but I think it's pretty, even if the rest of the house is not as decorated this year. As I was putting up decorations, we were chatting about how hard it is to believe it's almost December. In a strange way, it feels like our lives are back in September. Yes, we know time is passing, seasons changed and life has been happening, but there is a part of us that still can't comprehend all that has happened. That will come, but in the meantime, we will try to spread some Christmas cheer.

Tom is excited for two more "good" days before we start chemo again on Tuesday, as am I. More to come...

Grasping for Normalcy

Throughout the diagnosis, one of the hardest roles was managing all the love. Our family and friends were fantastic, but sometimes, the comments would puzzle me. We received so many care packages, gifts, cards, food deliveries and more, and I always wrote a thank-you note. Despite everything going on during this time, I made sure to design and send a Christmas card. People seemed shocked that I would be worrying about a Christmas card or sending thank-you notes. I received so many texts from people telling me not to send them thank-you notes. It was all lost on me. Those things were so important because they were normal.

I often had a simple question for myself – would I have done this before Tom was diagnosed? If the answer was yes, then it happened. I would never receive a gift from someone and not sent a thank-you note, so why would cancer suddenly be an excuse to not acknowledge someone? I have always sent out Christmas cards, so why would that change? I grasped for normalcy; I grasped for things that made me feel like cancer wasn't taking anything away from us. What people didn't understand was that sending a thank-you note was me telling cancer to take a hike. Sending Christmas cards empowered me and helped convince me that we would beat this.

There wasn't a circumstance in this world that would have prevented me from continuing to try to make people happy – and I'd be damned if cancer was going to take that away. I would never forget to celebrate the birthdays of family and friends because cancer wasn't going to take that away from me either. In fact, I threw my mom a little birthday party in the hospital room during one of Tom's chemo treatments. It was about creating a new, temporary normal so that we could make it through each day. It was about adjusting, but on our own terms. It was about adapting, but not letting cancer take control…it was about those damn thank-you notes.

Dec. 1 – Sixteen Down, Four To Go

So begins our LAST ROUND OF CHEMO! It's always a bit of a strange ride to the hospital when we are headed in for treatment – it's rather somber, and the week seems like a steep climb.

Anyway, we were especially curious about how this week would go, considering how weak his body has gotten and how it's been harder to bounce back. We headed in, and our moods were instantly lifted seeing our friends here at the hospital. From our transport guy to our nurses and support staff, everyone was eager to say hello and were excited for us that this is our last round of chemo. We are back in one of the smaller rooms because the oncology wing is completely full – but it's sort of like finishing off where we started, so

I'm all good with the cozier room.

We did the usual prep and got things moving right along for the week. Tom's blood work was done and he's continuing to kill the cancer, which is super important before surgery – all good news! However, unfortunately, he started to "feel" the effects of chemo this evening. Day One is by far the earliest he has ever felt sort of weak and tired from chemo – we've typically been able to get to Day Three or so before this point, but it's to be expected given the treatment. So, we hunker down for a challenging week – but at least we know it should be the last one. More to come…

The Last Week of School

I had unexpectedly become sentimental for the last round of chemo, and it caught me off guard. When I woke up in the morning, one of our favorite night nurses was saying her goodbyes. I woke up as she was finishing Tom's blood draw. She was telling him that she prayed for him every night and that she couldn't wait to hear about our success in beating cancer. I wasn't prepared for a goodbye so soon but had forgotten about the hospital schedules and that she would only be with us our first night. I started tearing up and lifted my head.

"Oh, I hope I didn't wake you," she said.

"No, it's fine, I was mostly awake. I'm so sad that this is your last shift with us," I said as I rubbed my eyes and fixed my ever-present hospital messy bun.

"I was just telling him that I have so enjoyed taking care of you guys and wish you all the best. I'm praying for you," she said compassionately.

"Thank you so much – you're a breath of fresh air. I'm mostly sad that we didn't get to chat more, given your night schedule, and I know Tom appreciated your Cubs scrubs too. Thank you so much, we can't say thank you enough." I was starting to get choked up and knew Tom wasn't far behind.

"Of course, it's my pleasure," she said. She gave us both hugs and was on her way.

"I wasn't ready for that this early in the morning," I said. "How are you feeling?"

"Yeah, that was tough; she was so nice to us. I'm feeling pretty shitty, but I love you a lot," he said as he stretched his arm out.

I knew what that meant; it had become a morning ritual for us. Usually, Tom had a very early blood draw, and it would still be rather dark out. I would typically wake up when the nurse came in. After the nurse left, I'd leave my couch bed and curl up in Tom's hospital bed with him. I crawled into his hospital bed and tucked myself in his side and shoulder that didn't have the port and IVs.

"I have a feeling this is going to be a long week of goodbyes. It's so strange because I never want to be back here, yet it feels like a weird farewell. It's like the last week of school growing up. You're excited to be done, but are going to miss seeing your friends every day," I said as I stared down at our feet with my head on his chest.

"Yeah, I know, this is so strange. They've become some of our biggest cheerleaders, seems weird that we won't see them. At least I hope we won't," Tom said, acknowledging what we never talked about, which was the potential for more chemo after surgery.

"As far as I'm concerned, this is it, and I'm handling it that way," not wanting to think about having to do two more rounds of chemo.

"I know, me too. It's going to be a roller coaster of a week," he said as he squeezed me closer to him.

"Roller coaster week? I'm pretty sure we've been on a roller coaster since September," I said.

Tom let out a bit of a laugh, and we lay there quietly – dozing off in bed. I felt so safe and comfortable lying there. Again, like the end of school – you're excited about the next grade, but the unknown is still a little scary, and there was comfort in the grade you were in. It was going to be a tough week of goodbyes and farewells to our new normal, and I realized it wasn't that I was sad to see these people and interim traditions go – the unease was that we were venturing back into the unknown.

Dec. 2 – Seventeen Down, Three To Go

What a Day. It's 1 a.m., and I shouldn't be awake, so I'm going to try to keep this one short tonight! This morning we started our day by saying goodbye to one of our favorite night nurses. She is off for the rest of the week so last night was our final night with her – she was standing at the foot of his bed at 6:30 a.m. to say goodbye. She, like Tom, is a huge Cubs fan and they bonded over the playoff run and he loved her Cubs scrubs! She had some incredibly kind words for us and wanted to be kept in the loop on his progress. She is a wonderful nurse, and we were lucky to have her the nights that we did – however, I'd be lying if I said a 6:30 a.m. goodbye didn't catch me off guard – even though we were awake I wasn't expecting it. As excited as we are to never return to this oncology unit – we will miss the people, so it creates quite the swirl of emotions. No one likes to start their day choked up!

Tom is feeling rough today and disappointed with how early the fatigue and nausea have set in – he is such a champ and I'm completely amazed by his strength, but you can tell this round has already been especially tough. I thought this last round would feel much faster due to our excitement of it being the last one, but it has been a bit of the opposite and seems to be dragging. Oh well – we carry on and keep working towards Sunday – his birthday! Tom will have a bit of an unfortunate birthday because it is one of his absolute worst days, but I told him that if one crappy birthday assures us that he celebrates many more birthdays to come, then in a backwards way, it's the greatest gift. Plus – he's thrown up on his birthday in years past for much stupider reasons.

So, fingers crossed that tomorrow isn't too rough on him…More to come…

Clothing Optional

We all do things we don't want to do; it's the nature of the beast when it comes to life. It can be extreme, like chemo, or less extreme, like sitting through a show. Some people are better at smiling through it; others, not so much. Tom had learned to smile through a lot when he married me because my adventurous spirit always had us headed in different directions.

We were on our way back from a visit to Cincinnati right after college, and I had recently downloaded a road trip app that notified you of unique places to visit. As we drove along, the icons popped up on the map, and I would check to see what we were near. There were historic sites and landmarks, and quirky things like the world's largest ball of yarn, the RV hall of fame, and a medical museum with a collection of brains in jars. Tom would shake his head as I excitedly read off all the things we were near. The problem was that I wasn't in the driver's seat.

"I don't understand why you don't want to see these!" I exclaimed.

"Because we've had a long weekend and I just want to get home."

"How about one? If I pick one, will you stop? I'll pick one that is quick, so it won't take a lot of time," I suggested. I had to play my cards right since I knew I was driving him crazy.

"Fine, one," he replied.

I was so excited and got to searching. A few minutes in, I found the winner.

"Alright, I found it. It's like thirty miles ahead."

"What is it?"

"A giant lady's leg sundial.... cross it off the bucket list!" I joked.

"What?"

"It's a sixty-three-foot-tall women's leg that is used as a sun dial," I said.

I kept reading and checked out the reviews. As I read, I realized where exactly we were headed – a nudist camp. I debated if I should tell Tom or not, and ultimately decided it was in my best interest.

"Okay, so just to prepare you, apparently this is part of a nudist camp. Which explains the need for a sundial, and justifies the humor that it's a women's leg," I said.

"You can't be serious."

"A hundred percent serious," I replied with a smile on my face. "That's hilarious, let's just pop off the exit and see if we can see it. According to most of the reviews, they let people see it with clothes on, but another review said you had to strip down." I thought for sure he wouldn't stop, but he did.

We got off the exit and didn't feel like we were in the greatest area. It was a remote part of Indiana.

"There it is! There is the turn-off!" I shouted, so excited that I had convinced Tom to do this.

As we drove in, a strange-looking man was coming the other way in a PT Cruiser. As I turned back to look at him, I saw a sign that was facing the other direction that read STOP: YOU MUST BE DRESSED BEYOND THIS POINT. This place was already amazing. As we sat in the car, I tried to bargain with Tom that we should just take our clothes off so they would let us in and we could see the sundial. Unfortunately, I couldn't convince him so we left before attempting to get past the gate.

We laughed so hard the entire way back to the highway as I grabbed the app to read more.

"You are crazy," he said as he shook his head and laughed at me.

"So, since we technically didn't cross if off the list, can I interest you in a collection of five thousand pencils a few miles up?" I asked, keeping my eye on the app so I didn't start to laugh. He looked at me with the most hilarious reaction, turned on the music and continued driving. He had humored me once, and while I know he would never admit it, we had fun on our little detour. His willingness to humor me and check it out was one of the reasons I knew I wanted to marry him. Despite not always being comfortable, he always trusted me for an adventure.

Dec. 3 – Eighteen Down, Two To Go – Let the Final Countdown Begin!

Chemo confusion is a real thing (much like pregnancy brain), and the regimen Tom has can make him easily confused or forgetful. He's joked quite a bit when he does something silly that it was just chemo confusion. Now I've got quite a bit on my plate right now, so I have jokingly referred to my own made-up caretaker chemo confusion several times when I've got too much happening at once and do something goofy (like when I looked for my cell phone for ten minutes and it was in my hand). Meanwhile, Tom has been pretending to play his chemo confusion card today by asking me what the Packers' record is and what happened during the Bears/Packers game last week. I don't think he appreciated my Packers sweatshirt for the game tonight – nor did it probably help with his nausea.

Anyway – on to more important things – we are over halfway done with our last chemo!! Tom rocked session three today but is feeling pretty rough. Last night was tough too – I was up quite late, and as he was sleeping he was making noises and sort of mumbling in his sleep, which led me to believe he was in pain. He said he doesn't have much recollection and luckily isn't in pain, it's just the nausea he's dealing with. It's tough to have to sit and watch someone you love be so sick and really feel helpless.

Despite that, we had some fun today too – for those that know my mother-in-law, you know she loves Christmas. I mean loves it at a whole other level than most of us. So today, we got a floral delivery, and sure enough, she sent us a baby Christmas tree for the room that even came with lights and ornaments since she felt it needed to be more festive in the room – it added a nice glow this evening.

Then, tonight, we coordinated treating the nurses to some dinner! A special thank you to my sister-in-law, Stacy, and brother-in-law, Michael. My brother-in-law is a proprietor at Outback Steakhouse and was kind enough to treat the staff to a whole spread of appetizers for everyone to share and enjoy. The nurses were so excited and very thankful. We've got some different treats coming for our day shift tomorrow too. I had a hard time figuring out what to get our nurses as a thank you this week so we figured treats and thank-you cards will have to do the trick for now. If I had millions and billions of dollars, I would do something completely over the top, but even with all the money in the world, there wouldn't be something that would adequately thank them for everything they have done for us over these four rounds of chemo. It's something money could never buy.

Two days of chemo to go and three nights in the hospital.... More to come tomorrow...

My Green & Gold Heart

I may only be twenty-eight, but my heart had years on it, and being a Packer fan didn't help. As I sat silently watching the Packer game in the hospital room one night, I couldn't help but laugh as I correlated how fast my heart was beating during a Packer comeback game and a funny moment from the beginning of our relationship.

Tom & I had met during a challenging time while my dad was sick. I was working an internship as well as the restaurant, and adjusting to the weird in-between of finishing my first year of college and being back under my parents' roof for the summer. It was non-stop, and I found myself at the doctor, getting a heart monitor because I was having weird pains. I was not the usual candidate to get directions on how to put on a heart monitor.

I had to have the monitor strapped on to my pants, and then there were four little stickies that were on my chest. When I felt the pain, I had to push the button for it to record my heart waves. If there was any unusual heart activity, the monitor would beep a few times and automatically record the heartbeat. I got it in the middle of July and would have to keep it for two weeks. It was a real pretty outfit accessory, to say the least.

The second week I had the monitor, I went to Tom's apartment to hang out. We were still very much in the beginning phases of our relationship, figuring out if this was more of a friendship or something more serious. We had a jam session at his apartment with his guitar and my fiddle and grabbed some takeout. It was relaxed, fun, and so awesome to hang with someone who shared my passion for music. Eventually, one thing led to another, and Tom kissed me. It wasn't but a few seconds later that we stopped and burst into laughter. My heart monitor had beeped and began recording my heartbeat. I was both embarrassed and surprised that it had gone off as I looked up to Tom.

"I did it! I made your heart monitor go off – mission accomplished!" he said with a grin on his face.

He did indeed; there was no denying that.

Dec. 4 – Nineteen Down – One To Go!

If there were cameras in our hospital room – I would be a YouTube sensation. Last night after I posted on the blog I was watching the end of the Packers/Lions game as I got curled up in my bed made for people that are five feet tall. I love my Packers – but our season was getting a little frightening, and this was a must-win game. So you can imagine my mood when we were getting beat 20-0, but then we slowly started to creep back into the game. Now, Tom had been sleeping for quite a while at this point, so I was here in a dark hospital room watching the game. I challenge anyone to watch the ending of that game to not SCREAM with joy – I almost imploded (it's like trying to sit still during Beyoncé's "Single Ladies" – not happening). Instead of screaming and waking up not only Tom but the entire floor, I proceeded to silent scream and jump up and down like a crazy person with no one to high five. What a game!

So anyway, today Tom and I were discussing the different chemo cycles and decided if we had to give each one a tag line, they would be:

Chemo #1: What The Hell Is Happening?
Chemo #2: Blood Shouldn't Clot.
Chemo #3: We've Got This – and Luxury Accommodations!
Chemo #4: Are We Sure There Is a Battery In That Clock?
I anticipate that the surgery tagline will be: Morphine.

Our day shift got the giant tower of cookies that we sent them this afternoon and they loved them. Then this evening we gave them a big popcorn tin that Tom's mom and aunt had got them too – I'm a little worried they are going to like this too much and try to keep us here longer!

Unfortunately, Tom had a rough day and evening. He was throwing up again, but we were able to get him some more meds quickly, and he has been sleeping pretty hard ever since. At least when he is sleeping, he doesn't feel the nausea, even if it takes strong medicine to do so. However, tomorrow is HIS LAST CHEMO!!!!! I'm hopeful that keeps spirits high throughout the day and then we can start our countdown to home. I don't think he really counts chemo as being "done" until we are on our way home, but I'm going to celebrate it either way – and I still have some of that Packer celebration to let out. More to come tomorrow!

The Anticipation

We were so ready to be home, and I was getting updates from my sister-in-law, Christina, on a birthday surprise I had been coordinating for Tom. She was collecting our mail during our hospital stays, and I had my sister Mame send out a note to ask people to flood our mailbox with cards for Tom, either a birthday card or a congratulations on chemo card. We really put Christina to work that week as our mailbox began to fill up with cards, goofy gifts and care packages. I knew we wouldn't have much of a birthday celebration, so I figured a stack of cards for him to open would be a great way to have some celebration without the exhaustion.

That night, we went on our nightly walk around the hospital and I kept squeezing Tom's hand and smiling at him.

"You're done with chemo," I said to him, as if he wasn't aware.

"I know, but it sure doesn't feel like it yet," he said. Our need to stay at the hospital until the next day, coupled with how terrible he was feeling as a result of the chemo, certainly wasn't the greatest celebration, but I was excited to see what had come in the mail and hoped it would be the best celebration possible.

Dec. 5 – Put Chemo In the Rear View Mirror!

Tom. Has. Finished. Chemo. What an emotional day for us! First of all, let me just say my husband a hundred percent rocked this treatment. I am in complete amazement at his attitude, strength and humor through this all – we have had some tough, tough, tough days here, but he continued to power through as best he could. Tom was sick during the night and woke up feeling quite rough. We were super excited when the last bag started to beep (the ONLY time I've been happy to hear that damn thing beep) – our nurse came in and took down the bag, and we celebrated.

It felt a little anti-climactic that we couldn't get up and walk out of the hospital but who cares – CHEMO IS DONE! There were some happy tears, but despite all that excitement, he continued to throw up this afternoon and still isn't feeling great. Luckily, he's been asleep for a while so hopefully all the rest tonight will do him good because tomorrow is his birthday! Unfortunately, we won't be doing much for his birthday. Typically, on our discharge day we are here in the morning, get discharged early afternoon and then we get home, he takes a shower and then is pretty much out for the rest of the day. But that's okay – we will just celebrate on a bit of a delay when he's feeling better.

Our oncologist was excited too! She has been so incredible, and we are lucky to have her. While this is a huge milestone – we do know that it is just the first of two huge steps in becoming cancer-free. Next up is surgery and we know that is an even bigger mountain – but we still need to celebrate this one – and she agreed!

We were thinking back today and counting silly things, so without further ado, chemo by the numbers:
One Port Surgery
Twenty Chemo Treatments
Twenty-Four Nights in the Hospital
Two Blood Transfusions
Sixty Bags of Chemo Drugs
Four Cafeteria Loyalty Cards Completed
Four Different Rooms
One ER Visit
Thirty-plus Doctors' Appointments
Twenty-plus Games of Uno (most won by Honore)
Two Business Ideas (I'm confident we will be on Shark Tank one day)
...and a partridge in a pear tree

There are plenty more things we could count, but it's amazing to think about how far we've come. We would not have been able to do this alone. We just want to say thank you to everyone who has helped us, stopped by for visits, or with food, sent us messages, cards, prayers, and care packages. You've helped us get through this first major milestone, and we know you'll be there as we start the next part of our fight. I mean it when I say we feel all the love, energy and prayers that have been headed our way - we are so so so so so so so lucky and are forever in your debt! More to come tomorrow...

I Don't Mess With Birthdays

I started planning for Tom's thirtieth birthday in late August. I had a crazy idea to get him thirty gifts and give him one gift for the thirty days leading up to his birthday. Tom was dreading turning thirty, but I was determined to make his birthday a great one.

I planned to have a gift and a small tag for each day and then one "big" gift every ten gifts, representative of each decade. The daily gifts weren't extreme but always had a clever tie. For example, the card read "I love you because you're so sweet" and it was a bag of his favorite candy. Another was, "I love you because I know you to a tee" and it was a bag of golf tees. In addition, I planned certain dates for certain reasons. We love a little breakfast diner near our house called TNT – so he got a card on a Saturday morning that said, "I love you because you're dynamite."

The first big gift was tickets to see Last Comic Standing on tour. We both love standup comedy and had gotten sucked into the show that year. I told him that he needed to come to a work dinner with me on a Friday. He was less than thrilled. He showed up to pick me up, and I handed him his daily card – it read, "I love you because you make me laugh."

"Wait, we aren't going to a work dinner?" he asked.

"Nope! We are taking a quick drive to Milwaukee to see Last Comic Standing on Tour," I excitedly replied.

"I'm so happy I don't have to go to your work dinner!" he exclaimed.

"What?! That's it?!" I said, jokingly.

"Oh, and of course to go to the show too," he replied as he pulled my hand and kissed it. "My birthday surprises are so much fun!"

The second big gift was a photo book that had taken me hours to create. It was an eighty-page book that documented our trip to Italy and Ireland earlier that year. I had spent hours laboring over all the pictures and images and making sure that it was a keepsake for years to come. We sat on the couch that night and went page by page, reliving the memories of that trip. It was as if we were taking the trip again for the first time.

The last one he got on his thirtieth birthday. It was a map and two tickets to Denver, CO. Tom had always wanted to go, and we were going to check that stadium off our list. Tom and I were on a quest to go to all the MLB parks and either see the Cubs lose or the Brewers win. The Cubs season opener was in Colorado, and we were going to be there. He was beside himself, he was so excited – and was such a great way to end the Thirty Days to Thirty.

His actual birthday landed on a Saturday. That morning, he got a card that said, "I love you more than I love steak." It was a dinner reservation for Chicago Prime – a fancy steakhouse we had both wanted to try. He was eager for the big feast, and I knew it would be the best dinner we had had in a while.

What he didn't know was that dinner was also to get him out of the house for a surprise party.

We sat at Chicago Prime that night and enjoyed an amazing dinner. I rushed us through dessert a bit because I was eager to get Tom back to the house. I had everything ready to go, and Tom's parents and aunt and uncle were going to quickly decorate before we got back. We had about twenty-five people coming, and I really thought I had him fooled. We wrapped up our leftovers and headed home – I was getting so excited.

"That was yummy, Happy Birthday!" I said as we drove home.

"Thanks, that was awesome. I'm ready to go home, take off my pants and watch the Hawks game," he said.

"Did you have a good birthday?" I asked, starting to worry that he wouldn't be very excited to have all these people at the house.

"Yeah, I really did. Thanks for everything," he replied.

"Is there anyone you haven't heard from today?" I asked.

"Actually, I'm really surprised I never heard from Nick. Lauren even texted me earlier, but I would be surprised if Nick forgot to text me on my birthday," he said. Tom was referring to his college roommate and one of his best friends, Nick, and his wife, Lauren.

Little did he know that Nick had driven in for his surprise party and would be at the house when we arrived. I had taken a wild guess when he mentioned not hearing from Nick that Nick probably avoided talking to him today to avoid any chance of ruining the surprise. Lauren couldn't make it down for the party, so it made sense that she had texted earlier. I laughed a bit on the inside.

"Wow, that would be really surprising. There is no way Nick would forget your birthday though," I replied. It took every ounce of control to not tell him Nick was back at the house.

We pulled into the garage, and I needed him to go into the house first since everyone would be right inside the garage door. I pretended to fix my jacket as he led the way. He opened the door, flipped on the light and immediately jumped back out and slammed the door. Not only did he just see people in our basement yell "surprise" but they had all held up the giant cutouts I had made of his face. Mission accomplished.

He hadn't had a suspicion that there was a party, and upon seeing Nick in the house looked at me and excitedly proclaimed that he couldn't believe I hadn't told him Nick was there. The party was a blast; the house was covered in balloons and photos of him growing up along with a huge poker-themed cake.

By the end of the night, I had been over-served by the bartender (I was the bartender) and was put to bed. The successful surprise party after thirty days of coordinating surprises had caught up with me. The next morning as I nursed one hell of a hangover, Tom rolled over and wrapped his arms around me.

155

"Thanks for such an amazing birthday, that was so much fun," he said.

"My brain is still celebrating because the room is spinning," I replied.

Tom let out a laugh as he grabbed me some water from the nightstand. "You were in rare form last night."

"Ugh, I know, hopefully I didn't make a fool of myself," I said as I gulped the water and some aspirin.

"Don't worry, my mom got it on tape," he said with a smirk on his face.

"Of course, she did. Let's erase that as soon as possible," I said as Tom snickered.

"I'm glad you had a good birthday, babe. I'm going to try to close my eyes again for a few minutes."

"Okay," he said with a sigh and a sad tone.

"What's wrong?" I asked, hoping it was nothing that required me to move my head too much.

"It's just kind of sad to not have a gift to open today," he said, trying to hold back his smirk.

I rolled over, opened one eye and gave him a look of complete disgust. Tom laughed and gave me a kiss on the head as he rolled out of bed and assured me he was just kidding. As he reached back to pull the door closed I softly heard him say, "I can't wait until I turn forty."

Dec. 6 – Home Is Where there are no IV Poles

I really don't even know how to write today's post. Today has been an incredibly emotional day – but an amazing day. First things first, HAPPY BIRTHDAY to my wonderful husband! I wish we had been able to celebrate more, but considering our situation, we did celebrate quite a bit! Tom was up bright and early getting sick, so our day started sooner than expected. The nausea and getting sick has been especially rough this round, so these last few days have been difficult. Tom said that since mid-Wednesday he has been focused on not puking – a lot of which is mind over matter. Even our doctor has said a trick to beating nausea is mind over matter, but unfortunately, there are points at which it is too much.

Despite that, I had a gift and two cards ready for him next to his bed for when he woke up. Once we got him all settled in again, he opened his gift and started feeling better. Then, our amazing nurses and doctor came in singing "Happy Birthday" with cupcakes they had made for him, sparking grape juice for a champagne toast (in foam cups - classy!!), a card from the team and a funny picture. Ironically, one of our nurses was the younger sister of a friend and bandmate of Tom's from high school. She had gone into her brother's vault of photos and found funny, embarrassing photos of Tom from his younger days. I know I've mentioned this many times, but we have gotten quite close with a lot of our nurses and doctors, so it really was so overwhelming and kind that they all coordinated a celebration and even baked for us.

We were on target to leave at 2:15 based on his final drip of medicines. Two p.m. felt like an eternity away – the celebration with our nurses helped pass some time and then I knew that some of Tom's family was planning to surprise him with a celebration. They came to the hospital with cupcakes and visited for, which was a great way to celebrate his birthday – and help pass more time! I curled up in the tiny hospital bed with him for the final twenty minutes as we stared at the IV pole and painfully watched it drip. Then….it beeped…and we could not have been happier. Back on September 16, we never thought today would come, and then suddenly our lives were a blur, and we are here. Our nurse was ready to go, got his port needles out and we got the heck out of there after a few more goodbyes.

We were both crying by the elevator and cried most of the way home – we aren't ashamed to admit it. It's the strangest, most overwhelming, confusing, and exciting feeling in the world, and it was like our minds froze and didn't know how to react. As we got home and kissed the floor, we had a giant stack of cards for his birthday/end of chemo in addition to some other gifts and packages. We didn't open them right away because we knew they would be overwhelming. We cleaned up – yay for normal-sized showers – and got ourselves situated and then spent time opening all the love.

Regarding his health, Tom's blood did not look good today – his white blood cells (the ones that fight infection) are the lowest they have been this entire treatment, which means he needs to steer clear of crowds, handshakes, kisses and general contact. Our doctor was very clear that we need to be very careful as he rebounds this time and gets ready for surgery. Tomorrow we will be back at the doctor for his booster shot, and then he will be lying low and trying to recover. I don't think it has hit me yet that chemo is over. I actually don't think it will sink in until we don't have to go back in three weeks.

I am so so so so so so so proud of Tom – this hasn't been easy – though he made it seem that way. This is just part one, but based on how he crushed part one, I have so much confidence that we will be ready to beat part two. More to come tomorrow…

Make You Feel My Love

I was at the grocery store. While we had previously been a "buy for the week" type of grocery shoppers, now I was frequenting the grocery store quite often to get whatever it was that Tom wanted to eat. The grocery store is just down the street from our house – it wasn't hard for me to jump in the car, get what I needed and be home in less than fifteen minutes – assuming, of course, I was in mission mode.

However, one night I only needed a few things and was lollygagging around the store. I got sucked into the floral department and was admiring all the flowers that were now somewhat seasonal for the upcoming Christmas holiday. The floral department is at the front of the store, by the checkout area and the piano. Our grocery store has a piano player at different times of the day. It's quite calming and a welcome distraction as you wait in line. As I roamed around the floral area, it took me a second to recognize the song, but when I did, I started softly singing the words.

"When the rain is pouring in your face, and the whole world is on your case," I started singing along, still not quite remembering how I knew this song. "I could offer you a warm embrace, to make you feel my love." There wasn't much of a line, and I was in the process of paying and walking out as the next verse started.

"When the evening shadows and the stars appear, and there is no one there to dry your tears," I softly sang. I started to cry with the words, "I could hold you for a million years, to make you feel my love..." I darted to my car and dropped the groceries in the passenger seat, then dropped my head into my hands.

Music had always been such a source of peace for me and yet it had just rocked me to the core. I sobbed. I hadn't cried in a while and there was something about the music, the lyrics and the whole dynamic in that grocery store that had broken the final straw. I had to figure out how I knew that song. I grabbed my phone as I sat in the dark parking lot and opened Google. I typed in the first line and the lyrics for "Make You Feel My Love" appeared.

As expected, I hadn't had the words right on the first line, nothing new for me. I switched over to my Spotify app and looked at my covers playlist. I had a cover of this song by Adele on my playlist; no wonder I had known the lyrics. I turned on my car so the Bluetooth would connect and tapped the song to play. Apparently, I wanted to torture myself. I sat in my car with tears rolling down my face as I listened to those lyrics. The last lyrics required a final sob before I took a deep breath and tried to pull myself together. "I could make you happy, make your dreams come true, nothing that I wouldn't do, go to the ends of the earth for you, to make you feel my love."

We were living and breathing the lyrics of this song. I was going to the ends of the earth; I was exhausted, and I knew that everything I was doing, including silly late-night trips to the grocery store on a cold night, was making him feel my love. As I turned down the street to our house, I took a few deep breaths and attempted to look like I hadn't cried as I pulled into the garage.

Tom was sitting in his usual spot on the couch. "You okay?" he asked.

"Yup – I'm fine," I said.

"I'm not stupid," he said as he put in so much effort to get up from the couch. He came over to the door and wrapped his arms around me as I put the groceries on the ground, wrapped my arms around him, and tucked myself into his shoulder and neck.

"I know you're not stupid, I just love you a lot," I said, into his chest.

"Trust me, babe, if there is one thing I know in this world, it's that you love me," he replied.

That was all I needed to hear. I knew it already, but I needed to hear it that night.

Dec. 7 – Wiped Out

Home feels wonderful! We are still catching back up but are so happy to be home. We were back at the hospital bright and early for Tom's booster shot, which will hopefully help make him bounce back faster. It's unbelievable how walloped he gets and the impact it has on his body these few days post chemo. However, the greatest part of this week is knowing this is the last time! It makes a world of difference to know that never again will we have to deal with chemo symptoms, managing post chemo drugs, or start to mentally prepare for chemo again. Amazing. For the most part, he is feeling pretty crappy, which we expected. This round has been especially challenging because he is feeling the impact of the compound effect of all the treatments, but like every other round he's got his eye on the prize and is being so strong.

I'm simply exhausted. A different type of exhausted from Tom, but exhausted nonetheless – it feels like the last thirteen weeks all hit me at once today (which almost resulted in a meltdown at the grocery store this evening), so I'm going to keep tonight short and try to catch up on some much-needed sleep. More to come…

Float Away

I never really took baths. They seemed so inefficient to me and given my track record of not being able to relax, it was hard for me just to sit there. On an especially challenging caregiver day, I decided to take a bath. I knew they worked magic for some people, so I thought I'd give it a shot. I left all technology, lit a few candles, and floated in the bath.

An hour and a half later, I got out, miraculously relaxed for a moment, and had a clearer head. I had spent about thirty minutes of the time in the bath figuring out if I could create something that kept bath water warm. While that wasn't relaxing for my mind, it kept my thoughts off our current situation, and that was a vacation for me.

I started taking them a few days a week from November on, and they were therapy, especially on tough days or nights where I didn't get much sleep. The day we got home from his last round of chemo, there was a package for Tom. He opened it and pulled out a brown box with a big blue bow on it. He handed it to me with tears in his eyes.

"This is for me?" I asked, assuming it had been a care package for him.

"Maybe…" he said, with a smile on his face.

"From you?" I asked, unsure of what exactly was happening.

He didn't answer and looked down for me to open the gift. I pulled the gift tag out from under the blue bow and began reading it. It read, "Thank you so much for always taking care of me. I couldn't get through all this without you. I love you so much and hope this can help you relax if just for 1 minute. Love, Your Soon To Be Cancer Free Husband."

I smiled as I read the card and looked up at Tom. I pulled off the blue bow and opened the small box. Inside was a box filled with goodies for the bath, some Epsom salts, a homemade soap bar and other bath items. It wasn't extravagant or over the top, but it was the sweetest moment in those first few hours we were home from chemo.

"Thanks, babe, you didn't have to do that," I said as I closed the box and leaned over to him for a kiss. "I can't believe with everything you're dealing with you thought to do that. I love that I can take care of you."

"I know, but it kills me that I haven't been able to take care of you like you deserve, and I wouldn't have made it to the end of chemo without you, and everything you've done to keep our lives together has been stressful for you."

"You take care of me just fine," I said as I leaned back in for another kiss.

"But just to confirm, you got me that because I've been relaxing in the bath lately right?"

"Of course, what else would it be for?" he asked.

I smiled as I replied, "Just wanted to make sure I don't smell."

160

Dec. 8 – A Lucky Break

I think it's safe to say we haven't had the best luck lately! However, today we caught a bit of a break, or at least we think it is a break considering the past twelve weeks of our lives. We were up all night because Tom was in an incredible amount of pain in his lower back area – he couldn't get comfortable; the medicines weren't helping, and he was only able to doze in and out a bit. Knowing what I know, and what I've been told to look for, my mind immediately went to kidneys. I assumed it would just be a matter of time before we were heading back to the hospital. I called the oncologist's office and talked to them, and they told us we were okay! The aches/pains he was experiencing is a common side effect with the booster shot he gets the day after chemo, so we were in the clear. For the record – that is the first time we've had an "issue" that hasn't resulted in us being back at the hospital. Woo hoo! Okay, in all reality it's about as exciting as finding out Kohl's is having a sale, but we'll take it.

Needless to say, a sleepless night is setting us back a bit in regard to exhaustion, but I'm just happy he is okay and thankful for heating pads! We are off to catch up on some sleep, but more to come...

Spinning

It felt like we were spinning a bit, waiting for all of the answers we wanted. The unknown was painful but at least understandable. While I wanted time to speed up, I also wanted it to slow down to put off the surgery. I had so much on my plate that it was easy to get lost in the days, but I worried about Tom and how much time he was alone with his thoughts. We were sitting on the couch and talking about where our heads were at. I wanted to make sure he was doing alright.

"I'm fine; I was built for this," he told me, which surprised me to hear so late in this whole process.

"Huh? What do you mean?" I asked.

"I was an only child for most of my life, I'm used to keeping myself occupied, and I'm more of an introvert as a result."

"Interesting," I replied as I thought about what he was saying. "I think you're right because I would lose my mind if I had to be as secluded as you have needed to be."

"Yeah, I'm fine to keep myself occupied. I mean, obviously this has been a lot, and intense, but I think my upbringing prepared me for this," he replied.

Tom was an introvert, and I was an extrovert, though I didn't always think of it that way. I always thought of an introvert as a quiet person in the corner who didn't want to engage with people, and that's not Tom at all. He's a bubbly guy who tries to make people laugh, but he described it so perfectly to me one evening back when we were dating. While Tom liked people, being in social situations and socializing was draining to him. I was the opposite; being around people and socializing energized me. Our situation stacked itself perfectly in this way; I had to deal with all the people, which was a great role for me. He needed to be an introvert –something he excelled at too – it was one of his favorite orders from the doctor.

Dec. 9 – The Money Questions

Now what? That seems to be the question of the hour – so let me give a quick update. When Tom has his chemo treatments – meaning we are in the hospital and he is on the constant IV – that is just his chemo infusion. His actual treatment cycle is three weeks, which is why we had chemo every third week. So while we are done with his chemo infusion (WOO HOO! Still very excited about that!), he is still technically in his fourth cycle of chemo. The drugs are still in his body and hopefully working their magic. What this means is that, unfortunately, we don't yet know the impact that chemo has had on the tumor. We continue our normal routine with blood work tomorrow and next week and then we will be doing the scans on the 21st and find out the results on the 22nd. The scans will ensure that the cancer didn't spread at all and determine how much the tumor shrunk – if at all. That second part is very important because that is going to determine how rough Tom's surgery will be.

When Is Surgery? Our other money question. Surgery won't be scheduled until (1) the scans are complete and we can get a plan of action (2) Tom's body bounces back. As our oncologist told us, this is a huge fight that Tom has ahead of him, and it will be critical that he is as close to a hundred percent as possible. Plus, in my dream world, we find out on the 22nd that it's completely gone and there is no surgery. I'm ignoring the less than 1 percent chance that this could happen. A girl can dream! In all seriousness, the best Christmas present ever would be to find out when surgery will be at our appointments on the 22nd.

So it's a bit of a countdown until the 22nd for us now. We will just rest easier knowing what we are dealing with and when we can deal with it. It's painful to have to wait, but it's only thirteen days away, and I bet that will go faster than the last twenty minutes of chemo did on Sunday. In the meantime, we will keep you updated as we always have and continue to blog as we get more information. Don't worry; I'm not done with all my rambling yet. More to come...

The Luck of The Irish

On the hardest days, we had to think of our happiest times. Talking about other things helped transport our minds away from our reality for a while. We would transport ourselves to trips, funny memories, awkward moments or smack talk about our sports teams. As he was recovering from this last round of chemo, I couldn't help but think about our road trip in Ireland. It was one of my favorite adventures with Tom.

We had flown into Dublin and planned a road trip up the coast into Northern Ireland, a place where I had spent almost a month a few years earlier. I was eager to take Tom to some of my favorite spots and drive through the Ireland countryside. We got to the rental car pickup and I was going to be the driver. We roamed through the parking lot and found our car, laughing out loud when we got sight of it. Thanks to my work travel, I had been upgraded to a brand-new Audi. Considering I was about to be driving on the right side of the car, on the left side of the road, the only thing I could picture was this new Audi floating in the Irish Sea in a few hours.

The next morning, we began our ride up the coast on the tiny Ireland roads curving around the sea. Despite almost a month of rain, we had the most picturesque day in Ireland: bright green hills around us and a clear blue sky above. Tom was squirming like a worm in the passenger seat, thinking we were always about to hit someone or that I was going the wrong way. It was sort of fun to torture him. Our main destination for the day was to get to Carrick-A-Rede Rope Bridge, a rope bridge made by salmon fisherman in 1755. It's suspended almost a hundred feet high, and once you cross the bridge, you are on a small island that has some of the best views of Ireland. On a clear day you can see Scotland. It's truly breathtaking. The whole ride up, Tom got more nervous about this rope bridge.

"Are there railings?" he asked.

"No, it's literally just wood and rope. It's a little scary, but you'll be fine," I said, weaving the corners of the coast.

"That's insane. I really don't know if I'll be able to cross it," he said.

"Well then, find your big boy pants, because we didn't come all this way for you to stand on the other side," I said.

"You don't think that's a little crazy?" he asked.

"Not at all," I said, laughing in my head, "They only let two people go at a time, so it's safe."

"That still doesn't seem safe," he said.

I could tell he was getting more nervous. "Why don't we stop for some lunch in the next town," I suggested.

A few minutes later we rolled into a small coastal town and parked the car. We found a takeout place and ordered some lunch to go. We walked across the street to the marina and climbed up a bunch of stairs to the top of a park. When we got to the top, there was a giant courtyard space with old concrete walls overlooking the sea. It was one of the most beautiful sights, and the empty picnic table was quickly filled with our food. We sat, staring out and eating our lunch in the perfect weather and salty smelling air.

"I don't say this often, but I think it's perfect right now," I said to Tom.

"This is unbelievable," he replied. Ireland has such a different pace and energy. It was a great reminder to us both to slow down and enjoy the simple things. We finished up and got back in the car for the final stretch to the rope bridge. We parked and began the mile walk to the bridge. I could tell Tom was getting more and more nervous as we walked. I tried to distract him with the amazing views, but he was more concerned about living. As we approached the bridge, I looked at Tom and smiled.

"It does have railings! Rope railings, but still railings!" he proclaimed.

"See, now there is nothing to worry about at all," I replied, hoping my psychology experiment of making it seem so much worse than it actually was would ease his mind.

"You drive me absolutely crazy," he said as we approached the bridge.

"I'll go first if you want, or second to make sure you cross," I said, joking with him.

I went first, and we made our way across. Once you cross the bridge, you have to hike up a few steps to get to the top, and then you get to see the view. Tom followed me up the path, and I turned back to him at the summit to see his expression.

"Wow," he said.

"I know, right? Worth almost dying on a rope bridge, right?" I said.

The entire island isn't very big, so we took a seat and chatted about how lucky we were to be there, and how much fun we were having on our road trip. We were in no rush, with no schedule and sat on that island for over an hour. Eventually, we decided to get back in line to go back across the bridge.

"You were wrong earlier," he said.

"Wrong about what?" I asked.

"You said earlier it was perfect, but I think this was perfect," he said. He grabbed my hand and we hiked back, smiling ear to ear as we took in the views.

"I don't even want to drive away," I said as I started navigating through the parking lot.

"Watch out!" Tom yelled as I narrowly dodged getting hit due to my focus on the view and a moment of forgetting to drive on the left side of the road.

"Whoops!" I replied as I gave him a cheesy smile.

"That would be our luck, survive the rope bridge but get hurt in a car accident in the parking lot," he said, shaking his head and laughing.

I pulled onto the main road. "I'll be honest; I'd recommend you take your chances with the bridge versus me driving on the left side of the road."

Dec. 13 – An Update

I've been a bad blog host the past few days! My apologies. Life has been a bit crazy with the holidays coming up and work, etc. On top of that, Tom has not been feeling well. He's not bouncing back at his usually speedy rate. He's feeling fatigued and still needing medication. Usually, as we turn the corner into Week Three, he is off almost all of the anti-nausea medicine, and we start a week of medicine as-needed only. However, this isn't anything we didn't expect since our doctors warned us that the compound effects of the four treatments would be especially tough this time.

Needless to say, he's getting a little restless and wants to speed up to next week so we can get results! This week will be relatively calm; he will have blood work on Thursday (fingers crossed we don't need a transfusion!), and we will meet with one of our doctors too. We really are just marching towards the 21st and 22nd. Best-case scenario this week would be that his blood looks good so we can maybe schedule the surgery next week. All good energy and prayers sent our way would be appreciated! More to come...

All I Want For Christmas Is Hair

"I really want to wear my hat," Tom said as we were getting ready.

"I know, babe, but I really think you shouldn't tonight. This is a nice steakhouse and you're among your work family. It won't matter," I replied, feeling terrible that he was having such a hard time with his baldness.

Until this point, we really hadn't been in too many social situations since he was just home sick so much and needed to be away from people. Even when we did venture out, he would have a hat on, and since it was winter, that wasn't strange. We were headed to his work holiday dinner, and he was very nervous.

"I look so sick," he replied as he looked into the mirror. "I don't look like myself."

"You look amazing, and let's think about it a different way. How awesome is it that you're starting to feel better and that you even have energy to go see everyone? They are going to be so excited that you're there, they won't care about your head," I said. I was trying to find the middle ground. I didn't want to minimize how he was feeling; he had every right to feel that way. However, I also didn't want those feelings to prevent him from being surrounded by all the love of his work family. It was a bit of a catch-22.

We got in the car and headed to dinner. Tom had his hat on in the car.

"You okay?" I asked, since he seemed a bit down.

"Yeah, I just hate being bald and it's a bit strange to be seeing everyone. I feel so guilty. I know my being out of work has created more work for everyone," he said.

"I know; you are going to beat it and be back in no time. Then they can pile all their work on you for a while. It can be an even exchange," I said with a smile on my face to try and get him to laugh.

He let out a bit of a snicker and looked out the window, I knew he was a ball of nerves and wanted to crawl back into bed. We pulled into the parking lot and began to get out. I was going to let Tom do what he felt he needed to do to be comfortable. He stood up, looked back into the car, pulled off the hat and tossed it on the passenger seat.

"You look great," I said as we grabbed hands and walked in.

We were one of the first to arrive and everyone was genuinely excited to see Tom and see that he was doing okay. They hadn't seen him since he started treatment, and I think they all felt better to set eyes on him. He wasn't fooling anyone; he was clearly very sick and weak, but we sat around that table and laughed and got caught up on everything.

When we left that night, the first thing Tom did was put the hat back on his head in the car.

"I feel better," he said as we quickly blasted the heat in the car.

167

"That was really nice. I think everyone was happy to see you, and no one mentioned your baldness," I replied.

"I know. I knew they wouldn't, but it's just still so strange to not feel like myself, to look in the mirror and not see myself," he replied.

As we drove home, Tom was exhausted; our adventure had been a lot for him. He started to doze off a bit in our short car ride home as I thought about his job. If everything went according to plan, the earliest he would be back to work was March. As I drove by the snow-covered trees, March seemed so far away. March, in a lucky year in the Midwest, was the beginning of spring. In that scenario, today was the midpoint of his fight to beat cancer. For some reason, that gave me comfort, but still, as I drove home, I felt that we had a long way to go.

Dec. 15 – A Very Merry Christmas Treat
Well, let me start with some great news. Tom started to turn the corner last night and managed to not need any of his really strong anti-nausea medicines today. This has certainly taken much longer than previous rounds of chemo, but we are thrilled that he is finally bouncing back. We were hoping he would, so we could make a special little adventure this evening.

As I've mentioned before, Tom is incredibly lucky to work for his company. He has the most wonderful group of coworkers who have been some of his biggest cheerleaders and have continually offered their support to both Tom and I – not to mention they are avid blog readers! They are truly a special group of people that I'm sure many would hope to experience in their careers. Tonight was their Christmas party, and they invited Tom – and me – to come if he was feeling up to it and take part in the annual celebration and Secret Santa exchange. Tom was hoping he would feel well enough because he truly misses his coworkers and all of the fun banter in the office. Some days this diagnosis can feel incredibly isolating, so he was eager to see everyone and catch up on everything he has been missing. To be fair to our day-to-day experiences, Tom was a little apprehensive to attend because of his hair loss, but as I had assured him, his coworkers thought nothing of it and agreed with me that he is rocking the bald head look.

As we have coped through this entire diagnosis, there are certain things that put in perspective the amount of time that has passed. The VP that Tom works under is retiring at the end of this year; when he returns to work she will already be gone. On September 15, when he left work, it never even crossed his mind that it would be the last day he would work with her. Truly, you never know what can happen or how quickly life can change. The day Tom was diagnosed, I had called his VP to fill her in on what was happening. From the moment I told her what was going on, she assured me that she and Tom's boss would do everything in their power to support us. Tom has learned an incredible amount from her and is very sad to see her go. It will be a bit strange for him to go back to work (though he is eager to do so), but especially weird for her not to be there. We wish her all the best and fully intend on celebrating with her when Tom is officially cancer-free.

Nights like tonight are reminders that despite a crummy situation, we are surrounded by so much love and support. I know I've said it before, but there are days where it is very overwhelming – in the best way possible. Tom's boss gave a toast tonight and was commenting on friends, family and how much time coworkers spend together – sometimes more than with their own families. I would say Tom is incredibly grateful to have such an amazing work family. More to come…

The Day I Broke

I was standing in the kitchen, making dinner after a long day. I had sobbed the entire way home. Tom was sitting on the counter chatting with me as I cooked.

"I'm so worried about you," he said when I was turned towards the stove.

"I'm worried about you too," I said, trying to deflect. I knew I was hitting a low point; I knew I was running out of gas. I was struggling because all of the "things" that needed to be done to keep our life afloat were easy. I could run on little sleep, make the meals, clean the house, get my work done, make Tom's appointments, manage medical bills, and more. I was running out of gas on the emotional side. The more we floated into the unknown, the more terrified I got. The closer we got to surgery, the more I had to try to wrap my head around all the possibilities, and figure out if I was going to be emotionally stable enough to handle all the possible outcomes.

"Don't think for one minute that I don't know this has been as hard on you as it has on me, chemo or no chemo. We both got diagnosed with cancer; your version just isn't in your body," Tom said to me.

It was an interesting point he was making and his continued recognition and gratitude for how hard this was on me too was something I was so thankful for. "I just want to cry," I said as I held back tears and focused intently on what I was doing at the stove.

"It's okay to cry. I cry all the time now. Damn cancer. I hate feeling all this emotion! I used to be so good at compartmentalizing," he said.

"You mean ignoring it?" I asked, to try and make myself laugh. I walked over to Tom sitting on the counter and stepped in between his hanging legs and leaned into his chest. He wrapped his arms around me and kissed my head. He didn't say anything and I was biting my lip so hard I thought I was going to bleed. I took a deep breath in and out to try to pull myself together. "I think I might try to find someone to talk to."

"I think that's great. I'm proud of you," he said as he hugged me tighter.

It wasn't that I was against talking to a therapist. I've always had a very logical approach to mental health. If you break your arm, you go to the doctor, get a cast, do physical therapy, and fix the bone. My mind was overwhelmed with trying to process this traumatic event. I needed to see a doctor, do some therapy, and get better too. It wasn't that I was depressed, but I needed to figure out how to cope with such waves of intense emotion as I worked through the reality, and the unknown, of our future.

"I don't want you to think that I don't want to talk to you about all this, but you've got your own cross to carry right now, and sometimes I feel like if I tell you certain things you feel guilt," I said, making sure he knew this wasn't going to create a barrier in our own communication.

"Trust me, it makes sense. If you want to talk when you get home, that's fine; if you just need a place to say everything you need to say, I get that too," he said.

"I think it will be nice to have a third party involved. I'm feeling such guilt for all our friends and family," I said, still nestled into his chest. I felt terrible unloading on my family or friends about everything. I didn't want them to worry, and I feared I might exhaust my friendships. Plus, none of my friends had experience with what I was dealing with. They were supportive, but none of them had been through this type of trauma, and they couldn't help me figure out how to deal with it. It wasn't like calling your girlfriend who had a baby before you to find out how they handled tantrums or sleepless nights; it was a whole different ball game.

"I agree. You should find someone that still uses the old school couch," Tom said, trying to make me laugh.

"Watch it with the jokes, you're next," I said to Tom as I pulled away and went back to the stove.

I knew that Tom was going to need to talk to someone soon too – but it wasn't the right time. He'd be on his own therapist couch soon enough. We'd be back on even ground for therapist jokes in no time.

Dec. 17 – Just One Of Those Days

Today is just one of those cancer days. Not because we got bad news or had an unexpected trip to ER because none of that happened. We are just worn down from this cancer fight and we are in this limbo that is brutal. Typically, we would know that we are four days away from his next round of chemo and know the plan. Now, don't get me wrong; we are thrilled that we aren't starting chemo again next week, but this unknown has just been tough, emotional, and quite frankly draining. We are looking forward to getting more of a plan next week after scans, but even that will only be one piece of the puzzle because the surgery is still a large unknown – one that will involve mid-surgery decisions so we truly cannot prepare. But we will continue to get as prepared as possible. We met with one of our oncologists today and Tom had blood work done – everything looked good, so that is great news as we go into next week.

Yesterday marked three months since his diagnosis. As I told Tom today, I feel that we are entitled to some rough days. However, our rule through this whole thing has been to not dwell and always try to have a better day than the one before. So on the positive side, we are getting out some bad days now, trying to just stay optimistic, and look forward to results and Christmas next week. More to come...

Attitude is Everything

I was walking to a conference room in my office building. My company has deep family roots, and still operates as a family company, and so there were always great artifacts, photos or quotes around the office. The Friday before our week of eves, I saw one I hadn't ever really noticed. It read:

Attitude

The longer I live, the more I realize the impact of attitude on life.
Attitude, to me, is more important than facts.
It is more important than the past, than education,
Than money, than circumstances, than failures,
Than successes, than what other people think or say or do.
It is more important than appearance, giftedness, or skill.
It will make or break a company...a church...a home.
The remarkable thing is we have a choice every day
regarding the attitude we embrace for that day.
We cannot change our past...
We cannot change the fact that people will act in a certain way.
We cannot change the inevitable.
The only thing we can do is play on the one string we have,
and that is our attitude...
I am convinced that life is 10% what happens to me
and 90% how I react to it.
And so it is with you...We are in charge of our ATTITUDE.
-Charles Swindell

As I read, it was like a symphony. The words flowed like a song and every word made a little sunshine break through the clouds of the unknown in my head. It was going to be a long few days, but I knew we had control of how we reacted. Our attitude was that laughter was the best medicine, and we made the choice to see our situation with as much of a positive outlook as possible. Because the adage was true, and we knew it now more than ever, attitude is everything.

Dec. 20 – A Week Of Eves

We've got lots of eves this week – tonight is Scans Eve! We will be up bright and early tomorrow to get to the hospital for a few tests. We kick off with the CT, then right into the MRI, and then blood work. Then we should, in theory, have a little break to go home, and then we will come back in the afternoon for a pulmonary test. I say "in theory" because usually this stuff moves at a snail's pace and is lots of waiting and moving around to different waiting rooms. So we are planning for a long day and setting the bar low by assuming it will take up most of the day...and we will be delighted if it doesn't.

Tomorrow is a bit of a tease because we will not get any results, but step one is getting the tests done. That's what will give us all the answers we need on Tuesday. Which brings me to Monday night – Results Eve! I will be shocked if I sleep much tomorrow but we've got appointments with both our surgeon and oncologist Tuesday morning. Thank goodness I managed to finagle all the morning appointments; otherwise, that would have been a long morning waiting to find out the results. Tom is feeling alright, still not quite where he would like to be, but he's starting to get more color and be more active, which is great. As you can imagine, he's ready to get these tests and the results.

Wednesday night is Going Home Eve – another night that I anticipate little sleep! Tom and I rotate holidays so it is our year to do Christmas with my family in Wisconsin. When Tom was first diagnosed, we didn't even know if we would be able to be in Wisconsin, if he would be in chemo or how he would be feeling so I didn't get my hopes too high. However, since he is feeling better, we will be heading home for a very brief trip, but a trip nonetheless. I haven't been home since early September and with everything I've been dealing with that has been an especially tough part of this all so I'm super excited.

Then of course Thursday is Christmas Eve! It will certainly be a low-key Christmas, but I'm looking forward to Christmas and all the traditions that come with it. So, lots more to come this week...stay tuned.

Crazy Loves Me

I would estimate that in any given month there are at least two moments where I question if I'm on *Candid Camera* – the show that pulls pranks in normal social settings. I've gotten so used to being surrounded by strange situations, circumstances, and people. I suppose you could argue that I'm the commonality in the situations, but I don't think it's that – crazy loves me.

Tom and I were laughing hard as we were in the CT waiting room because we were again surrounded by crazy. It was a delightful distraction in that moment. We floated through the hospital that day and tried to grin and bear it all. Tom's last test of the day was the pulmonary test in the basement of the hospital – the only floor we hadn't been on yet – we could officially say we knew the hospital well, something I never wanted to be able to say.

We walked into a small waiting area with three chairs around a TV and coffee table and a small desk. We were the only ones there. I approached the desk and rang the bell. From the back came a woman who acted like we had been friends for years. She took Tom down to the testing room and told me I could sit and wait in the chairs, but to not change the channel, she was watching *Family Feud*. I should have known this was going to be a fun forty-five minutes right then and there.

I sat down, grabbed a magazine, and began thumbing through the pages while listening to *Family Feud* in the background. Tom and I watched *Family Feud* during his chemo treatments, so I was well versed in the game. About ten minutes into my wait, the woman returned and sat down right next to the TV in the waiting area with me and began yelling out her answers.

Steve Harvey said, "Name a word that most people yell at their dogs…"

Without missing a beat, she yelled "WOOF!" at the TV, looked at me with a big smile on her face and then looked back at the TV to see if she was correct.

I had caught the giggles and was trying to not be rude. She continued to be shocked after each answer that wasn't "woof". The number one answer was "No" and the second was "Sit". I had a little trouble understanding her *Family Feud* excitement, but I felt like this show, both the one on the TV and the one in the waiting room, was a great distraction from the day.

The next question was asked: "Name a bad sport for someone who is afraid of the water."

She quickly yelled "Bath!" and again looked back at me with the same expression of glory as with her first terrible answer. I had to look away as I was visualizing what a bath must be like for this woman that she thinks it's a sport – I couldn't contain my laughter. She looked back and smiled at me, so excited that I was obviously enjoying this game show too.

Once again, the crazy, or should I say unique, had plopped down right next to me, and it was exactly what I needed to get through that day. As crazy as she was, she would play an important role in the biggest day of our lives down the road.

Dec. 21 – Is It Morning Yet?

Well – scans and tests are complete! We had quite the day of chaos, but we made it through. I, of course, was attracting every weirdo in the waiting rooms (story of my life), including an old couple who thought that Steve Harvey was O.J. Simpson, thought Donald Trump running for president was a movie preview and giggled at a Viagra commercial. Then there was a woman who kept telling Tom and me that she smelled like pasta sauce, and then of course a woman who wanted to celebrate with me every time she took a sip of her pre-CT cocktail. The good news is all these people kept the day interesting for me.

We were up before the sun and at the hospital for our day of fun. We started with the MRI... once that was done, Tom had to drink his pre-CT cocktail. They can't do the CT until an hour after the drink is consumed, so we had to sit in this waiting room along with several other people who were drinking and waiting like us. Think of an incredibly awkward bar – and that's where we were trapped except with way uncomfortable seating and no jukebox, which was unfortunate because I think Journey's "Don't Stop Believing" would have helped the whole waiting room have more fun. Once the time had passed, they took him back for the CT. When that was finished, we had to go up to the oncologist for some extra blood work. Our oncologist called us on Saturday concerned about some of Tom's counts, so we had to go and do another check. Essentially the blood thinners made his blood too thin – or, Tom was being an overachiever. So we had to get that all checked out – that was another waiting room, another blood test, and another wait for results. Blah.

Our last adventure for the day was his pulmonary test. There is a chance they will have to remove a part of Tom's lung in surgery, so they have to figure out how much they can take if they need to. That required him to do these different breathing tests for an hour or so. Quite the day of fun, which was topped off with a trip on the "Care Cart." These are little hospital golf carts that we've never ridden on before. It was especially funny when we almost got in an accident with another Care Cart driver (I stand firm that we had the right of way)!

We made the most of our day at the hospital, but we are eager to go to sleep because tomorrow morning we will spend several hours with our surgeon and oncologist to find out the results. It goes without say that there will be more to come tomorrow....

The Balance

There are many things that require balance: work and personal life, relationships, and more. It's a delicate dance that can be exhausting, and that balance was challenging as we were waiting for the results. It's the balance of being positive but not being naïve. It's what I called cautiously optimistic. In my heart I knew he was doing everything within his power to beat this, but the human body is crazy, and science isn't foolproof, so we knew that many different outcomes were possible.

The alternative would be to assume the worst and then be happy when that didn't happen. The old under-promise, over-deliver approach. I could never get to that place, though, because it felt like if we took that route in some way we were allowing "the worst" to be an option. Also, it was just a negative approach to the situation. That wasn't our style thus far, and that wasn't about to change.

Our cautiously optimistic approach worked; we were on cloud nine with our initial results. Despite there still being so many lingering questions, it was a moment of bliss for us. To celebrate I ran out to pick up some sushi for Tom because he had been so excited to get his sushi restrictions lifted. I went to a place near our house and had him call in his order, since as a non-sushi eater I wouldn't know where to begin.

In fact, I don't eat seafood at all. I can't wrap my head around the fact that seafood floats around in this big body of water with human waste, animal waste, animal reproduction, human fluids and so much more. It gives me goosebumps just to think about it. For the record, the argument that pigs roll around in mud is an invalid one; my bacon isn't in that mud.

I walked into the dimly lit restaurant and told the hostess I had a pickup. She returned a few minutes later with a huge bag and a bill for just under $50. I laughed as I saw how much he had ordered; apparently, I had been cautiously optimistic that he was going to order a reasonable amount of sushi.

Dec. 22 – Boom!

What a morning we have had – I know I usually post at night but I figured I'd post a bit earlier today. I'll give the punch line right out of the bag – the tumor has shrunk more than they expected!! We were up at the crack of dawn this morning anxious for our appointments. I was a hot mess – by the time we got to the surgeon's office I thought I was going to throw up. Tom was actually much calmer than I was – I was staring at the shadows that appeared by the door when people walked by our room and got eager if I thought one was the doctor.

Once he came in, we got the great news. Now, there is still a mass there, but it shrunk in such a way that it is no longer touching his heart, which is so important for surgery. Our surgeon is so happy with the results. The surgery may even be less invasive and will be done at our local hospital now rather than us needing to travel for surgery. This is HUGE for us. This surgery is still going to be quite a doozy, but the fact that we no longer need to have the bypass team on call and don't have to mess with the heart increases the success rate big time. Plus, given the size of the tumor, the surgeon will try to make fewer, less invasive incisions to get it out. If he is able to do so, it will dramatically improve Tom's recovery time. However, we won't know that until they are actually in surgery.

Then we met with our oncologist who was equally excited for us and walked us through all the actual scans and size reduction. We went over what Tom can and cannot do, and one of the best parts of his day was finding out he could eat sushi again – yes, totally crazy, but something Tom was eager to have again and has been craving. So we are celebrating tonight with some sushi for dinner for him. It's the little things!

We were honestly both in shock today – it feels like all the sleepless nights, pain, nausea, and emotions have actually all been for something. We still have to process this all – but we both have smiles on our faces today.

So while we had great news today, we won't really know our status until after surgery. While the tumor has shrunk, it doesn't necessarily mean there is no active cancer. Two things can happen after surgery:
1. They remove and inspect the tumor and determine that there is no active cancer and he is considered cancer-free. If this happens then all we have left is the surgery recovery.
2. They remove and inspect the tumor and find active cancer cells and then, unfortunately, we would have two more rounds of chemo.

We are hoping for #1 with every ounce of our being but a lot of people end up needing additional chemo. However, we will deal with that when it comes – and Tom has beaten the odds so far, so I'm cautiously optimistic that we will be cancer-free after surgery. For now, we get ready for surgery and do what we need to do within our control.

Surgery will be on January 19th –Tom's body needs to recover as much as possible before surgery. Thank you to everyone for all the prayers, good energy and love that have been sent our way – we know that we could not have gotten this far without everyone's love and support. I don't even know what else to say today...so more to come tomorrow...

Christmas Chaos

We were sitting in my parents' bookstore when his phone rang. It was one of my favorite places to be during the holiday and my parents had the store for our entire lives. I was reveling in the glory of being home – we hadn't been there for more than an hour.

"It's Doctor Sobol," Tom said as he stood up, surprised to be getting a call from her late in the day on Christmas Eve. We were sitting in the back of the store, visiting with a friend of mine since third grade, Caitlin.

I tried to keep the discussion going while eavesdropping on Tom's conversation in the other corner of the room. I finally just stopped talking with Caitlin and looked over at him. His face didn't have the happiest look.

"Okay…okay…alright…Thanks for calling…Have a Merry Christmas…" I heard him say. I hated that I was only hearing one side of this conversation.

"I'm so sorry," I said to Caitlin, realizing I had stopped in the middle of my own sentence toward the end of Tom's conversation.

"It's okay," she said patiently.

Tom hung up the phone and looked at me. I knew it wasn't good news.

"Everything okay?" I asked.

"She got the blood work back from Monday. The tumor markers are still showing active cancer. We should prepare ourselves for more chemo after surgery," he said.

"I'm so sorry, babe," I said, as I got up and hugged him.

Caitlin sat patiently, bearing with us. I'm sure she probably wanted to disappear in that moment. Tom didn't really say much and sat back down as we continued visiting. I felt like Tom and I were having an entire conversation with our eyes. Shortly after, Caitlin had to head out to begin her own Christmas celebrations. I walked her out and Tom stayed in the back of the store. She said goodbye to my mom and was on her way. For a moment, the store was quiet. I walked to my mom and softly told her what had just happened.

"The doctor just called, still active cancer in the tumor, so we should plan for more chemo," I said to her, trying to hold back my own tears. She reached over and hugged me.

"Is he okay?" she asked as she motioned her head to Tom.

"Doubt it," I said as I turned and walked towards the back.

Tom was sitting on the couch staring up at one of the shelves of books.

"This sucks," I said, not for a moment thinking to ask him how he was doing. I already knew the answer to that.

"Yup," he said.

"Why don't we head downtown and pick up those last few things we needed for gifts tomorrow," I said.

"Okay." His lack of engagement worried me.

We walked to the front of the store as my mom was restocking a shelf.

"Hey, Mom, we are going to head to Public Market to get some Kehr's candy and a few other things. We will see you back at the house."

"Sounds good," she said. She knew not to question.

We got in the car and headed downtown. The minute his door shut he had tears coming down his face.

"I can't do more chemo; my body can't take it," he said, completely defeated.

"If it happens, we will take it one day at a time. It could still be elevated levels. She warned us when we saw her that it was a possibility," I said, trying to hang on to hope that the cancer would miraculously be gone after surgery.

"I wish she hadn't called until next week," he said. "Should I call my parents? I don't want to ruin everyone's Christmas."

"Yes – just tell them and tell them to not bring it up at the Christmas Eve festivities tonight," I said. I had tears rolling down my face too. I had been feeling so great. I was finally home for the holiday, but the wind had just been sucked out of our sails.

We drove downtown squeezing each other's hands, tears rolling down our faces. My heart broke for him.

We grabbed our few things at the market and headed back home. We walked into the house and unloaded our bags. My dad was standing there to give me a hand. Tom went to the bathroom and I told my dad the news.

"Dammit!" he said. My dad wanted things to be better for Tom and was angry at the cancer.

"I know. Let's not talk about it. We want to keep the focus on Christmas and have a happy night, no dwelling on sadness," I said, hoping to salvage what I could of Christmas. My dad nodded to acknowledge what I had said, shook his head and walked out of the room.

Later that evening, we headed to church. With all the germs, people and kids, it was not a good place for Tom to be so we had planned for him to hang at the house instead. I walked into church and wanted to cry. I had driven separately from my family so I could leave if needed; I had become a professional at making sure there was always a backup plan or way for me to get out of a place quickly. I saw family friends, old school mates, and people that I grew up with at church. I listened to the music, gazed at the decorations, all the kids in their Christmas outfits, my nephew in my arms, and tried to process what we had heard this morning. I was very emotional.

I was sitting in the pew and everyone was there, except Tom. I knew he was at home, but it suddenly hit me that if something happened to him, this would be my reality. I didn't want this to be the future. As I looked up at the altar, I thought about when I walked down this exact aisle a few years earlier to marry him. I grew up in this church; I went to the adjoining school from K-4 through eighth grade. I graduated from grade school in this church; I did concerts in this church; I got married in this church; I met lifelong friends here. In fact we were still close with my principal who was having the school kids pray for Tom every morning. This church embodied so much of who I was and how I had become that person. There were so many emotions swirling through me, I almost went to the bathroom because I thought I was going to throw up.

While I was connected to the space, the smells, the comfort of growing up here, I felt disconnected. I hadn't lost my faith during all of this, but I was certainly looking at it from a different point of view. I hadn't been in church since Tom was diagnosed since our lives were so chaotic. It was forcing me to really acknowledge where I was with my faith, and the confusion of it all was a lot to comprehend. I made it through mass and quickly left, wanting to get back home; I just wanted a hug from Tom.

I walked into the house, which smelled amazing. There was a fire in the fireplace, and Tom was chatting with some other family who had arrived. I sat down next to him and leaned in.

"How was mass?" he asked.

"Fine, just a lot more intense than I thought it would be," I said.

"Really?" he asked.

"Yeah, just a lot to think about. Lots of babies to remind me that we don't yet have a family, lots of things to consider given the news this morning…" I tapered off since family was walking closer to us. Our conversation ended abruptly, and we proceeded to have a great Christmas dinner and evening, but we were smiling despite what we were feeling.

As we climbed into bed later that night, we curled up together. "I love you…Merry Christmas…" I said.

"Merry Christmas, are you okay from mass? We got cut off," he asked.

"Yeah, just a lot to process, but I tried to stay positive," I replied.

"What a day…" he said as he took a deep breath.

"I know. I'm still hoping that the levels are just elevated," I replied, trying to end our night on a positive note.

Tom's eyes were closed; he was exhausted. He took another deep breath and softly replied, "We will see…"

Though strange, that was the best response I could have expected from him. He was such a realist, and usually was the one reminding me about facts with my pie-in-the-sky hopes. He could have told me I was being too optimistic, or been irritated that I was ignoring the facts, but he said *we will see*. His response implied that he wasn't resigned to the fact that there was more chemo ahead – and that was the best Christmas gift he could have given me.

Dec. 26 – One Step Forward, Two Steps Back
We've had quite the rollercoaster the past couple days – and took a break for a few days from blogging for reasons which I will explain shortly…So what have we been up to?

Thursday morning we headed up to Milwaukee, which was one of the best feelings in the world. I haven't been home since September – we went right to my parents' bookstore. Once I walked in and heard the Christmas music playing and saw customers bustling about, it officially felt like Christmas. My heart was calm – we've had some incredibly long days and nights through this, and I had been envisioning Christmas at home to get me through some of those tough days. However, this is where our holiday took a bit of a turn – our oncologist called around 1 pm on Christmas Eve. We got some unfortunate news – the final results we were waiting for confirmed that there is still active cancer in Tom's tumor. So while it shrunk significantly, and the surgery is now much better than we expected…. there is a higher chance that we will need to do more chemo after surgery, which is exactly what we didn't want. So how do we know this? There is a blood test that measures Tom's tumor markers, which help detect and diagnose certain types of cancers. The number has steadily dropped throughout chemo, but unfortunately is still outside of the "normal" range, which is correlated to cancer still being present in his body. There are no words to describe how we felt after this call…the wind was taken right out of our sails. Suddenly the chance of finding out at the end of January that he's cancer-free was potentially moved to March/April. Tuesday was the highest of highs and then suddenly Thursday was back to one of the lows. Plus, we were so excited for the holidays, and my family was so excited to see Tom too – so we were trying to just keep smiling despite a crushing blow.

Christmas Eve and Christmas Day we tried to stay positive. It was my nephew's first Christmas, which was super fun and we got to spend the day with family and around good energy. So given the news, we figured we wouldn't post anything until today to keep the holidays positive. We've come so far, we will certainly continue to fight this as best we can, but I will admit this has been tough to swallow. We are planning to do what we've always done and stay positive and deal with facts, so while our road has gotten a bit longer we will figure it out, try our best to stay positive, and still kick cancer's ass. I figure this post needs to end on a positive note so I hope you all get a kick out of one of Tom's Christmas presents from me…. a Chia pet – so he can race his Chia in hair growth ;-) More to come…

181

A Germ-Infested Haven

For as much as Tom loved to take care of me, I loved to take care of him too. He thanked me every single day during his treatment and I knew he meant it with every ounce of his being. Until his cancer diagnosis, I always gave him a jokingly hard time about the greatest caretaking I had ever done until that point. I had come into town to see Tom while we were dating long distance, and his apartment was disgusting. It was his senior year, and he and his roommate were less than eager to make cleaning a priority. They were on the top floor of a walk-up, which resulted in a heap of garbage bags in the kitchen that hadn't been taken down in weeks.

Ground zero was the bathroom, though. The muscles in my legs had gotten stronger since we started dating because I had mastered the hover that I needed to do to use the bathroom and not actually touch toilet seat. It was gross. I had come in late on a Thursday night, and Tom was going to be in class all morning on Friday. One option was to sleep in and lie low until he was done, but I thought I would do something sweet and clean the apartment.

I hauled over twenty bags of garbage down the stairs to the garbage bin in their parking area. I scrubbed the bathroom while wearing two pairs of gloves and plugging my nose. I mopped the entire apartment, scrubbed the kitchen appliances, organized, tidied up his room, and did it all in record time.

Tom's roommate Nick got back from class first and did a double take as if he had walked into the wrong apartment. He couldn't believe his eyes and was especially shocked to see that the bags of garbage were gone. Tom followed and looked equally as shocked. I was so happy to see how excited he was and felt like I was taking care of him.

"Why on earth did you do that to yourself? You were supposed to hang out and relax," he asked.

"It was 90 percent for you and 10 percent because my legs just hurt from hovering over that toilet."

Dec. 29 – Limbo

Well, yesterday was a bit of a strange day – a bit of a bizarre world for us. Tom went into work! He only went in for the day to help train the new person, but for him that is quite a lot of activity/energy, considering his life for the past three months. He was thrilled to see his coworkers, help the new guy get acclimated and feel productive. Plus, he can rest a bit easier knowing that a lot of the year end stuff was taken care of – it's been very weird for him to be away from work so I think it did him good to go in for the day.

Of course, the one day he goes into work we get hit with an ice/snow storm during the commute home. I had quite a harrowing commute only to end up in a snowbank in my driveway. It took me a solid twenty minutes to get myself out, but I used some of my tricks (car mats!) and was able to rescue myself. Of course, Tom pulled up right as I had just dug myself out, which actually is for the best because I wouldn't have let him help anyway and he would have gotten frustrated watching me try to get myself out. I cleaned up with the snow blower until it ran out of gas and then finished up with some shoveling. These types of things are what really drive Tom crazy because he hates that he can't help – but he needs to lie low and recover.

It's a bit tricky for him right now – while he feels stronger each day, his body is still recovering from quite the beat-down over the past twelve weeks. We are definitely on track for him to feel great by surgery – but it is a weird limbo to be in where he is feeling better but still needs to be very careful. However, this has afforded us more "normal" days, which has been great for both of us. The other thing that this "limbo" has created is an opportunity to take a deep breath and realize what the heck just happened for the past three-plus months – and more importantly, start to figure out what lies ahead and get our heads wrapped around the new normal. Admittedly, we had to make decisions and move fast, so I don't think we processed a lot of what happened. These waves of emotions are just starting to hit and it is a lot to process while still trying to keep our heads in the game and prep for surgery and the likelihood of more chemo. So, despite us not being in the thick of chemo or yet at surgery, it's still a day-by-day process, but we're doing the best we can. More to come...

A Hangover-Free New Year

We were on the couch in our pajamas at 8 p.m., eating take out and watching a show on TV. How different this New Year's Eve was for us – there was an element of hesitancy going into the New Year, but for the most part we were determined to relax and enjoy the evening. In previous years we either hung out with friends or went to his aunt and uncle's house for a party. One of the traditions with his family was to do predictions for the year. Each year we would open the predications from the previous year and determine the winner.

Questions were dependent on the upcoming year, but they would always include predictions of the Super Bowl Winner, the cost of gas or a gallon of milk on Dec. 31 of the next year, the first lady's inaugural gown color for an election year and many more. While the questions varied, the first question every year was the same –celebrity deaths. You had to select three celebrities that you thought would die in the year. It's pretty dark, but not mean-spirited. However, it did create quite the chain of text messages throughout the year as celebrity deaths hit the news.

Tom and I sat, eating our takeout, as we chatted about how strange it was to be holed up at the house this year.

"It feels weird to not being doing predictions– wouldn't those be interesting questions for our life this year?" I asked Tom.

"Ha, I don't think my family would answer any questions about me," he replied.

"Well, I know the answers for all of them already anyway," I said.

"Oh, yeah?" he asked, curious to see where I was going with this.

"Yup. When will you beat cancer? January. How many rounds of chemo will Tom have in 2016? Zero. Will Honore cry when you beat cancer? Of course."

Tom laughed and shook his head at me as he often did. I usually wasn't this confident about my predictions, but I truly believed all of these could be true. I needed them to be true to make it through 2016.

Dec. 31 – Happy New Year!

So today has been an interesting one as I've been thinking about 2015. The change to a new year is really an insignificant moment – the clock ticks like it does any other day and suddenly we change the year. It doesn't require any effort on my part other than to keep on living the way I do – but regardless, there is something momentous about a new year. It's a reason to pause and reflect on the past and think about the New Year. Some people choose to make resolutions; others just try to implement new habits. It's a moment to reflect.

There is a part of me that wants to say to hell with 2015; it was one of the worst years of our lives. However, the cancer diagnosis and last four months of 2015 is just fresh – not defining. I got angry with myself as I realized how much I was taking away from the rest of the year if I had that mindset. Tom and I took some wonderful trips in 2015; we added a nephew to our aunt and uncle duties; some of our closest friends had the most beautiful babies; I got a new job; we had the majority of our first year in our first home (including an awesome wine cellar project), and so many other great things. Certainly, I wish cancer wasn't on our list of things that happened this year, but we fully intend to celebrate being cancer-free, and I know that will bring us a lot of great moments in 2016. While we had some of our worst days in 2015, we had some great ones too, and I refuse to let our current hell define eight other wonderful months.

As I've mentioned, we've been in this weird limbo – however, a few days ago Tom said he felt the best he has felt in four months. He made dinner this week, was running errands and doing work from home. I'm thrilled he's feeling better – however, it's a bit of a tease that I know we will be back at square one in just a few weeks. But – we aren't going to dwell on that; instead, we will make every effort to enjoy these few weeks of "normal" before surgery and make the most of the time we have while he's feeling better. While we are still cautious, we certainly have more ability to be out and about, which is awesome.

So I wouldn't say I have any resolutions this year – I never quite understood that to be honest – why limit yourself to one time a year to reflect and improve? I anticipate that our first few months of 2016 will be the toughest, but it's my hope that each month gets better. We have every intention of continuing to be as positive as possible and tackle this one day at a time – and that to me is the only resolution we can make going into 2016.

For everyone that helped us get through 2015, from the bottom of our hearts, thank you. We wouldn't have made it this far without you and feel better knowing you'll all be behind us going in 2016. Happy New Year!

Baby Tonner

I had been tossing the idea back and forth to surprise Katie for her baby shower. Her shower was New Year's Eve weekend in Cincinnati. I had told her parents I was considering it but knew it would be a last-minute decision. I kept talking in circles about it with Tom, agonizing over leaving Tom for a night. I gave him his nightly shots, so we would need to coordinate someone coming to do that. The guilt either way was all consuming. Leaving Tom felt impossible, but not being at Katie's baby shower and seeing all my girlfriends seemed impossible too.

"You're going to the shower," Tom said to me, trying to be stern.

I was sitting on the floor in the living room, looking up at him.

"No, I can't. It's too much, and I'm already running on empty. She will understand." The minute I would make a decision the alternate option would flood in my mind and make me feel guilty.

"What if I take you?" Tom asked.

"Ha – good one," I replied.

"I'm serious. I'm feeling much better, we could both use a change of scenery, and I know you want to see everyone. We can make it quick and leave super early and then leave after the shower," he replied, having thought this through.

While Tom was feeling better and trying to distract himself from surgery, I wasn't sure if this was our best option.

"I don't know, babe, that's so sweet, though," I replied. I saw in his eyes the guilt; he didn't want this to be another thing that cancer took from us. I would have gone in any other circumstance, and he couldn't stomach the thought of me not being there. While I knew this was good for me, it could be good for him too.

"I'm serious – we are doing it. I need this; you need this; I want to see everyone, and it will be quick," he replied.

The "everyone" he was referring to was the group of girls that were my "people." The six of us had met in Husman Hall at Xavier University – all of us were on a "substance-free floor," which was ironic because we all excelled in drinking. All five of my girlfriends were going to be in town for the shower – four still live in Cincinnati, and one in the Chicago area. I wanted to go and see everyone so badly. I felt so disconnected. Two of my girlfriends had had babies in August that I had yet to meet due to Tom's diagnosis. They had all been so supportive, sending messages, cards, care packages and doing everything they could from afar; I wanted to see all of them. We would be there just a few weeks before his surgery, and I'd have been lying if I said I didn't want us both to go just in case something happened. I knew realistically that Tom would be okay, but the thought of a potentially bad outcome was starting to really wear down on my mind. If we didn't go, I would regret not going, regardless of the outcome.

"We are leaving at 5 a.m. on Friday. I'll drive!" he excitedly replied since he was off all of his major medications.

"We will see about that," I replied with a smile on my face. "It certainly is an interesting way to spend the first day of the New Year, and we could use a final in-person push for Tonner." Tom and I had been trying to convince Katie that a combined version of our names was the perfect moniker for the baby. Tonner had a nice ring to it, though she seemed to come up with so many polite reasons why that might not be the best name – just like my girlfriends Becca and Angie had done with their little ones a few months earlier. I thought some in-person persuasion would help our cause.

Tom wasn't kidding – he was up and ready to go at 5 a.m. on Friday. We got into the car, and I even let him drive. I knew this was as important to him as it was for me. We drove along, watched the sunrise and got more and more excited about the surprise. As we got close, I texted her mom to make sure our surprise was set – she had told Katie to be ready to run errands around twelve.

We walked up to the house and I rang the doorbell. Tom decided to hide in the bush next to the house for a double surprise. Minutes passed with no answer. I knew she was home, so I grabbed my phone and called her mom to let her know she wasn't answering. She called Katie, who had been blow-drying her hair and hadn't heard the doorbell, and told her to come downstairs and that she was at the door. While this was happening, we heard a voice.

"Um, excuse me, can I help you?" a man asked Tom.

Tom hiding behind the bush had concerned a neighbor and he wanted to make sure we weren't up to any trouble.

Tom started laughing as he replied, "We aren't breaking in – we are in town to surprise her."

The neighbor half smiled as he saw my head peer around the corner but lingered to make sure we weren't lying. Finally, I saw movement, and Katie pulled open the door in her bathrobe.

"What are you doing here?!?!?!" she replied as I jumped in the door and gave her a hug.

"It's your baby shower – what do you think I'm doing here?" I said as I hugged her and tried not to cry.

"I even have a special guest with me," I said as I pulled away and looked over my shoulder. Tom popped up and walked in to give her a hug too.

In hindsight, I suppose it was kind of mean to not give the seventh-month pregnant woman an emotional heads-up that her best friend and her cancer-stricken husband were going to show up, but you live and learn. A few minutes later, as we were chatting in the living room, we heard her parents walk in and I was eager to give them hugs too – they had been so supportive of us and we were very close with them. We chatted for a while and then they headed on their way with plans to see them later that evening.

As that was happening, I texted my girlfriends to see where everyone was and let them know we had made a last-minute decision to come to town. They were all at my girlfriend Becca's house, so we headed that way. They had no clue that Tom was in tow.

We pulled up to her house, rang the doorbell and Katie and I walked in. I looked down the hall into the kitchen to see Becca's husband look up and then say, "Tom?"

Everyone looked shocked that we were both there. My girlfriends were giving me hugs and it took every ounce of my being to not burst into tears. But I didn't want this to be sad; I wanted it to be happy, so I swallowed the lump in my throat, blinked away the tears, and tried to stay positive.

I got to snuggle the babies, chat, and hang out with everyone for several hours. It was perfect; if we had to turn around and go home right then it would have been worth it. I needed that little bit of time with the whole gang together. After a few hours, I could see that Tom was fading a bit, so we decided to call it a day and head back to Katie's house. We spent the rest of the night at her house. It was a strange visit to Cincinnati. I'd never come to town and not been out and about for the entirety of my trip in town seeing people, but I knew that wasn't the reality of our situation. Katie's parents came over and made soup and sandwiches and we chatted around the table that night. It was another one of those rare moments where I forgot our reality for a moment.

The next morning was the shower, hosted across the street from Katie's parents' house, and I got to hang with all my girlfriends and shower Katie with baby love. Tom was having lunch with Katie's dad and brother during the shower, though for brief moments I wish he had been in the room. So many people were asking about Tom and saying such kind things to me, I wanted him to hear them all. As the shower wrapped up, I said goodbye to my girlfriends and prepared to head home with Tom. The goodbyes were gut-wrenching. I felt so lost as to when we might be back, what the next few weeks of our life would be and wanted to stay in this twenty-four hours of reprieve that we had so badly needed.

As we drove the 350 miles home, just over twenty-four hours after arriving, I smiled and squeezed Tom's hand.

"I'm so glad we did that. Thanks for coming with and forcing me to do this. I hope you had a good time," I said.

"I did. We needed that; it was a good way to start the New Year. It's a good omen that we are going to get our lives back this year. 2016 will be a good year," he said, looking over at me.

188

I dropped my hand from the wheel and he grabbed it and kissed my hand.

"We get a pretty cool sunset too," I said, as I pointed out the window.

We were in the middle of Indiana driving through a long stretch of solar-powered windmills. It was a unique sunset with so many pinwheel monstrosities turning about.

"Yup – 2016, here we come," he said.

We didn't say much for the next stretch of miles, but held hands the whole time. Tom would randomly squeeze my hand or vice versa. I couldn't dwell on the fact that we were going back to square one in a few weeks, but instead watched that sunset and knew that while some rough days were still ahead, better days would have to come.

Jan. 3 – On The Road Again

Happy New Year! It's hard to believe that January is our fifth month of fighting this darn thing – but hopefully we are closer to the end than the beginning at this point. Tom and I decided to kick off the year on our terms and took a little trip. We got away for a night and were able to surprise and meet up with some friends and feel "normal" for a moment.

We were gone for less than thirty-six hours, but even in those thirty-six hours we felt like we had our lives back a bit. Tom is feeling much better and stronger each day, so that was the only reason we decided to get away for the night – in fact we didn't even make a final decision on if we would go anywhere until late Thursday night. We are so glad we did. To feel normal was one thing, but to know that we are already living life a bit differently because we've had it taken all away was another thing. I've said this before but I'm very excited for our post-cancer life.

We've got sixteen days until surgery and I'm hopeful that he continues to feel stronger each day until then so he can have an easier recovery once surgery is done. In the meantime, we will continue to enjoy our brief brush of normal even though we know there is an asterisk to the normal right now.

One thing that helps is the lack of doctor's appointments! We will meet with the anesthesiologist next week, but other than that, we won't be back in the hospital until the day of his surgery. This is a real treat for us since – it's the little things! More to come this week...

The Initial Meeting

My poor therapist has no idea what he signed up for when he agreed to see me. I had come so far to this moment, but I didn't know how to begin filling him in on me or my life for the past five months. There were so many layers to it – the actual diagnosis, everything that had happened as a result, but also the most important part in my mind – how Tom and I were somehow prepared for it, given the adventures we had experienced together. He sat there patiently taking notes as I attempted to explain to him what was going on with my life. I'm sure he wondered what took me so long to get my butt on his couch.

It was a bit of a word-vomit session, as I was detailing what had happened, what I had been doing, the blog, and how I was balancing everything. I felt like I had so much to fill him in on before he could even attempt to help me, yet the entire time I was talking, I couldn't believe I was there. I trusted that it was where I needed to be, and more importantly trusted that I could tell him what I was thinking. He asked me questions from the get-go, I felt so comfortable, and trusted that he was going to help me.

By the time I got him up to speed on how I had ended up in his office, it was almost the end of the session.

He looked up at me, put his cap on his pen, and asked, "Why are you here? You seem like you have things under control. I'm impressed with everything I've heard and what you've done."

"I'm here because what you said is exactly what everyone thinks, and it's not true. I'm falling apart," I replied, holding back tears.

Had I fooled another person into thinking that I was doing okay? I had been pretty honest about everything as I was getting him up to speed, but I think I unintentionally painted a rosier picture so that I didn't seem negative. My attempts to remain positive were once again coming off as ease and control. It made me feel even more confused. We agreed that we would meet again next week and work through the fears and anxiety about the upcoming surgery – the most immediate need. I knew there would be so much more to work through, but for now I needed to keep myself as composed as possible.

As I walked out to the car, I felt lighter. I hadn't said much that wasn't just stating facts, so I'm not sure why I felt as light as I did. I sat in the car and felt incredibly proud that I came to the session, despite almost backing out multiple times. It was a new year, and it was going to be a hard one, but it would be a year of mental and physical health for me. I needed that more than ever. I was committed to this therapy and wanted this entire situation to make me a better person in some way; I just needed help figuring out how it would manifest.

There was one thing I took away from that day that made me believe I could do it, and that I could handle the unknown of our future. I had told him that I was struggling, that I felt broken, and that I was at my lowest point - and he had said that was okay.

Jan. 6 – A Month Out of Chemo!

It's officially been a month since chemo! That is actually hard to believe because some parts of the past month have felt so slow, and yet all in all it has moved relatively fast. I think the holidays helped with that too, though! Regardless of speed – we are headed in the right direction – towards a cancer-free life!

We are officially under two weeks until surgery – thirteen days to go! Really, that just means lots of calls and paperwork – we have to get all the insurance updated and make sure everything is ready to go for surgery. Our doctor sent us some prep videos today (nothing with too much gore!) and we are continuing to do research ourselves. Each day closer we are excited to get this next phase done, but at the same time the nerves go up a bit too.

Tom is feeling much better than he was a month ago. His strength is coming back and dare I say some of his hair is trying to grow again too. Each bit of strength puts some more chips in our favor going into surgery, so I'm so happy he's been on the upward trend! I'm looking forward to a month from now, when we are two and a half weeks out of surgery...More to come...

The Sweet Life

I had to give it up – cold turkey. Cookies, cake, candy, ice cream, sweets of all kinds were going to be gone. A few days into the new year, I decided to do "No Sweet 16" – the entire year of 2016 without sweets. I had been using sugar to keep myself going for months. I would have cookies at the hospital almost every day, mostly because I timed it so I went down when they were hot out of the oven. We had so many care packages sent to the house filled with sweets and I was using sugar as fuel, the worst possible thing to do. At one point, I was standing in my kitchen and wondering if the cookie I was eating was my second of the day, or second of the hour. I had no idea; I had just thrown everything aside when Tom got sick, and my waistline was feeling it.

At the beginning of the year, I had gained almost fifteen pounds from when Tom was diagnosed. I would chalk a few of those up to the winter months – I needed to stay warm – but the rest was what I was eating combined with little activity. We were so lucky to have people who made meals and dropped off food, but often these were lasagnas, or heavier types of meals. I had chosen to not worry about it and just focus on getting myself, and Tom, through each day, but it eventually caught up with me. Beyond my physical health, I knew it was affecting my mental health. I wasn't feeling good, and I had promised myself that 2016 would be a year of good mental and physical health. I needed to put my money where my mouth was and give it all up.

The first few days were rough; I found that in moments of stress or in moments where I felt like I needed a hug or encouragement, I wanted a sweet of some sort. If ever I had doubted that I was using food, or specifically sweets, as a coping mechanism, it was now obvious. I had headaches for the first few days and felt lethargic, which wasn't surprising in the least considering the quantity of crap I had been putting in my body. But as I anticipated doing for the rest of 2016, I took it day by day. Making this change was a big one – and I reminded myself each day that nothing changes if nothing changes.

Jan. 10 – The "Normal" Life

Hello there! I know it's been a few days and I haven't been too active on the blog – the good news is that's because we haven't had any major updates or shots out of left field! The bad news is – the posts will be picking up again in regards to frequency as we get back into the thick of this cancer fight.

It really has been delightful to have a few weeks of normal – Tom mentioned today he feels the best he has in five months. He has said that before, so the fact that it's continuing to get even better is awesome. We had a relatively normal weekend, saw some friends and family, watched some great football (GO PACK GO!) and relaxed. We have been trying to strike a good balance of

192

"normal" while still making sure there is plenty of time for him to relax since doing activities still wipes him out more than usual. I think we've found a decent sweet spot and are enjoying these last few days before surgery.

We officially begin surgery prep this week – we have an appointment with the surgical team and anesthesiologist on Wednesday and will go over the plan for next Tuesday. While I'm sure the reality of the surgery and all the info we get on Wednesday will be a lot to process, we would rather know all possibilities and prepare accordingly than be surprised during or after surgery. Tom has never gone under before, and he's got some nerves around that, but I'm hoping once the anesthesiologist explains everything that he will feel a bit better and at least know what to expect. Nine days until surgery!

Speaking of Wednesday, we are planning to be the lucky winners of $1.3 billion dollars. I actually got one regular ball and the power ball for a big old victory of $4 – but hey I only spent $11 on tickets so that's not too bad, right?! I've got a whole list of things I would do with the money – and I feel like with a billion dollars I can try to cure cancer too. Because along with any debt we have – I want cancer gone with my billion dollars too so no one else would ever have to deal with this! More to come...

Back On The Couch

I was back for my second therapy session with Dr. Crane. It had occurred to me in the time since my first session that he had the same name as the doctor from the show *Frasier*, and that made me happy. I was eager to have another session. It seemed he always started the sessions with the same question.

"How are you doing?" he asked.

For some reason, the way he asked it always made me feel like he already knew the answer. "Surgery is six days away, and my anxiety is out of control," I replied.

"Anxiety about what specifically?" he inquired.

"Well, of course the main anxiety is the surgery; I want this surgery part to be done. We met with the doctors today for all the prep and it was terrifying. Then there is the question of whether the cancer is gone. I know I have no control over either of those. The third one is managing the day and the people," I said. I was figuring it out as I talked.

"What do you mean by the day?"

"I tend to worry and take care of others. Tom's parents and aunt will be there, and my mom will be there too. To be honest, I know I'll worry more about making everyone else comfortable, and I sort of just want to be Tom's wife that day. Isn't that silly?" I asked.

"No, that's actually very self-aware of you," he replied.

I was so worried about how the day would go, the fact that I would be in the waiting room with a bunch of other people who love Tom, and that all of us would be a mess. I didn't want to make light of the situation and try to pretend the reality wasn't there. I explained every possible scenario I was worried about. He patiently listened and looked up to me.

"Why are you overthinking this? Is there something wrong with just letting the day happen and taking it as it comes? Create open communication on how you're feeling and just let the day happen," he said so simply. "By doing that, you're just being Tom's wife."

He was right. I told him that I was fully aware that my anxiety with the day and the waiting room was partly my mind distracting me from the much darker potentials of the day. Talking to Dr. Crane gave me a sense of calm. I was able to tell him what I was feeling without the guilt of worrying him that I had when I told Tom everything I was thinking. At the end of the session, we scheduled my next session for a few weeks after the surgery. He wished me the best and told me to call him if I needed anything. I hoped that if I got desperate, his offer included wine delivery.

Jan. 13 – Let's Get Ready To Rumble

A friend and I were chatting this week and she remarked that I have a lot of fight in me. Kind words. I replied yes, but that I feel like my punches are getting weaker – this has been a long five months. Her reply was simple, but perfect – even professional athletes need a half time. Amen to that. It's a great point – while I have felt like we are a bit weak right now, this really is our "half time." The second part of this fight is going to be rough – we know that – and in some ways probably tougher than the first part. Regardless, we are gearing up to kick butt in the second half of this fight.

Today we had our pre-surgical meeting and prep. Really, not a whole lot happens, and quite frankly I wish we had gotten more answers – and it wasn't for lack of trying. First, they did some blood work – which Tom didn't realize would happen today. I was thinking that we had overcome some of the blood obstacles, but the minute the blood draw started....cue the profuse sweating, extreme paleness and blood pressure drop. I think it was a combination of a few things – but mostly I think it was because it has been a few weeks since he had to give blood and he got out of the "routine" of it.

Anyway, the nurse talked us through the day of surgery – asked tons of questions to confirm we won't have any issues – and then we figured out all of Tom's medicines between now and then so we can get him off anything that could cause danger or issues during surgery. Then our anesthesiologist came in and talked through the procedure from his viewpoint and again asked questions, looked over Tom, and made sure that he will be ready for Tuesday.

So here is what we do know:
1. Surgery is Tuesday, but will not start until late morning.
2. We should plan for surgery to be about six hours (dagger in my heart).
3. They are using a robot to start and then will make decisions from there (I YouTubed videos of the exact system they will be using and eventually had to turn it off because I started to gag – hence my lack of a medical career!)
4. Many parts of this procedure are very ambiguous. They will be making decisions as the surgery unfolds and they get a better understanding of what they are dealing with. The number of sentences that started with "Well, that depends..." was killing me today.
5. Tom will have some help breathing until they know he is stable but should be breathing on his own by the time he leaves recovery.
6. Our stay at the hospital depends (that damn word again!) on how the procedure plays out, but we are planning to be there for a few nights at a minimum.

I am very confident in our doctors and nurses and am eager to get this show on the road. We want the tumor out, so we can get a final verdict on if the cancer is gone and either deal with more chemo or deal with surgery recovery and move up that finish line to getting our lives back. Regardless, this is a huge milestone for us and I'm ready to add it to the list of things Tom has conquered. More to come...

Tough Guy

"Right this way," the nurse said as we walked through the intake room and into the next waiting area of the emergency room.

Tom and I were both exhausted, and the fact that we were back in the emergency room with a potential to impact surgery had our stomach in knots.

"Tell them you need to lie down," I said to Tom, knowing that this next corral waiting area was for blood work.

"I'll be fine, I'll just sit in the chair," he said as he handed me his jacket.

"No, there is nothing wrong with telling them you need to lie down."

"I'm really fine. I just want to get this done," he said, in a frustrated tone. It had been hard enough to get him to come to the ER, and I knew he was thinking about every possible scenario. "I'm tough, don't worry."

Moments later, his name was called, and we stood up. Tom sat in a chair in the hallway area where they took blood and I stood near the privacy screen holding our stuff. I smiled at him as they were getting the needle ready. The nurse stuck his arm and began the blood draw. Within seconds his face went pale, his lips lost color, and I knew what was about to happen.

"Are you going to throw up?" I asked as I looked directly at the nurse instead of Tom to give her the hint.

"You okay?" The nurse asked as she grabbed one of the puke bags.

Tom took it from her hand and began throwing up. It was a new record, only a few seconds from when the needle was in the arm to when he was tossing his cookies. I ignored the instruction to stay to the side since the needle part was done and grabbed a paper towel to wipe his face and rubbed his back.

Tom took a few minutes to get himself back together and we chatted with the nurse. She told him that next time he should tell her right away about his reaction so she could get him into a room before doing the blood.

"I told you so" was trying to burst out of my mouth as the nurse turned to the computer.

Tom looked up at me. "Don't even say it."

I looked down with a smile, "I'm not saying a thing, tough guy."

Jan. 14 – We Missed The Emergency Room
Today was one of those fun days in our life of fighting cancer. I must say one of the hardest things about the past five months has been the inability to trust any moment in time. We can have a great morning where things are going well, and by the afternoon we have major problems. It's almost like in the back of our minds we are always waiting for the other shoe to drop. Today was unfortunately one of those days – Tom was up during the night with some pain but was feeling okay by morning. By mid-morning, he was experiencing the same pain, including pain from breathing, in the same location where he had

his blood clots. Uh oh. While it is unusual to have blood clots while on blood thinners, it can happen when someone has cancer.

I called the doctor and she told us we should head in to the ER just to be safe. The real concern was that the pain was in the same spot as the previous location. So I packed up at work, headed home and got Tom, and off to the ER we went. We were on such a streak of not being at the hospital!

Tom didn't think he would have an issue with blood despite his wife telling him he should lie down before they take blood. Now, I really hate to be right when it comes to this stuff, but fast forward five minutes and he is pale as a ghost, dripping with sweat and just to top it all off....cue the puking. Once we got him all taken care of and situated, it was a matter of a few hours before we got the scan done and the results....NO BLOOD CLOTS!

We were thrilled to say the least. Not just because blood clots are dangerous, but if there had been a blood clot, our Tuesday surgery would have been at risk of cancellation. It's a bit of a catch-22 because if there was a clot, then he needs blood thinners, but you can't be on blood thinners before surgery. Luckily, we don't have to deal with that nightmare, but it certainly was weighing on our minds the entire time we were at the ER.

So while it was another one of those days that was a roller coaster of emotions, we are happy that we are sleeping in our own beds tonight and that there weren't any major issues. Perhaps this is the change in luck that we've needed (the lottery win didn't pan out) and is a sign of more good things to come going into Tuesday's surgery! More to come...

One Year Old

My nephew's first birthday was January 11th and my sister was having his party the weekend before the surgery. I was going back and forth about making the trip to Milwaukee, but I wanted so badly to be there and to be surrounded by my family since I knew the upcoming surgery would keep me away from home for quite a while. Plus, it would be a distraction, and we were in desperate need of being distracted.

Ultimately, we made the decision to go to Milwaukee for one night and be there for the party. The "kid" party was Saturday afternoon, and the family party would be Sunday morning. On Saturday morning, I got a call from my mom who informed me that both she and my dad had a cold. She wanted us to know because we couldn't risk Tom getting sick before surgery. Luckily, we had bid on and won a night at a brewery hotel in Milwaukee at a charity auction months earlier and they had a room available so we decided to stay there for the night to avoid the germs at my parents' house.

We had a great Saturday afternoon at the kids party and headed down to the hotel later that evening. The hotel was new and built in the old Pabst Brewery so there were giant brew kettles in the middle of the hotel and a very chic and modern atmosphere. It was freezing cold outside, but we had a rustic suite with a unique ambiance and layout. I loved it. As we curled up that night, I was very grateful that we ended up in the hotel. We hadn't been anywhere but the hospital or our house, with the exception of a few nights, for months, and the change of scenery, the calmness of the hotel, and this time together was refreshing. For quite a while we chatted about the day and the reality of the next week as we dozed off to sleep. It was so special in such a unique way.

The next morning, we once again braved the cold and headed to my parents' house for the family party. The calm from the previous night was gone and I wasn't sure why it happened so suddenly. Perhaps it was because my extended family would be there, and I knew they were all eager to see us before Tom's surgery. However, I think the real reason as because it was the Sunday of the week of surgery and we knew we were getting closer to the big day. I could tell Tom's anxiety was increasing along with mine. We enjoyed the party but decided to leave right when my nephew finished opening presents.

When we started our goodbyes, everyone in the room got quiet and somehow stood up in unison. The joy that we had just had watching a one-year-old open his birthday gifts was gone. No one really knew what to say or what to do, but Tom and I made our way around the room giving hugs and accepting well wishes. There were almost twenty people, and I managed to not cry during the hugs. It felt like we were in a funeral line. I should have just waved at the doorway and told everyone we loved them rather than go through that because the anxiety continued to build up within me.

As we turned out of the living room, I looked up at my dad. He had a tear rolling down his face. I gave him a huge hug and he then he gave Tom a hug. I knew this was tough on everyone. We headed into the kitchen where my mom and sister were with the baby, said our goodbyes, and started putting our shoes on in the foyer. I looked over at Tom, who I knew was about to cry too, and then looked up at my sister holding the baby. I walked back into the kitchen and gave him a kiss on the forehead and squeezed his chubby legs.

"Your auntie loves you," I said as I burst into tears. I quickly hugged my sister because I didn't want everyone to see me crying and grabbed Tom and headed out the door. I walked to the car with my head down, crying, and heard the back door open and my mom yell out.

"MOTHER LOVES YOU!" Knowing my sister had probably just told her, I burst into tears.

We got into the car and I looked over at Tom. "That was awful," I said as tears continued to roll down my face.

"Definitely a strange vibe," he said as he looked out the window.

"How can so much love feel so sad?"

"I have no idea…" he replied.

Our hour and twenty-minute ride felt like it took a month, but we eventually made it home and talked through most of our ride. Tom didn't cry; he just listened to my stream of consciousness as I tried to figure out my emotions. I knew he was being strong for me, and I knew that this was my last chance to lean on him for a while since I would need to be strong for the both of us for the foreseeable future.

Jan. 18 – Comedy of Errors

You know how things never seem to go as planned when you need them to? We were hoping to have a bit of calm before the storm to kick off our week but that failed. Yesterday I was a bit of a crazy person getting ready for the week ahead. It's sort of like getting ready for vacation, but the worst vacation ever that yields no hotel points or fun. I was trying to get ahead of some work stuff, figure out all the insurance/preauthorization calls that needed to happen today, cleaning, laundry, etc. Laundry was important because there is nothing quite like coming home and knowing that there are clean sheets on the bed (there will be no infections on my watch!) and that things are clean and orderly. It's surprisingly calming when the house in good order when we come home. Anyway, I say all that to explain that last night at 11 p.m. when my washer decided to die on me after only one load of laundry, I about lost it. Water is a very important part of laundry and the washer disagreed. The verdict? Frozen pipe. Lovely.

We are both a bit overtired already because we haven't been sleeping too well, especially these past few nights. The anxiety and nerves are real, different for each of us, but present nonetheless. The back and forth of wanting this to be over yet not wanting to deal with it all is a real struggle. We know we've got some long nights ahead but are ready for the second half of this fight to start so we can declare victory as soon as possible. And we will declare victory.

As I've mentioned, the surgery is not starting until mid-morning. I'll be sure to update the blog throughout the day. Let me just take a moment to say we are completely aware and in awe of all the love and support that has been coming to us and will be headed our way tomorrow. We feel it; we love every text, email or message, and appreciate all of the support and love that we have received. This would be impossible without support, and I don't use that word loosely. Impossible. Part of the reason we are confident going into tomorrow is for that exact reason – we know this cancer isn't just fighting one person, it's fighting all of our friends and family – the most amazing network of friends and family – with an enormous amount of prayers, energy and love. A lot more to come tomorrow...

A Hole In His Heart

I was a woman on a mission. We had just been told we could go upstairs to the recovery unit and wait for a nurse to come and get us. We had so much stuff and snacks with us and we packed it up and headed upstairs. The receptionist downstairs had said there would be a family waiting area to the left of the elevators, and to wait there. I was done with the waiting game though. Tom's parents, aunt and my mom walked in to grab some seats, and I told them I was going to go on a hunt. I couldn't handle waiting and there were no receptionist desks in sight.

I followed the twists and turns of the hallway and walked towards a big nursing station. I didn't think I was supposed to be roaming the halls, so I tried to blend in. A woman looked up and peered from behind her screen and gave me a big wave and smile. It was the *Family Feud* enthusiast from a few weeks prior – I never thought I would be as happy to see her as I was in that moment.

"I remember you! The nurse needs you," she proclaimed.

"Am I allowed to see him? Where is he? What does the nurse need? Is everything okay?"

"Technically, you can't see him yet, but we could use your help with some questions," she replied as she motioned for me to follow her.

As I turned into his room, I was taken aback. It was terrifying to see how sick he looked. Tom was hooked up to so many machines. I knew he was okay, but it took my brain a second to be certain when he looked the way he did. I introduced myself to the nurse and proceeded to help her with some of the questions that Tom was trying to answer but was confusing the nurse. I was surprised they relied on the patient to answer some of these questions in the first place. Everything was moving slowly; it didn't seem real. I was trying to talk with Tom and I suddenly snapped back into reality.

"Is it okay if I go get the rest of the family?" I asked the nurse.

"Yes – if you can just answer these last two questions for me," she replied.

I answered her questions and then told Tom, whose eyes were still closed, that I was going to get his family since they were anxious to see him. I stood there frozen for a few more moments; I was scared to leave his side. The nurse walked back in the room and I looked up at her. I'm sure she's dealt with plenty of concerned wives and read my face immediately.

"Are you okay?" she asked.

"I think so. This doesn't seem real," I replied. "I don't want to leave him."

"I know. I'll stay here until you get back; I've got to draw some blood," she said with a smile on her face.

"Thank you so much," I replied as I rushed out of the room.

I took a few deep breaths and tried not to cry as I found my way back to the waiting room. Tom's mom was standing up towards the front of the room; she could immediately read my face.

"Did you find him?" she asked, concerned.

"Yes, luckily, I ran into a woman who remembered me," I said to her, trying not to cry.

"Are you okay?" she asked.

"Yeah, it is hard to see him in so much pain, but you can come back."

My mom looked over and said she would sit with our stuff. My mom was still dealing with a cold and didn't want to get Tom sick. They followed me back and I'm sure were equally relieved to see him, but terrified at how serious his situation looked.

The afternoon was a blur. Time didn't seem to be moving, and I felt like we weren't making any progress. Tom would rarely open his eyes and wasn't saying much, which was okay – he needed to be resting. In the early evening, the doctor came in to talk with us again. He was pleased with Tom's progress post-surgery and would be back to see us the next day. The doctor walked out and I looked over to Tom's aunt and mom on the other side of the bed.

"Shoot, I forgot to ask him if they saw a hole in his heart when they used the camera in his chest today," Tom's mom said, disappointed. Tom's mom had had a stroke about twelve years earlier due to a hole in her heart. She had always wondered if Tom had one too, but there was never a reason for them to explore in his chest.

Tom hadn't said anything in hours, and he opened his eyes a tiny bit, looked over to his mom and mumbled, "There isn't a hole in my heart. I married Honore."

I looked up at his mom and aunt, who were holding back tears. Tom closed his eyes and moved his head back to the middle. My gut reaction was frustration – had he been awake this whole time and wasn't saying anything?! I was dying to know he was okay, but then I realized what he had just said, and I almost burst into tears.

What a day he had gone through and yet that was at the top of his mind and the tip of his tongue. It was such a special moment. In the days leading up to this surgery, Tom had told me he was fighting this for us, and that we had some rough days ahead, but he was going to knock out this surgery, be done with cancer and get back to spending the rest of his life with me. As he lay in that hospital bed withering in pain, heavily medicated, he was still focused on the end game – beating this and getting on with the rest of our lives. I had even more gratitude for him, his fight, and how much he wanted our happily ever after – no matter how many bumps in the road, we would get there.

Jan. 19 – What. A. Day.

I don't even know how to begin the post this evening, so please excuse me if my writing is sub-par today. First, and foremost, Tom is doing well. In an incredible amount of pain but doing well. I suppose as Julie Andrews once said – let's start at the very beginning.

Last night and this morning were tough. Last night we had to have some hard conversations about "what if" scenarios and didn't sleep well. We got here at nine this morning and they they took Tom back for prep. Unfortunately, he had to go back by himself for prep so I had to sit in the waiting room for about forty-five minutes. Tom's folks were here and his Aunt Paula and my mom. Once he was settled in, we were all able to go back and see him until they wheeled him to surgery. Unfortunately, they were about an hour behind, which was brutal because Tom was so nervous. The cardiac anesthesiologist came in and talked about her plan for the day, and quite frankly it scared the crap out of us. While we appreciate being told all possible scenarios, it's a bit tough to hear where IVs are being placed and hearing things like "IVs in your arm or hand aren't lifesaving." Certainly, we realized the severity of the surgery, but when you are so close to an operation, panic comes easily.

More panic set in when the doctor came in to chat and said that he had concern about one artery near Tom's heart. If he put in the camera and didn't feel like it was safe, they were going to stop the surgery and reschedule for another day with a different team and different equipment. I about lost my cool. The thought of walking out of here today without this surgery being done almost made me physically ill, and based on the look on Tom's face he was feeling the same way. Suddenly the focus became less on the surgery's results and more on if the surgery would even happen. The doctor said he would call out to the waiting room phone and let us know his decision once he got the camera in so we'd know exactly what the plan was even though we were confined to the hospital waiting area. Eventually, the nurses came in and we had to say our goodbyes, and they wheeled Tom away. That was a tough few minutes, especially after all the scary talk from the doctors, but I was eager for them to get things moving.

We hunkered down in the waiting area and kept our eyes on the reader board that shows surgical progress. We had a number assigned to Tom and were able to see what stage he was at in the surgery. About an hour into the waiting, one of the receptionists came over and told me I had a call. I followed her to the phone, hoping they weren't about to tell me that they couldn't do it, and thank God, they said they were going to take a run at it but would have to open his chest. The relief of knowing that they would be getting the tumor out today was so great. Then we braced ourselves to get our next progress call. Early afternoon, as I was walking out of the bathroom, I got pulled into the post-op family room and our surgeon was standing there with an update. I was shocked that he was already done! He said that the tumor was "ugly" and about the size of a softball. This thing was no joke.

Unfortunately, because it was a gnarly son-of-a-gun, it didn't leave with ease. They had to take 10 percent of Tom's lung along with his phrenic nerve. That will be something he deals with for the rest of his life but is a small price to pay to have the sucker out, and we had known there was a chance that would be necessary.

You know when you read a book and aren't focused and you get to the end of the page and then think, "What in the hell did I just read?" That's how I felt processing everything the doctor was saying. It's like my mind was racing 1098745098 times its normal pace and all I wanted to do was get to Tom. Dr. C gave me a hug, and I swear to you it was one of the biggest, tightest and sweetest hugs ever. We have gotten to know him during this process and I hugged him back just as hard. He commented to my in-laws that he just hates to see this happen to "young kids" like us. Thank God I'm only twenty-eight and still classified as a young kid ;-) I can't say enough about the doctors we have been fortunate enough to have – they are unbelievable – and we are forever in awe of their abilities and dedication to their work.

Anyway, as we were walking out, he told me that it would be about two hours before I could see Tom – say what?!?! It was almost worse knowing that it was over and I couldn't be with him than when he was in surgery. I was counting down the time to when we would be able to see him, and finally (as I hovered near by the receptionist's desk looking at the reader board for his progress), she told me she had just gotten a call that we could move to the ICU waiting room. We moved up to ICU, and I hunted down a receptionist to find out how long we would need to wait. She recognized me from another part of the hospital and took me to his nurse who then took me into see him because the nurse had some questions that Tom wasn't answering clearly.

His initial appearance took me back – he was visibly in pain and hooked up to so many machines. Oxygen, 3 IVs, a blood pressure IV, two blood drain tubes and much more – meanwhile the nurse was asking me a bunch of questions. There was a lot going on at once. As Tom and I were talking last night, he made me promise that the first thing I would tell him when I saw him after surgery was what ended up happening with the procedure. Since we knew there were so many variables, he wanted to know what had actually happened regarding the cuts they had to make. So he and I made a deal last night – I would tell him about the cuts first, but then he had to tell me a joke so I knew he was okay. So it went something like this as I was squeezing his hand:

Honore: I love you; it's done; you did so great; the doctor is very happy, but they did have to open up your chest.
Tom: Everything hurts.
Honore: I know. They are getting you some more medicine for the pain.
Then I start answering the nurse's questions....
Tom: Why did Adele cross the road?
Honore: Why?
Tom: To say hello from the other side.
Honore: Solid and timely joke, babe, great work.

So I knew that despite his agony and pain that he was okay, and things could only go up from here – it was a huge relief in our own goofy way. The rest of the afternoon/evening he came in and out of it and mostly rested. We were having a tough time getting his pain under control, but dare I say I think we are getting that problem solved, and he's starting to actually rest. There are no words to describe how tough Tom has been today; despite being scared, he just crushed it. His anesthesiologist came in tonight and said as they were taking him out of the room, he gave two thumbs up to the entire surgical team. I'm so very proud of him and the fact that he has continued to be positive and full of gratitude, through it all.

So now what....in the immediate future, tomorrow, there will be more scans, the drain tubes should be removed and hopefully he can try to tolerate some food. I'll keep posting updates on our progress. In the longer term, we now wait three to five days to find out if there is active cancer in the tumor. We still need all the prayers, energy and love sent our way for this. It would be a miracle for there not to be any active cancer in the tumor, but dammit, I'm not giving up hope until they tell me one way or the other.

I'm beyond exhausted, so I'll just close with the biggest thank you I could ever send via a blog. The number of texts, messages, calls and emails we received today was unbelievable, and so appreciated. They kept smiles on my face all day and reminded me how lucky we are. Thank you, thank you, and thank you. More to come tomorrow...

Ice Ice Baby

It was, no doubt, the longest night of my life. I hadn't slept but a few hours in days, and the night was long in the ICU. I slept in a chair pulled up next to Tom's bed. The back of my chair faced the door, and I faced Tom. If he woke up, I wanted him to look over, know I was there, and be able to tap me without having to move his arm very far. Nurses were in and out all night, and the machines beeped and buzzed. Even if I did fall asleep, it was short-lived, as I would continually wake up, worried about whether he was okay.

I hadn't gone out to the car to get my things the night of his surgery because I wouldn't leave his side. I was still wearing my clothes from the surgery day. I had a blanket that a nurse had given me and one of those paper pillows that do nothing other than slide around on the chair. My height made it a challenge to be completely covered by the blanket, and I couldn't get comfortable. The worst part of the night was the temperature in our room – it was freezing. Tom was the only patient in the world to come out of an operating room sweating. He ran hot before this all happened, and surgery didn't help. He had two – count them – two fans on him; the temperature in the room was low, and it was January in the Midwest, so the beautiful views from the windows in our corner room were a reason I was shivering all night. At one point, I got up and turned off the fan that was facing my chair. I figured one fan would be fine. Half an hour later Tom woke up and asked me to turn the second fan back on because he was hot. I smiled as I got up, hoping he wouldn't notice the icicles forming on my eyelashes, and flipped the other fan on. I felt like I was in a bad *Saturday Night Live* skit. When I closed my eyes, I dreamed about the sweatshirt and slippers I had in the car to make myself warmer.

At 4:30 a.m., two technicians arrived to take a mobile x-ray of Tom's chest and I had to leave the room to prevent me from being exposed to the x-ray. I got up and walked into the hallway – it was like stepping into a cup of hot chocolate. I couldn't believe how warm the hallway was compared to our room. The technicians were in the room for five minutes, and I was hoping they would need to be there longer. I stood in the dimly lit hallway moving each of my toes and warming up. The techs walked out, said it was okay to go back in, and mentioned how cold it was in his room. No kidding.

When I walked back into the room, Tom looked at me with a half-smile on his face. It was the most alert I had seen him since surgery.

"I love you," I said, smiling, "Do you need anything?"

"I love you more – no, I think I'm okay – just so much pain," he replied as he started to close his eyes again.

"You're maxed out for now, but you can have more in the morning," I said as I squeezed his sweaty hand.

"Your hands are cold," he said as he dozed off. "That feels good."

I couldn't help but laugh and fell back asleep holding his hand.

A few hours later we woke up again to a nurse coming in for morning rounds. It was about 7 a.m. Tom was alert and seemed to be much more aware of what was happening. Once the nurse completed all her tasks with Tom, she told me to order him some breakfast, but that he could only order from the liquid menu. I ordered him the liquid breakfast and hoped there was something on the tray that he would want to eat. A while later the tray showed up with a random selection of items for him to choose from.

"Hey, babe, the food is here. Do you think you could try a few bites of something?" I asked as he opened his eyes.

"Sure," he said as I moved his tray onto the wheeled table in his room.

"Anything look good?" I asked.

"Maybe the Italian ice?" Ninety percent of me thought it was a very cute full circle moment that he wanted to have Italian ice like we had enjoyed so many times during our late-night chemo picnics on the hospital bed. Ten percent of me was dying on the inside because he picked the only frozen item on the tray and I already was numb.

"Good choice," I said as I grabbed the napkin and wrapped it around the Italian ice so I could hold it and not feel the icy cold cup on my already freezing hands. I dug the spoon into the Italian ice to feed him his first bite. Tom took small bites, but I assured him I wasn't in a rush… I knew there was no chance the Italian ice would melt in this room.

Jan. 20 – A Whirlwind Day

Boy oh boy, we've had a whirlwind of a day – but Tom is doing very well and already out of ICU! We had a very long night last night in ICU – we had nurses and doctors coming in all the time, we had x-rays at 4:30 in the morning, all the while Tom was feeling terrible and still in pain. We didn't get a ton of sleep – but we were making progress.

The morning continued to be tense, as Tom's blood pressure remained high (usually indicates pain level), and there were so many tubes still attached to him. While ICU provides wonderful care, it's a very scary place to be has tense feel. We got two of his huge IVs taken out mid-morning, which required lots of work – then they wanted to get him up in a chair to sit upright. This was quite the feat for Tom. It took a while and a few nurses, but we got him up and moved to the chair. It's very painful for him to get up and down, but he did great!. Going back to the bed a while later was equally as tough and painful, but he powered through, followed all the directions, and made it safely back to bed.

While he was sitting up – we saw some familiar faces peek around our door.

Nancy and Lisa, two of our day nurses from his chemo treatments, had found us and had come up to see us! It was the sweetest gesture and they were so excited to see Tom had conquered surgery – we didn't even know they knew we were back at the hospital. We love our nurses and were so incredibly touched that in the chaos of their day they saw Tom's name on the hospital list and came to say hello. Like I've said before, they really have become friends.

After he conquered the chair, they were able to take out one of his chest tubes. I'll spare you the gory details, but it was not pleasant. The only upside was it was one less tube going in his body. Once this was all done, we got the all clear that he had graduated from the ICU! Let me just say – Tom continues to amaze me – he was leaving the ICU just shy of twenty-four hours after his procedure finished, and they had originally told us to prepare for several days. INSANE.

We got to our new home in the cardiac unit– which was quite the process, considering Tom is still hooked up to oxygen,IVs, drain tubes, etc. We got him settled and then were able to relax. Our new unit is one floor above our chemo floor. We are familiar with this area of the hospital and in a weird way being in one of our typical rooms made us calmer since it felt familiar and has way less equipment or tension than the ICU.

Tom rested most of the afternoon until it was time for a walk. Once again, quite the production – it requires two nurses to carry everything that he's hooked up to – but he conquered it. The walking is mostly pain-free for him – it's just the up and down that is tough. After a few walks today, he really was done for the night and has since been resting.

He did perk up this evening for our oncologist because we hadn't seen her yesterday. She was pleased with the surgery and is hoping to get us some preliminary results by Friday. Plus, she showed us a picture of the tumor, which blew our minds. I won't be posting it, for many obvious reasons, but this thing was huge and gnarly, and I'm so glad it's out! To round out an absolutely insane day – I walked into the hall this evening to see Kevin and Julie, our night shift chemo nurses, coming up to see Tom. We just love them.

Despite the chaos of the past thirty-six-plus hours, we are so grateful for our nurses and doctors and every single person in this place who had a hand in this going smoothly so far, no matter how small a role they may have played. So tomorrow will be considered a success if we can get more of the tubes out of him, get his blood pressure down and his pain more tolerable – so that's the plan! More to come....

The Weight of The World

I was almost disappointed with Tom's reaction. I had to snap back to reality and remember how medicated he was, how in shock he was, and how cautious we were both being with the information we were hearing. When our surgeon had walked into our room, Tom was sitting in the big recliner next to his bed. They had laboriously moved him there in preparation for a walk. I was sitting on the edge of his bed holding his hand and we were chatting when the doctor walked in.

It felt like a slow-motion dream. It was like when the sounds from a TV are a few seconds behind the picture, creating a disconnect between what you're seeing and what you're hearing. Our doctor first asked how Tom was feeling and then asked if our oncologist had been by to see us yet. We told him she hadn't come by yet, and a big smile came across his face. He was eager to be the first to tell us the news. As I listened to the words come from his mouth I remember slowly turning my head towards Tom to see his reaction. He closed his eyes and put his head back on the headrest of the chair. I wasn't sure if tears would be pouring from those eyes when he opened them or not, but I squeezed his hand and looked back at the doctor.

"Wait, so we're done, it's all gone, no cancer?" I asked, trying to replay what I had just heard.

"Done, you guys did it, no cancer. I couldn't wait to get up here and tell you. I actually was on my way to a procedure and had to take a quick detour up here," he replied, with the biggest smile on his face.

I just stared at him until I heard Tom's voice and turned towards him.

"Wow," Tom said, without an ounce of emotion on his face. He had to have been in shock.

The rest of the conversation was a blur. The surgeon checked on his tubes and gave me a hug before leaving.

I leaned in and gave Tom a kiss on the cheek. "You did it. I'm so proud of you; We are done! We just need to get through this surgical crap and we are done. We get our life back, we get our family one day, and you did it." I felt like I just wanted to scream from the mountaintops.

"Wow," he replied as he squeezed my hand. He was so physically exhausted already and now the news had created a mental workout that I don't think he was prepared for. It must have been an hour that we just sat there, me squeezing his hand and smiling, and him giving an occasional smile back and making a comment or two.

About 1 p.m., we snapped back into reality when the nurse came in. Tom went for a brief walk, no small feat and the first of two that day, and he got settled back into the hospital bed. We had been in our own world and in complete shock for the last few hours when it occurred to me that we had exciting news to share.

"Do you want to make some calls?" I asked him. "Or I could send a text and see if your parents and Aunt Paula and Uncle Rick would come up for dinner. It seems like it would be more fun to tell them in person," I said.

"Yeah, I'd rather tell them in person," he replied.

"Okay, I'll send them a text and tell them we are hoping it's your last night in the hospital and see if they would bring up dinner. We can finish this the way we started that first night," I replied.

"Perfect," he replied.

We weren't expecting the pathology until the next day, so I was pretty sure they wouldn't catch on to us trying to lure them to the hospital. I texted his mom and aunt and told them that Tom was eager for some company and invited them for dinner. They both immediately replied that they would all be up later that evening.

As I was coordinating all of this, Tom had fallen back asleep. I sat there, staring at him, unable to process what had happened in the last few hours, so I did the only thing I could, started writing. I wrote what I was feeling and also started working on the blog post for that evening. I wanted to call every single person that had been rooting for us to tell them the good news but knew that wasn't feasible. I typed and typed as I tried to process what I was feeling. The first page was a stream of consciousness that I didn't even remember writing.

It's over. He beat cancer. I want to tell the world. I want our life back. We are getting our life back. I am so thankful. He did everything he said he was going to do. He defied every timeline or odd that they gave him. HE BEAT CANCER.

I stopped writing as a nurse came in to take out his final drainage tube. Once they had that awful process taken care of, I sat hanging off the side of Tom's bed.

"I got a text back; your aunt, uncle and mom will be up later tonight, probably around five or so," I said.

"Awesome. That seems so long from now," he said as I turned over my shoulder to look at the clock.

"Only a few more hours," I said. It was 3 p.m. and so we only had a short stretch to go.

"Can we call my parents and tell them since we can't tell them in person?" I asked. It had been killing me to not call them right away, but we had been dealing with nurses and Tom trying to sleep.

"Of course," he said. He was the most awake I'd seen him in days.

We called my mom and dad and told them the news. My dad was driving when we told him and almost drove right off the road. My mom thought we were pulling her chain at first, but quickly realized from our voices that it was real. They were elated, and shocked, which I figured most people would be feeling – just like us. I swore them to secrecy until we told Tom's family in just a little bit. Next, we called my sister and told her the good news too. I thought she was going to cry; otherwise it was our sister ESP that she knew I was holding back tears on my end. It was so exciting to say the words out loud. As we wrapped up those calls, we had about an hour until his family would arrive. It was painful to wait; the clock didn't seem to be ticking at all.

"Maybe we shouldn't have told them in person," Tom said. "I just want them to know."

"Do you want to call them? We can just call people if you want," I replied.

"No, I do want to see the reactions," he said as he smiled.

He still hadn't seemed to be processing it all yet. I knew that was mostly due to our location, his pain and the shock.

"I need to pee," he said. It was the first time since they had taken the catheter out.

"Oh boy," I replied. "Do you want to try and get up or use the urinal jug?" I asked.

"I might use the jug if that's okay."

"Of course, I don't blame you. By the time we get you up and out of that bed, you would need to pee ten more times," I replied.

I walked around his bed and got the jug from the floor. "Here you go," I said as I handed him the jug.

He flipped off the blanket and started taking care of his business. I turned and walked to the bathroom to get him some paper towels and make sure the curtain was pulled back. As I came back to his bedside he smiled at me.

"What's so funny?" I asked.

"Nothing," he said, giggling.

"I feel very uncomfortable having a conversation with you and looking you in the eye while you're peeing in a jug," I replied as I laughed.

"This is what you pictured when we got married, right?" Tom replied, laughing hard.

"One hundred percent. I prefer this ten times as much as romantically walking down a beach like those fairytale marriages," I joked.

"See, you're so lucky," he replied as he pulled the jug out from under his hospital gown, still laughing.

"I'll trade you," I said as I reached for the jug and handed him some toilet paper. "There'll be no shaking in that bed, if you know what I mean."

Tom grabbed it from my hand and handed me the jug.

"I can't believe I'm standing here holding a jug of your pee," I said.

"It can still get worse," he said as he smiled and handed me back the paper towel I had just handed him.

"Well, that's very true," I said as I grabbed it from him and took both into the bathroom in our room. "But it could get even worse than that," I replied as I came back out.

"How so?" he asked.

"I could be holding your pee and you could still have cancer," I replied as I leaned down and kissed his head.

We continued to laugh and go back and forth with stupid jokes. It was the first time in days that I felt like I had my husband back. He was still medicated and a bit loopy, but our banter made me know that he was bouncing back.

A short while later, his aunt and uncle appeared in the doorway as we were about to take Tom on his evening walk. His aunt came with us on his walk as his uncle set up the food in the room. Tom was still moving slowly and requiring help, but we made our way around the recovery unit. His aunt couldn't believe that he had been lying motionless in the ICU less than forty-eight hours before and was now up and walking around. We got back to the room, and waited for his mom to arrive. It was only about fifteen minutes or so, but it felt like an eternity. Tom's aunt and uncle were asking what had happened all day, and we danced around topics and tried to avoid screaming out that we were done. We had talked about how to tell them earlier, but I told Tom it was up to him when, and how, he wanted to bring it up.

Tom's aunt and uncle were sitting on the couch near the windows on one side of Tom's bed, I was on the other side in the recliner near the doorway, and there was a chair at the foot of Tom's bed too. When Tom's mom walked in she gave hugs and sat down in the chair at the foot of his bed. Tom's aunt stood up to hand her the food order and Tom blurted out his news.

"I can't wait any longer, so I wanted to tell you guys that the doctor came in this afternoon and told us that there is no more cancer. We are done."

This was another slow-motion moment. Tom's aunt turned and looked back at Tom as she was still trying to hand off food. I couldn't see his uncle behind her, but his mom shot up, gave me a hug, and then immediately turned to give Tom a hug. There were hugs, some tears, and everyone settled in with their meals as we told them what had happened. His mom called my father-in-law to tell him the good news since he couldn't make it up to the hospital that night, and everyone sat in shock as we told them what had happened earlier that afternoon.

Seeing their reaction helped make it real but it still hadn't sunk in. Later that evening, after everyone had left, I got up from my couch bed and went over to Tom's bed like I did most nights when we were in the hospital.

"I'm so proud of you. Thanks for fighting so hard for this," I said as I grabbed his hand.

"It's easy to fight when you have something to fight for," he replied.

"And what's that?" I asked.

"You, and our future, and our future family. It was worth everything if I still get to have all that," he said.

It was the only time he almost cried that day.

Jan. 21 – Five Months In the Making

There are no words. There are no words. There are no words. Except for these simple ones:

Tom beat cancer.

Let me say that again, Tom beat cancer.

Okay, one more time in caps…TOM BEAT CANCER.

My heart is full; I have goosebumps as I type, and I sort of want to puke. That's what happens when your surgeon comes in and tells you and your amazing fighter of a husband that there was no active cancer in the tumor and the fight is over. We do not need to do anymore chemo; our last and final step is this surgical recovery.

The only emotion I can put around this is shock. It's almost the same type of shock we had when we first found out it was cancer – just a much happier type of shock. When he walked out of the room, Tom and I just stared at each other – had the biggest smiles come across our faces and couldn't believe what we had just heard. If Tom wasn't in so much pain or hooked up to so many tubes, he would have flown out of that chair – it's truly unbelievable. The odds were not in our favor that this would be the end – but as I've said many times – this cancer picked the wrong person to mess with.

This has been a fight; we are not naïve enough to think we don't still have a tough road ahead as he recovers from this surgery, but what a difference it makes to know that each day he feels better is actually a better day rather than a good day before the bad days of chemo return. This fight has knocked us down so many times; it has been the hardest thing we've ever had to do, but we got back up every damn time because we were not going to let it win. I couldn't have done this without the fight in my husband – he kept a smile on his face, which in turn kept a smile on mine. Proud doesn't even describe how I feel about Tom right now – I will forever be in awe of what he managed to do over the last one hundred twenty-eight days of our life, and I know he will finish out his surgical recovery strong.

214

We will get a lot more updates tomorrow from our oncology team and are eager to find out how this will all finish up – so more to come on that tomorrow. After reading my post so far to the Editor-In-Chief (Tom), I asked if he wanted to include anything in the post this evening. His reply was exactly what I was going to close with – a thank you. I feel like I've said it a hundred times, but this would not have been possible without our doctors, nurses, techs, friends, family, and coworkers. In line with our fight analogy – we needed people in our corner, and we had an army of them. Like I said in the beginning, there are no words...More to come tomorrow...

Do You Believe In Miracles?

I had hardly slept a wink; I couldn't stop my mind from racing, celebrating, trying not to cry, and comprehending everything that had happened in the past seventy-two hours. While my faith was an important part of everything, I was having a hard time understanding what exactly had happened. How did we go from active cancer in the tumor and planning for chemo to miraculously not having any active cancer cells? I was thrilled with the outcome, but the lack of concrete answers couldn't help but make me wonder if they would come back and say they had messed up the results.

I could apply logic and say that perhaps his levels were still too elevated, and his markers were out of whack during Christmas week. I could apply faith and consider that every prayer, thought and good ounce of energy sent our way made a difference – and I believe it did. But did that mean it was a miracle? I wasn't sure. To me, a miracle implies that another power created an outcome. In a sense, that seemed to minimize what Tom had been doing. He had worked so hard to beat this, listened to everything the doctor said and had one focus – beating the cancer. To me, that couldn't be a miracle because he was working hard at doing it too.

One other potential influence was the medical marijuana. After Tom's chemo, he switched to a high cannabinoid strain of marijuana, proven to slow or even shrink tumors in cancer patients. Could that have made a difference and helped continue to break down the tumor and get him cancer-free? It was certainly a possibility. There were so many variables and I wanted there to be an answer.

The reality was that I wasn't going to get that answer. The doctors didn't even really have one, and I would need to be content with that. I think I was getting lost in wanting the answer to the "how" because if we ever had to do it again, we'd know what worked before. Yet the reality was we would never get that crystal-clear answer and I had to let go of wanting one – regardless of the answer, we had achieved the outcome. Tom was cancer-free.

Jan. 22 – It Wasn't A Dream
I woke up this morning and turned towards Tom's hospital bed to tell him about the craziest dream I had – we had been told he was cancer-free and that this was going to all be over soon. When I looked over at him, he gave me a certain smile that all of a sudden made me realize it wasn't a dream – yesterday really happened. We are STILL cancer-free. Whoever said that winning isn't everything obviously never had cancer. The icing on the cake today – WE ARE HOME!!!!!!

As we were preparing for surgery, they told us that depending on how surgery went and how he did recovering that we should anticipate three to five days in the ICU and then a few more days in surgical recovery. We are home after only three nights in the hospital total – take that, cancer!!! During this whole fight, we never denied the diagnosis, but we did try to defy the verdict of what "should" happen and the timeframes they gave us. Our doctors came by this morning and told us that we could go home once we got Tom off the IVs and made sure he was okay with the pain and without oxygen. He passed with flying colors and actually felt the pain was better once the IV was gone and he could use the oral pain pills. It was a little crazy that we were just waiting for the doctor to come back to give us the all clear – usually we knew exactly when we would be able to go home because of our chemo timer!

While we were waiting for the okay to go home, our oncologist walked into the room – there was a part of us that was going to wait for her to tell us we were cancer-free before we told anyone, just to be sure. In a sick way, over the last five months we got so used to not catching a break that we were waiting for the other shoe to drop. Our oncologist has been with us since day one; she is one of the best doctors we've ever seen, and for her to come in and smile and tell us we beat the cancer was an unbelievable feeling. She acknowledged that she did not think the tumor would be cancer-free, and either did the pathologists.

She gave us the biggest hugs and said to focus on his recovery. We will see her in about a week and get a plan for the future. In the short term, we will get his port out; in the longer term we will be getting scans and blood work done every three months for the foreseeable future. Given the aggressive type of cancer Tom had, we will work hard to stay ahead of any problems that could arise.

Before we left, some of our oncology nurses came up to our room to celebrate with Tom since they heard the news. It's so cool to see the full circle of this diagnosis – and it must be awesome for the nurses who put so much into their patients to see a patient beat cancer too. They thanked us for letting them be a part of this, and our lives – I couldn't even believe that – if anyone is owed any thanks, it's them. I about cried! They truly are part of the reason we were able to beat this.

Tom is feeling well, all things considered, and is moving well. It's amazing to see the progress he has made in just a few days. On Wednesday morning, it took multiple people to get him out of bed and to a chair, and today he was able to get up and down, though slowly and in pain, with my help. We also had a good chuckle about his departure. Once we got the all clear, I got us packed up and went to go get the car and bring it to the door. Meanwhile, they called a *transport volunteer and he wheeled him down to the door where we could then get him in the car. Tom's transport man was easily eighty years old, rolling a thirty-one-year-old out of the cardiac/surgical unit. I literally laughed out loud, and this sweet man could hardly believe that Tom had been so sick. You would think in a more "normal" situation the two of them would switch places. We smiled the whole way home. I really think being home also helps lift the spirits – we spent twenty-seven nights in the hospital in the past few months and are excited to avoid another stay for as long as possible!*

We received so many amazing messages and calls filled with excitement about our news – but I must say, it hasn't sunk in yet. Whether we knew it or not at the time, when we got the diagnosis back in September, we chose to be survivors, an option that some cancer patients are not lucky to have. It wasn't a conversation, but a mindset that we both immediately had – and I think that is part of the reason we are still in shock. It's not shock that we did it – that was always the plan – it's the shock that this finish line danced around like a drunken person at last call, but we made it. More to come…

I Love You Because...

A few years back we received a gift from Tom's best friend's wife May. It was a craft she had made for us and I loved it. It was a 5x7 frame with two felt roses on the top left and a pattern inside the glass with the text "I Love You Because..." and then the rest of the area was blank. She gave it to us with some whiteboard markers so we could write on the glass, and it was immediately up in our house. Sometimes we would put silly things on there; other times serious ones, and sometimes passive-aggressive statements. We didn't change it every day; occasionally it would be on there for a week or so at a time. We changed it when one of us felt compelled.

During chemo, I would change the sentiments to be silly or encouraging. "I love you because you look like Mr. Clean" or "I love you because you have a special relationship with needles" or "I love you because you're a fighter; I love you because you amaze me every day." Tom would rebut with sweet nothings like "I love you because you are the most kind and amazing person in the world" – which would make me feel bad for a moment that I had called him Mr. Clean.

In the first few days home I was running around like crazy taking care of him but slowed down for a moment to change the I love you because frame. I wrote, "I love you because you beat cancer!" Tom had been sleeping, but it was at the foot of his bed on the TV stand so I figured he would see it when he woke up. Later that evening as he was slowly moving around the house I got him all situated in bed and crawled in next to him. As I curled up next to him, I noticed he had changed frame. It read, "I love you because *we* beat cancer." A smile came across my face as I read his edit to the frame.

"Why did you change the I love you?" I asked.

"Because I couldn't have beaten cancer without you. We beat cancer," he said to me.

It still felt strange to hear him say that we had beaten it. This recovery was so intense it was easy to forget that we were headed in the right direction, back to our normal lives. As I lay there, curled up next to him, I took a deep breath, looked up at him and smiled, "We did beat it, didn't we..."

Jan. 24 – The Cancer-Free Roller Coaster

It's been an interesting few days here in our cancer-free household. There has been so much to process, and all the while Tom is in the first, and toughest, days of his surgical recovery. He is doing incredibly well, but he does require quite a bit of assistance in moving around, which we expected. Also, our nights have been a little tough because he has to sleep on his back and that just isn't a comfortable way to sleep – I think we figured out the appropriate pillow situation to get him as comfortable as possible but it still isn't as natural, or relaxing, as he'd hoped.

Tomorrow is a big day as all of the bandages will come off and hopefully that will help with his mobility a bit. His large incision is already uncovered and very large, but the other ones we will get eyes on for the first time tomorrow. That should be interesting since there are no stitches – just holes in his side. The doctor said it's normal for him to "leak" from these open holes this week. I disagree; there is nothing ever normal about leaking from a hole in the side of your body. I've got a pretty strong stomach for medical stuff now, but this particular situation will be interesting. Plus, I assume if I had two holes in the side of my body, red wine would come pouring out, or something green and gold.

Throughout this experience, there have been many unexpected situations. Yesterday and today was one of those – we both sort of crashed. Between the tension and anxiety of the days leading up to the surgery and then four long days with little sleep and lots of emotions at the hospital, we were both just beat. Tom obviously more so because he also has the recovery, but we allowed ourselves a few days to just relax, recover, and sleep. I guess I thought we would be running more on adrenaline knowing this was going to be over soon, but I think we finally were both able to take a deep breath. We just needed to let our bodies – and minds – recover.

I can't tell you how many conversations we have had since Thursday about this still not feeling real. I thought being home would help make it feel real, but it really hasn't. I think over the next two weeks as we get a plan for scans, get the port removed, and figure out when we can stop nightly shots then perhaps it will start to sink in. Heck, there is a part of me that still hasn't processed the fact that Tom even had cancer. I think it will take a while, which I hear is normal, and then I think it will be the simple things that help us process, like going to a restaurant again, or going to a movie, or taking a trip. Even silly things that were put on hold because of his diagnosis. For example, right before we got Tom's diagnosis, we were planning to invest in a good mattress – versus the nice but lower quality ones we've had since college. So as silly as this example is, I think it's things like this happening, which we've talked about all through treatment, that will help this all start to sink in. We certainly are excited to get him feeling better and starting our post-cancer lives. More to come tomorrow…

Who Is That?

We stood in the mirror looking at his scars. Tom had gotten queasy but was feeling better and willing to look at his chest. I was standing in our bathroom looking in the mirrors. It was a badly bruised and a scary landscape.

"It doesn't feel like I'm looking at my own body," he said.

"I know, babe; the only thing that will make this more normal is time. Time heals on this one," I replied.

"I know, but it doesn't feel like this could be my body," he said, staring into the mirror.

I knew the disconnect between his mind and body was going to happen. He had gone to sleep on the day of his surgery and woke up with so many stitches, holes and bruises; how could a brain reconcile that? As we stood there, staring in the mirrors, what was even more frightening was that I didn't recognize myself in that mirror either. I was exhausted, I was on empty, and I had gained fifteen pounds since he was diagnosed. I hadn't put on a lick of makeup in a week, and there were bags under my eyes. I didn't recognize myself and it was partly body, and partly mind.

Jan. 25 – Ground Zero

Well, today was a bit of a strange day – we took off Tom's bandages – and that didn't quite go as planned. Tom's big scar was already uncovered so he has had time to adjust to that. However, he has had bandages on his side since we left the hospital and had been instructed to keep them on until today. Two of the bandages were covering the holes from where the tubes had been – as I mentioned, these didn't get any stitches or anything – just random holes in his side. Then, there was a third one that was used for the camera that had helped guide the procedure. Have I mentioned lately how insane science is?

Anyway, the goal of today was to get these bandages off (cue my nurse glove snaps), so he would have a little more freedom in movement and could get cleaned up. I knew better than to have Tom looking in a mirror as I was doing this, so instead I turned him away from the mirror and started to remove the bandages. As I was pulling them off, I realized it didn't matter if we had a mirror or not because Tom had looked down and boom – the reality of this war zone on his chest hit him. I came pretty darn close to calling an ambulance as I got him seated, put a wash cloth on his head, held his head up and made him converse with me to ensure he was staying with me. I think it was a bit much for him to see it all, see blood-soaked bandages and reconcile that it was all from the surgery. I'll be honest – it was tough for me to even see and it's not on my body. Needless to say, we took a break after that first bandage removal and will take care of the rest tomorrow.

In a strange way, Tom doesn't feel like it's his body he is looking at. It's not like when you break a bone and you are completely aware and can associate the pain with a moment in time. He really can't. It's a strange disconnect his brain is having with his body – and I think that was a big part of today. It really put into perspective everything that happened in the past week.

Speaking of the past week – I have NO idea where the time has gone. If I put myself back to this time last week we were an absolute mess of emotions and nerves getting ready for surgery. Tom is feeling a bit frustrated that he isn't getting better "fast" enough, but I told him the fact that we are home and that he is on the mend a week after surgery is a complete victory to me. It feels like there is more progress being made when there are these tangible targets in the hospital like leaving ICU or removing tubes, but I really have been amazed at his recovery so far.

Despite his awesome recovery, Tom is feeling pretty icky and still on a heavy medicine regimen, but it's getting us headed in the right direction where his pain is manageable and he can feel better. I can't wait for this all to be a distant memory. More to come tomorrow…

Recovery at Home

It had been a long week and a half. I was sitting in the living room working from home and taking care of Tom. He was sleeping in the bedroom and I was quietly taking calls and getting work done. I looked up from my laptop at the gallery wall in our living room and looked at all the pictures and keepsakes up on the wall. I had recently added one to the bottom right. It's pastel yellow with black writing on it. It reads, "There's nothing half so pleasant as coming home again" – Margaret Sangster. I had purchased the quote plaque at the hospital gift shop during one of Tom's chemo sessions that felt especially long. Now, I sat in my living room still trying to juggle everything that was on my plate, but I was home, and most importantly, home with Tom. The caregiving post-surgery was a different kind of caregiving and was both physically and mentally exhausting. I was Tom's upper-body strength to get in and out of bed and helped him move around. I had to find the balance of support for him, without letting him get too used to my support. He needed to challenge himself so he could get better.

As I was sitting there thinking about the last week of our lives and how happy we were to be home, I heard the channel change down in the bedroom so I assumed Tom had woken up. I slowly went down the hall and peeked my head around the doorframe, hoping to not wake him up if he was still asleep.

"I'm awake, no need to tiptoe," he said with a smile.

"I didn't want to wake you up; I lose caregiver points for that," I replied.

"You could never lose a caregiver point; you've been amazing, babe. I couldn't have done this without you," he replied, much more romantic than I would ever be if I was waking up from a nap.

"Oh, hush," I replied as I headed to the kitchen to replenish his water and grab his pain medicine.

As I was filling up the water, I was thinking about the people in my life who had a similar caregiver role. My Aunt Joyce had taken care of my Uncle John for two years through a terrible esophageal cancer; I couldn't imagine what she experienced in those two years as I was still struggling to wrap my head around the last five months. My Aunt Jody had taken care of my Uncle Freddy for almost ten years through a rollercoaster ride of cancers, her unwavering love and compassion through that many years was mind-blowing now as I was experiencing such intensity. They were both humbling examples to me, and in some way had prepared me for our own fight.

As I headed back to the bedroom to give Tom his medicine, I felt grateful. I knew realistically that this was as tough of a situation as any twenty-eight-year-old could manage. I felt like I had handled it well, or as well as I could have, but I was thankful in those moments that I had good examples. I wish it hadn't been because cancer had been in my family, but both uncles didn't get the same outcome as Tom and ultimately passed away. I only wish they knew that, even though cancer took them, their niece was still in awe of what they did, how they fought their cancer, and the women who were by their side. By being such strong examples, they had helped us beat cancer. I am forever grateful.

Jan. 27 – No News Is Good News!

Happy eight days past surgery! What a difference eight days can make! Tom is doing quite well and is on the mend. Yesterday he was able to get cleaned up, we reapplied bandages and he is moving around very well. He is still dealing with quite a bit of pain, but that's to be expected when you have as many large incisions as he does on his chest. Overall, he is such a champ. I'm blown away by his positive attitude and desire to push himself each day despite the pain.

I'd say we are very happy with where things are at – we certainly had prepared for the worst going into surgery. I don't think we would be having the same recovery if we knew we were recovering to just march ourselves back into chemo. Admittedly, before surgery, we were really on our last leg as it relates to keeping our spirits up and feeling like we could beat this thing. I am so thankful that there isn't more chemo because we probably would have been expending all kinds of energy just to stay positive. I know we would have found a way – but I'm just grateful that we didn't have to go down that path.

I am in complete awe of patients and caretakers who must fight this awful disease for years – some of which I've seen firsthand within my own family. We are not blind to the fact that we only had to deal with the active cancer for one hundred twenty-eight days, and for that we will forever be grateful. Cancer touching our lives will extend well past a hundred twenty-eight days; it will be with us forever. It's part of our story now, and I know it will shape the rest of our lives for the better. More to come...

The Hair Color Asterisk

"I remember my uncle's hair coming back curly after his chemo treatments," I said to Tom in the hospital bed.

"That's just so crazy that it could change texture or color," he replied, lying in his bed.

It was during our first chemo cycle, and we were learning a lot about the different symptoms and changes that patients experienced. One of the greatest things about our nurses was that they have seen just about everything so could prepare us for many situations. They mentioned, as had our doctor, that often after chemo treatments, a patient's hair will come back a different color and texture. The texture would revert over time, but it was a potential side effect.

"Remember when we had our wedding vows, and I promised to love you through sickness and in health, and for richer and poorer?" I asked, with a smile coming across my face.

"Yeah...." he replied, hesitantly.

"I'm here for all of that. I'm here for the long haul, but don't be coming back as a redhead," I said, starting to laugh. Tom and I both had redheads in our families and have always joked we would have redheaded kids. I think they are adorable, and I love redheads, but our joke about this has gone on for years. "No offense, but your skin tone isn't a good match for light hair. You're more of that Italian olive skin, dark hair look."

"Wow," Tom said, as he began laughing.

We had that conversation so long ago in that hospital bed, and now we were watching the strangeness of the hair growing back. Back then, we hadn't realized what it really meant to lose all his hair –Tom lost everything, including the things we never even thought of. Eyebrows, arm hair, nose hair, and one that was especially tricky – eyelashes. I remember him being outside for a few minutes one day in December and he got back in the car with tears rolling down his face and his eyes red. I couldn't figure out what had happened as he yelled out, "I miss my eyelashes!" He had nothing to help protect his eyes, and the wind and cold had immediately made his eyes water. It's easy to forget that everything has a purpose on our bodies.

As things started to grow in, I became a petting monster. The hair on Tom's head was coming in like baby hair, that super fine and soft texture. I couldn't my hands off his hair.

We were sitting on the couch the evening that we planted the Chia Pet and he looked over at me. "I bet it's going to come back curly."

"That's okay," I replied. "I bet it will be cute."

"You have to say that, you're my wife."

"No, I don't, I think it could be cute, and I'll handle any texture, but you know the rules about color..."

Tom laughed. "You act like I have any control over it."

If there was one thing I knew, it was that we hadn't had control over anything in a very long time.

Jan. 30 – Ch Ch Ch Chia

Houston – we've got hair coming back! Tom's hair is coming back fierce, and unfortunately, we didn't time it well with the Chia race. Tom wanted to hold off on the Chia Pet until he knew for sure he didn't have more chemo. However, by the time we found out we were cancer-free, the top of Tom's head had some growth.

So the race has started a little late – but the Chia is making up for lost time and Tom is on a mission to get his hair back! Surprisingly, his eyebrows have come back very quickly and they were the last to go. Our oncologist told us that it's not uncommon for the texture or color to change, but so far it looks like not much has changed. The color seems a bit lighter to me, but that may just be because there is still so little versus when he had a full head of hair.

While it may seem insignificant – Tom is so excited to start to have his hair back because it makes everything seem more normal. Plus, he's thrilled that it's coming back now so he can potentially go back to work with a full head of hair versus the patchiness as it grows back. Beyond the hair growth, life is slowly getting back to normal, in a strange new way. More to come on that tomorrow…

Career Change

"I've been thinking about my post cancer life and what I want to do career wise," Tom said as we were hanging out at home during his recovery. We had talked about this a few times during his chemo sessions, and I had a feeling I knew where this was headed. "I think I should be a standup comedian; I'm funny," he said with a grin on his face.

"You go right ahead. I just will have to sit in the back of the room," I replied, with a grin right back at him.

Tom and I loved standup comedy. For my last birthday, he had gotten us tickets to see Chelsea Handler, a comedian I loved. Her opening act was another comedian we both loved, Josh Wolf. Josh had started a bit on how ridiculous the reality show *The Bachelor* was, and that he went crazy listening to his wife complain about how he didn't do all the nice things that the bachelor did. Now, I am a closet *Bachelor* fan and enjoy getting lost in someone else's reality for a while; it's one of the only ways I can relax. Tom would often make similar jokes to the ones Josh was making and Tom kept whispering loudly to me during his set, "That's my bit!! That's my bit!!"

I leaned over to him and whispered into his ear, "You're not getting paid for this bit, so I'm pretty sure it's his."

As we sat there on the couch and I thought about the comedians we've seen and how much we enjoyed it, I encouraged Tom. "If you want to try it, then by all means, go right ahead. I just want you to be happy. Go explore every career option."

"Maybe I will. I've already got my bit list in my phone," he said as he grabbed his phone with a smile on his face.

A bit list? I threw my head back and laughed. That was the funniest thing he had said all day – maybe Tom was funnier than I thought.

Jan. 31 – I'm So Funny It Hurts
The good news – we've been laughing hard lately.
The bad news – it hurts Tom quite a bit to laugh.
The worse news – I'm funny.

So Tom cracks all his silly jokes – and of course laughs hardest at his own jokes – and then proceeds to keep laughing because it hurts and for some reason that becomes funny...more on that in a minute. We had lots of laughs this weekend and quite an eventful weekend, but we are certainly still trying to figure out Tom's limits. I'd say Thursday night into Friday was the turning point for Tom. Up until then he really needed quite a bit of help (I've essentially been functioning as his upper-body strength), and that's when he really started to have some strength back and was continuing to challenge

227

himself to push it a little more each day. I continued to help quite a bit, but I also let him try to be independent where it makes sense.

Friday night, we ventured out for one of the first times since surgery. As I mentioned in a previous post, Audrey, the VP of Tom's department, retired at the beginning of the year. Friday night was her retirement party, and Tom really wanted to attend. We originally thought there would be zero chance that he would be able to be there since it was only eleven days after surgery, but since he had turned the corner a bit and had a bit of energy, he decided to give it a try. I told him going in, if he could only handle being there a short time that it was okay; I was more eager for him to get out of the house a bit and socialize with people who have been rooting so hard for him through this all.

We surprised everyone (except the host who knew we were coming), and they seemed very excited to see Tom. We were able to catch up with them, hear about all the fun Tom has been missing and of course celebrate with Audrey. Also, I got to meet many of his extended coworkers who have been reading the blog and had so many kind words for us both. It was a fun hour and a half, but then Tom gave me the look that it was time to go. It was getting close to when we needed to give him his shot so we made our way out. We were about twenty minutes away from home, and mid-chat, I realized that Tom had dozed off. Considering the last eleven days of his life, that hour and a half took the wind completely out of him in the best way possible :-) Tom is eager to get back to work and we will find out more about when that will be this week after we meet with the surgeon and the oncologist.

We had some visitors on Saturday, which was fun – in the afternoon his cousin and aunt and uncle stopped by for a visit. They were quite surprised how well he was moving, which was great to hear. Tom hears me say how amazing he is doing all the time, but I think hearing it from outsiders who haven't been with him constantly is additional affirmation. Earlier in the day on Saturday, my sister, brother-in-law, and nephew came down for a visit, which was fun, but a little frustrating for Tom. My nephew adores Tom so he immediately reached for Tom when he got here, and sadly Tom couldn't hold him because of his lifting restrictions and the continued pain from his incisions. Dagger in the heart. We figured out other ways like putting him next to Tom on the couch etc., but Tom is eager for his lifting restrictions to be lifted – no pun intended.

Speaking of, I caught him in a lie today! So, I dragged all the groceries in today and got everything upstairs. One of these items was a twelve-pack of green tea. Tom can't lift anything over eight pounds but he came waltzing into the kitchen wanting to help. I told him I had it covered and to not pick up a thing. As I was unpacking the bags, I realized the twelve-pack of green tea was in the fridge. It went something like this:

Honore: Tom! Stop lifting stuff! Go sit down!!!
Tom: I didn't lift it!
Honore: Then how did it get in the refrigerator?
Tom: I moved it with my mind.
Honore: No you didn't.
Tom: It's under eight pounds.
Honore: No it's not.
Tom: Yes, it is!
Honore: (Grabs twelve-pack out of the refrigerator, walks it into the bathroom and pulls out the scale)
Tom: (laughing/in pain) There's the stubborn Irish wife I love!
Honore: (puts twelve-pack on scale) Thirteen pounds! Now go sit down.

Remember the laughing part at the beginning of this blog? We were laughing quite hard during this entire exchange, and so I think he went and sat down mostly because he made himself hurt quite a bit from laughing. Plus, if he had telekinetic skills and is just telling me about it now, I'd be irritated. He could have helped me a ton with those skills over the past five months! ;-)

So all in all – a great weekend – we are starting to get glimpses of a "normal" life again, and it is incredibly refreshing. As I mentioned earlier, we have doctors' appointments on Tuesday morning and will hopefully know more about when we can stop shots, when we will get the port out and plan for the coming year to monitor Tom. We are so eager for these last few steps where we can really start to feel like we beat this thing. More to come...

Holy Crap. That Was Awesome.

I was walking up and down the card aisle looking for good thank-you notes for our doctors. I wanted to get a thank-you note for our surgeon and our oncologist, but I was looking for the surgeon's card first.

I couldn't find the right card. I didn't want lovey-dovey thank-you notes; I didn't want something too dramatic; I wanted something in between. I saw a card that looked promising and pulled it from the cardholder. On the front it read "Holy Crap. That Was Awesome" and the inside was blank. It was perfect. What this surgeon did was awesome. He had opened Tom's chest, perfectly maneuvered a bunch of tools and a robot in his body, and removed a tumor so we could declare Tom cancer-free. There are days when I can't keep a serving of lasagna on the spatula long enough to make it to the plate so that kind of precision is not lost on me.

When we were in the appointment with the surgeon, I grabbed the card out of my bag. I had written a long note in the card and left a few tear drops.

"It's just a card, but I hope you know how appreciative we are for everything you did to make this happen. We can never repay you, but please know that we are forever grateful for you and your work," I said.

He paused and took the card from my hand with a very sincere look. "That's awfully sweet of you. Thank you for letting me be your doctor," he replied as he gave us a hug and walked out of the room.

It was bittersweet. In his lifetime as a surgeon, we were just a blip on his radar, but his name, face, kindness, and compassion would stay with us forever. He would never be forgotten.

Feb. 2 – Did You Have Surgery?

I'm going to let the cat right out of the bag for today's post: Tom is completely crushing his recovery. We had a fun morning of appointments, but all yielded great results. There was a small part of me that worried they would see us today and say they read the pathology wrong, or while we were cancer-free, they highly suggested a "clean up" chemo. Thank goodness none of that happened – my heart couldn't have taken that.

Tom started the day with an x-ray of his chest. Given that they had to take part of his lung, they wanted to check to make sure that the lung was recovering and expanding the way it was supposed to. After the x-ray, we went right up to see our surgeon for the post-surgical checkup. Tom's surgery was exactly two weeks ago today, and when the surgeon's physician assistant, who also worked with us post-surgery, came in to the room, she said Tom looked "awesome" and was so impressed with his attitude, the color in his face, his ability to move around, and how all the incisions were healing. She remarked that she has lots of patients who come in two weeks after surgery and are still very weak, in a bit of a slump, and have a much harder time. As of today, Tom is almost completely off the strong narcotic painkillers and just using the prescription-strength ibuprofen. Plus, his ability to move and get up and down on his own is getting better and better each day. I'm so amazed by how well he is doing and admire how much he is pushing himself.

Next, the surgeon came in, closed the door behind him and said, "Did you have surgery?" with a big smile on his face. He too was very pleased with Tom's recovery, checked on the incisions and gave us the rundown of what to expect next. Tom needs to recover for about four more weeks and will continue to have lifting restrictions – but he got the all clear to drive. After four weeks, he is good to start going back to work and all restrictions will be lifted, but of course he will need to be careful as he gets back to his new routine and not try to do too much too fast. We will see the surgeon in about four months, but so far things are looking great.

Next we met with our oncologist and got a plan for all the pieces of that puzzle. Tom's port will be coming out next week, and I can promise you he will not miss it one bit. He doesn't even go under to get it out since all they need to do is pull it out versus the intricacies of it going in and getting in the veins. It will be quick and mostly painless. There will be another incision on his chest with stitches that will need to heal, but at this point, given the tumor surgery, another small incision doesn't seem like much. Right now, if you played Connect the Incisions (a derivative of Connect the Dots), you'd have a strange-looking hexagon. If you add in all the bruises from the daily shots, then you've got a first-grader's art piece – lots of chaos. Regardless, another incision is one step closer to the end of this all, so he doesn't even care – let's get it out. Obviously, the next year is still going to involve lots of doctors. For at least the next year and a half we will do scans and blood work every three months. Certainly that's not fun, and there will be nerves before we get the results, but I'm honestly glad that we need to do them this frequently because I think it will provide some peace of mind knowing that we can catch any problems. That said, our oncologist said today that Tom has been cured of cancer. He is not considered to be in remission; he is considered cured. I get goosebumps just typing it.

For both of our appointments today I had thank-you cards for our doctors. Thank you doesn't even begin to scratch the surface of what they've done for us, but they really became such an important part of our lives. Tom promised me he would grow old with me, and there were moments in all of this that I thought that might not happen. Without this team of doctors, I'm not sure he would have been able to keep his promise. The insane amount of dedication our doctors have to their practice and patients is unbelievable and inspiring. Today felt like a bit of a "goodbye" because we won't see them nearly as frequently (we are 100 percent okay with that!), and it was the first time we'd seen them since he was declared cancer-free in the hospital. For the first time in six months, we really had joyous appointments with all our doctors and their staffs, with lots of hugs and smiles. We even had various staff who have worked with us through this whole thing pop into our exam rooms to celebrate because they too were rooting for us. The only word I can use to describe today is grateful. Grateful for our doctors, their staff, their patience, our friends, our family and so many other things. After a very long six months, it was incredibly energizing to know that we are so close to the end of the fight. More to come…

Scar

For needle-phobic Tom, a tattoo was never in the cards, but in a way he got a free one from his scars. He hated the scars, mostly because they made him feel like a foreigner in his own body. I knew he was struggling with the scars, the pain around them, and how intense they looked. They would get better over time, but less than a month out of surgery, they were still looking pretty gnarly.

I was at work and saw a post on Instagram that I copied and sent to Tom. It read, A SCAR SIMPLY MEANS YOU WERE STRONGER THAN WHATEVER TRIED TO HURT YOU. I sent it to Tom with the text, "I love you." A few minutes later I got a reply from him, "I really like that..." I knew it wasn't going to solve all his issues with his scar, but it was a step in the right direction. I also tried the humor route a few times and suggested that Tom get a tattoo around the scar to blend it in. The scar was big, straight down his chest, an inch and a half wide. I suggested using it as the middle of a butterfly, but he quickly vetoed my suggestion. To this day I don't understand why.

In a way, the scar is important; it marked an important time in of our lives. I'm sure he would have chosen other ways to mark that history, but it is a daily reminder to me. When he would get out of the shower or be changing, I'd see the scar and remember how far we've come, or that something I'm annoyed about at work isn't a big deal. It was, and would continue to be, a constant reminder of perspective. He always thought I was lying to him or just being nice when I said that his scar was badass and that I liked it, but I meant it. A scar was not ideal but was a badass reminder of the craziness of our life, all the love, and most of all the victory of beating his diagnosis.

Feb. 5 –Trading Places

Well, as I predicted weeks ago, the last six months just ka-boomed on me. As things are starting to wind down, my brain caught on and decided it no longer needed to use all my adrenaline or run on empty, and my body crashed hard. I've got a double ear infection, sinus infection, fever thing going on – lovely, just lovely. I'm on the mend now, but it's been a crappy few days.

Tom was frustrated and remarked, "I hate seeing you so sick – I just want to make you better." I lifted my head and said, "Multiply that by a hundred and that sums up the past six months of my life." Tom has said through this whole thing that he would rather be the patient versus the person who has to helplessly watch/care take and keep it all together. I take the other stance; the entire time we were going through this, I would say I wish I could do this for him so he didn't have to suffer. Certainly there isn't a "right" answer, but I do find it interesting that we both wished we could be in the other person's shoes for his/her sake. Both positions are different, have different levels of risk/danger, and have their own challenges. I wish we hadn't needed to experience either of them – but we did, and I think we did quite well.

Tom has been such an amazing patient through all of this, though in this conversation he admitted there were days where he may have worn a fake smile so as to not worry me. My reply was "I did the same." I can't tell you how many times I cried in the shower or cried in the car – the same for him. Not because we were trying to hide any feelings from each other but because we didn't want to bring the other one down with us. I had terrible and great days, as did Tom, but by our count there was only one occasion where both of our terrible days landed on the same day. We needed to balance each other out to make it through, and we did. So regardless of role during this whole fight, our roles now are much more similar – husband and wife living life cancer-free.

Tom is feeling great and getting stronger each day. He gets on the treadmill every day to help build back lung capacity and pushes himself to do a few minutes longer each session. It's not an easy task for him, but he knows it will get better. His scars are also healing quite well, and we both were shocked at how faint the scar will likely be when it finishes healing. There are parts of the large incision that have already had the glue come off and look great – or as great as a scar can look. Tom is still working on the harrowing tale that he will tell about his scar – originally, he was thinking a shark bite but the line is far too straight for that! More to come....

Our Identity

I will fully admit that, in a non-sadistic way, I was sad to see the nightly blood clot shots go. I was so happy that we were turning the corner into more normalcy, but for five months they had been part of a daily routine. We had to make arrangements based on the timing of the shots to make sure that we had them with us wherever we were, or were home in time to do them. It had been a task that we had learned to fit effortlessly into our lives. As we inched towards normalcy, giving the shots felt like a reminder for Tom that I was still taking care of him. It was a sign of love.

What was hardest to accept was that we were saying goodbye to something that had become part of our "normal" during the cancer fight. I was happy, but I was terrified, because the further we got into recovery, the closer we were to having to figure out our new normal, and I didn't know what that would look like or feel like. With the shots no longer needed, we were starting to move away from patient and caregiver back to husband and wife. The irony was that our time as patient and caregiver had transformed us into an even better version of husband and wife. For all my doubts, I couldn't wait to see how it all transpired.

Feb. 7 – Super Shot Sunday

Today was a big milestone for Tom – his last shot! Tom is thrilled, as am I, but I think for different reasons. We've had to plan around these shots for the last sixteen weeks, so I think it will help in feeling like our normal is coming back. His last shot was tonight (and the glove snap was on point!) because he has to be off the blood thinner for a full day before the port removal. Then, after the port removal on Tuesday, he will go back on blood thinners but in pill form instead of the shot. In mid-March, he will do all his final blood work, and we hope at that time he is off the blood thinners completely

For those living under a rock...today is Super Bowl Sunday! As I mentioned, I have been sick and was feeling much better yesterday. Today? Not so much, I took what feels like five steps back and literally did almost nothing today...which is very unusual for me. Tom kept telling me I needed to just lie down and rest and due to how crappy I felt. I listened. So as a result we didn't do anything for the Super Bowl other than watch it here together – which was A-OK by me because I feel so awful. On a positive note, Tom is feeling better and better each day. I can't say enough how impressed I am with how far he has come in the past nineteen days!

As we were watching the game (and disappointing commercials), I pointed out to Tom that this all began after the first week of football. Tom and I love football – different team allegiances – but love football nonetheless. It's part of the reason I love fall so much, and we have always looked forward to our football Sundays. We usually have something in the crockpot all day and get things done while we relax and watch football. We were discussing tonight how distinctly we remember the first Sunday of football this year – it was three days before Tom was diagnosed. We had gone for a run that morning and I remember us eating dinner that night. We had smiles on our faces that fall was coming, and we were discussing landscaping stuff that we needed to figure out before winter since we are still novice homeowners. We were so content and so genuinely happy. We'd created a life we both loved and felt like we had a great day – I remember thinking how lucky I was. Seventy-two hours later, our life was flipped upside down and needless to say our fall Sundays that we so treasured were out the window.

So in a way it seems fitting that Super Bowl Sunday landed today. The day of his last shot, and the first day of the week where we get the port taken out – one of our last big milestones. I think about all the time, energy, effort and heart that football players put into getting to the Super Bowl and I think Tom matched that times ten to get to where he did over the past weeks. I still consider myself lucky – for a whole slew of new reasons. If I keep the analogy going – Tom is the MVP of this whole thing – and I would be Beyoncé during that halftime show. More to come…

Kill Me With Curiosity

I always wondered what was happening around us in the hospital and I had a front row seat to figure it out. For Tom's chemo sessions, with the exception of his Hercules room, we always had a room on the main path of the unit, and the couch always was parallel to the door. We would leave the door open and I would see all the comings and goings of family, friends, patients, doctors and more.

It was a real-life reality show around me, and the curiosity I had about all the characters was a distraction, though sometimes hard to watch. I'd wonder if someone was coming to say goodbye to a loved one or rekindle a broken relationship. I'd look at a doctor and wonder if they were about to deliver good or bad news and try to understand how they handled the emotions of a day.

The day of Tom's port removal, there was something going on in the room next to us and I never quite figured out what it was, but as I sat there it occurred to me that I wouldn't be part of this world much longer. I wasn't going to have to live, or have a front row seat, in this nightmare anymore.

Feb. 9 – Peace Out Port

The port has left the building! Three weeks to the day since Tom's surgery and he is cancer-free, and now the port is out. Talk about progress! We headed to the hospital at nine this morning and got Tom checked in. It's technically day surgery so they have to get him in a gown, check his vitals, and ask the same registration questions they have asked us a thousand times. Short of my bra size and political views, I think they know just about everything about us.

It was quick and easy (Tom's words), and he was awake the whole time. They gave him some meds to "relax" him and then used a topical numbing agent. Here's what's weird about that – he could feel everything happening on the inside of his body since that wasn't numb. I say that only because the port had gotten a little too comfortable in there. Since it was surgically implanted, it's pretty deep to begin with and since it's been in there for six months, it went even deeper. They said they had to "dig" a bit to get it out (gag), and Tom could feel all the pulling and prodding (gag again). As a result, he is actually having quite a bit of pain in that area because they really had to dig around and there are stitches there now. The positive side? Tom said his big incision didn't have any pain because there was so much pain around the port.

They monitored him for a bit afterwards and then we were free to go. If only everything had been this easy! On our way there this morning we were talking about how strange it felt to be going to get it removed and how little we knew when we had it put in six months ago. We had no idea what we were about to do, how we were going to manage to do it, and the toll it would take on us both. His port was put in the day before his first chemo and within that same week he had five days of chemo, five nights in the hospital, throwing up, pain, a seizure in my lap that will still haunt me for the rest of my life, and I think I slept four hours that week. Today? Quick and easy and our only appointment of the week! Plus, today's removal was symbolic of the end of this journey versus the beginning – thank goodness.

Speaking of the end, we are planning on having a big 'ol "Tom Beat Cancer" Party! All will be invited, but we are thinking we won't have it until early summer for a few reasons. First, we want Tom to be feeling better so he has a little more strength for a party. Second, for some of our non-local friends and family, it's a better city to visit in the summer. And lastly, you can never trust the weather in the Midwest so we want to hedge our bets a bit on that one. More to come...

The Simple Things

Valentine's Day has always seemed a bit silly to me, but I can appreciate the sentiment of taking a moment to tell the people you love that you love them. People don't do that nearly enough. Usually, Tom and I don't exchange gifts as much as we do something together, but we always exchange cards – and we always each get two cards for each other, one "serious" one and one funny one. We had agreed to just do cards for Valentine's Day this year – or so I thought.

I rolled over Valentine's morning and reached for my phone to see what time it was. My hand bumped into an object. I lifted my head to see what was there: a small box on top of a card. I smiled as I put my head back on the pillow and Tom rolled over and gave me a good morning kiss.

"What's that?" I said as I pointed to my nightstand.

"Oh, nothing…" he said with a grin on his face.

I rolled over onto my back and scooted myself up on my pillow and the headboard of the bed. I looked over at Tom. "Happy Valentine's Day."

"Happy Valentine's Day," he replied. "There might be something over there for you" – as he peeked around me to look at the nightstand.

"I thought we agreed to just do cards and go see a movie?" I asked.

"I know, but I couldn't help it. You deserve the world, especially this year, and I just wanted to get you a little something. It's only half for Valentine's Day," he said.

"What's the other half?" I asked, confused.

"A thank-you for helping me beat cancer gift," he said.

"Oh, for goodness sakes, that's not a thing," I said.

"Yes, it is, and I had cancer, so I get to make it a thing," he replied.

I knew it wasn't worth arguing, but I did feel terrible that I didn't have anything for him other than the two cards. I reached for the card and box. I opened the card, and it was the serious one – far too emotional for a woman who had only been awake for about five minutes.

"Well, that was very sweet," I said as I closed the card and kissed Tom.

"Just wait until the gift, it's even sweeter," he replied with a cheesy smile on his face.

I laughed as I started to unwrap it. A jewelry box was inside. I opened it and immediately knew what this gift represented. It was a shiny silver heart, with another heart inside of it, and within the second heart was a diamond. It was Tom's heart and my heart. The "hole in the heart" from the day of his surgery was a diamond.

I looked over at him. "You're right, it was even sweeter. Thank you so much. You didn't have to do that."

"Stop saying that and just know how much I love you. I know you aren't big on material things, but I just thought it was perfect," he said.

He was right; it was perfect. We lay in bed and were chatting when he looked over at me and smiled.

"What's that sneaky smile for?" I asked, knowing he was up to something.

"I have one other gift and I'm too excited to wait to give it to you," he replied.

"Tom! You weren't supposed to do any gifts and now two?!" I was actually getting a little frustrated because I didn't want him spending too much with all the medical bills, and I certainly didn't want him to spend it on me.

"Remember how I told you to stop saying that?" he said as he jumped out of bed and went to his hiding spot for the gift. He returned to the room a few minutes later with another card and another box.

"Oh goodness," I said as I took it from his hand. I read the card, thank goodness it was the funny one, and proceeded to open the second box. This time a unique silver ring was shining back at me. It was the infinity symbol, but on one edge of the loop was the squiggly line of heartbeat. Tom must have heard me mention that I had wanted an infinity ring, and found this unique one that also symbolized the last few months of our life.

"You are ridiculous," I said as I looked up at him, smiling. "Thank you so much; you didn't have to do any of this."

I felt like a broken record, but I knew that these gifts were just as important to him. He felt like he had just been "taking" for the last few months, and he wanted to finally feel like he was giving something too. He wanted to feel like he was doing something special, and he had succeeded.

Feb. 14 – Happy Valentine's Day!

Eek! It's been a few days since I've posted! Happy Valentine's Day to all – we enjoyed ourselves and as per usual my very romantic husband went above and beyond. Tom is feeling well, though I must say I am shocked at how bruised he is from his port. There is a very thick and solid ring of yellow bruises around his port, and it looks like it hurts. You can tell it's tender and that he is moving very deliberately so that it doesn't hurt as much. However, he didn't complain for the last six months, so it's no surprise that he hasn't complained about this either.

We started working on our post-cancer bucket list this weekend and got ourselves a new mattress! We had the most wonderful man assist us. He helped us figure out what we wanted and, even better, was able to deliver it same day. Though silly, it was very exciting to be buying an item that we had talked about doing once this was all over – and quite frankly what I dreamed about when I was sleeping on the tiny uncomfortable couch at the hospital. As with any new mattress, it takes a few days to get used to, but I'm already sleeping better than I have in months, and it's only been one night! Another thing we did this weekend was go to the movies – another silly thing – but we hadn't been able to be in a movie theater for months because the crowds made it a risky place while he was going through chemo. It's truly the little things that put smiles on our faces. We feel like we are getting our lives back and starting to feel "normal" again.

Despite these exciting milestones, it has been a strange transition for us both. When we were told Tom had cancer, we had to adjust to our situation quickly but had a list of things we had to do. Meet with doctors, get second opinions, get the port in, start chemo, etc. While it was chaotic, we had a plan that we had to follow to beat cancer. Coming out on the other side has so many happier feelings, but has been a bit more ambiguous. There is no real manual on how to adjust back to life, but we are doing our best to figure it all out as best we can.

Since we hate to go too long without a doctor's appointment, we will be back at the hospital in the morning for Tom's port follow-up. It should be quick and hopefully then we will have a break for a few weeks before any more appointments – woo hoo! More to come tomorrow....

128 Days & Counting

I knew I needed to translate what had happened to us into a book; it always seemed like part of the purpose of this fight. The white pages and blinking cursor had become my therapy of sorts, complemented by Dr. Crane. Yet I was desperate to end the blog. It felt like it was getting to be the right time to end it, and I seized the opportunity. Tom was heading back to work; I was starting to see glimpses of "normal" and feeling like I had less to report. If I was staying true to the purpose of the blog and sharing Tom's progress, it felt like we were starting to level out.

When I hit "OK" on the final post, I felt relief, and expected a few angry texts from some of our more loyal readers. When it posted, I looked at it on the page. This little haven of the internet had our story in it, the good, the bad and the ugly, and as I scrolled down that page, I reflected on the number of months down the side in the archive. I knew we were lucky to only see six months there, yet it felt so much longer. I felt such accomplishment as I scrolled. I had not only taken care of Tom all these months, I had tried to take care of everyone who loved us by keeping them informed, and even trying to make them laugh some days. Yet the person it helped most was me.

Feb. 17 – The Farewell...To The Blog

I think it's time. I've been tossing it back and forth, but I do think it's time to retire the blog. Back in September, a bit panicked, I was trying to figure out a way to keep everyone informed of our progress, but this blog transformed to so much more than that. I've said it a thousand times before, but the comments, the encouragement, and the love we felt are part of the reason we were able to beat cancer. In a bit of a strange way, the blog became my sidekick of sorts, a bit of a crutch and way for me to process everything that was going on in a simple way because I had to find a way to communicate it simply.

Writing this blog I always tried to be fair to our situation while trying to maintain a positive perspective. Perhaps some days I wasn't as fair to it as I should have been, as some people have said we made it look easy. Trust me, it wasn't easy – but there were reasons that some things went unsaid. There were moments of this whole cancer fight that I just didn't want out in the world – I didn't want anyone to have to go where we had to go to – it was a tough place to be and where we could prevent additional worry, we did.

Tom's diagnosis and subsequent caretaking role for me was like adding another full-time job to my plate. A job I truly feel lucky to have had. There were days where the blog felt like the "homework," the proof that we were making progress and doing what we were supposed to be doing. There were nights I was simply exhausted and didn't think I had it in me to write, but we wanted people to know what was happening so they could keep praying for us. In a weird way it became our acknowledgement – our way of saying we know you are all there rooting for us. I know some days the writing wasn't eloquent and most days it lacked perfect grammar or punctuation but hopefully you recognize that it was just raw – it was what we were feeling and experiencing.

Obviously, this isn't all over yet, but the bulk of the "fight" has passed. We've got a way to go in regard to getting back to our lives, not being nervous of scan results or going down the "what if..." spiral, but we will deal with that like we've dealt with everything else – one day at a time and with a positive attitude.

So what's next? I was talking with someone recently about the pressure to do something earth-shattering now that we've beaten cancer. Certainly, we will live life differently moving forward, and I know we will make decisions differently as a result of this. Maybe that will be in the next few weeks, or maybe that will be years from now. The possibilities are endless. Are we going to quit our jobs and go live on a beach with Aruba? Nah – not yet anyway.

Speaking of jobs, Tom will be headed back to work in just two short weeks. He will be back in the office the first week of March and will obviously be careful as he eases back into work. He is still on lifting restrictions, but for the most part we can see "normal" getting closer and closer! Tom is feeling great, he has defied the odds once again, and for people that aren't aware that he just had such massive surgery you really wouldn't know. He is eager to get his restrictions lifted and get back to the golf course!

We both agree that the one thing that is a non-negotiable is that we want to pay it forward. If we can do anything for the next cancer patient to make it easier on them, we certainly want to help. That is currently manifesting itself in many different ways, and again, time will tell how this all plays out. For me, one thing I'm in the process of doing is pulling this all into a book. As I mentioned above, I didn't blog everything, but I wrote along the way in addition to the blog. My goal is to pull it all together and tell a story that can help people, make people laugh, and perhaps teach some life lessons that Tom and I had to learn all too soon.

So to close, we want to say thank you. A few people have referred to this blog as a love story – and I loved that reference because as terrible as this all has been, it's been so surrounded by love. Our love, the love of our friends and family, and most importantly the power of all the love, energy and prayers. We are so very proud of everything we accomplished in the past six months, and we certainly tried to do it with as much grace and gratitude as possible. We will continue to keep everyone in the loop, but if you are worried about missing out on all my profound wisdom, sarcasm or jokes, give me a call...or stay tuned for the book that will hopefully be hitting the shelves soon.

We love you all SO much, and from the bottom of our hearts, thank you, thank you, thank you.......

Part 3
February

Of high importance was naming the single chest hair that had popped up next to Tom's scar.

"What about Kevin Costner?" he suggested.

I burst out laughing. "Because of *The Body Guard?*" I asked.

"Yup!" he said with a smile at his clever quip, "The Scardian!"

"Scardian it is," I said as I laughed.

Beyond the important task of naming the chest hair, the dust continued to settle. I was getting back into the groove of working a "normal" schedule, and Tom was preparing to head back to work at the beginning of March. His recovery was still our number one priority, yet more priorities started to creep back into our life. For months, we had one focus, Tom beating cancer. He solely focused on that. I had so much more to handle, but my focus was still the same; everything I was doing was to enable Tom to beat cancer.

I wasn't sure how I had made it this far, or the intensity of what had happened, but one priority I had was finding a way to channel my strong desire to help others who might be going through the same situation. I had heard about a non-profit, Imerman Angels, which provides one-on-one cancer support for both patients and caregivers. I loved that this organization knew caregivers needed help and could learn a lot from each other. Also, what made this organization so unique was that it matched people with someone with their exact type of cancer and/or treatment. It was a differentiator because someone who had gone through breast cancer wouldn't have had the same experience as Tom. I figured I had nothing to lose and signed up as a caregiver mentor, or angel, as they called them.

A few days later I received a call from the agency wanting to have an intake discussion about all the specifics of our cancer diagnosis. I talked with the woman for about thirty minutes and found myself stalling in my answers, not because I didn't know the answers, but because I hadn't really said them out loud before. She was one of the few people I had talked to who didn't seem fazed by my answers or my youth; she heard about the chaos of cancer every single day. As we wrapped up our conversation, I felt better than I had in months. There was no timeline on when I would get matched with someone, but knowing that I might be able to help another person in our situation made me feel like I was doing something productive with everything we had gone through.

Another priority was to start to get our lives back and reenter the world. While Tom was still fragile from his surgery, we were able to start being in public places and had to worry less about him getting sick. One of our first big events was something Tom had been eagerly awaiting for months: attending a

Chicago Blackhawks game. One of my best friends, Andrew, has had season tickets and often took Tom to games during the season.

Andrew and I had met in college and quickly became close friends – he was like a brother. The last two years of college we lived in the same house and I gave him endless relationship advice. He got along well with Tom from the first day they met, and they quickly became friends. They had a shared love for all things Chicago sports and always had fun together. In fact, at one point in college, Tom and I had almost broken up. Andrew had come into my room after class and could tell I was mad. I explained everything and said I thought maybe things just needed to be over. Andrew told me it was a terrible idea and tried to be an advocate for Tom, while still acknowledging my anger. Ever since that day, Tom has always said that Andrew was *his* friend now. Andrew had been anxiously waiting to hear that we could to go a Hawks game with him, and we set a date in late February. I picked up Tom after work and as we drove down, we were giddy that we were headed to the game.

"Are you excited?" I asked, with my own overenthusiastic excitement.

"So excited. I can't wait to be at a Hawks game," he said.

"Me too. Are you feeling okay? I'm worried about the crowd with your scar. I can be your bumper if you need!" I said, trying to acknowledge my concern without ruining the excitement.

"I'm fine…" he said, rolling his eyes, as he grabbed my hand and kissed it. "I know you want to take care of me, but I'm going to need to keep doing things on my own," he replied.

"So…yes to being your bumper?" I said, ignoring his statements.

I was nervous about him being in the crowds but figured I would subtly try to buffer him a bit if I could. As we walked into the United Center, the crowds were buzzing and the excitement was building. I did the most important thing first, which was to buy a 50/50 raffle ticket. I was bound to win one of them one day if I played enough, right? Tom laughed as he saw me beeline for the raffle vendor.

"Don't laugh," I said as I walked back with my tickets. "We've got medical bills that could be paid!" I joked.

"You know the odds are so slim, right?" he said, pragmatic as usual.

"Right, but the odds were slim with your cancer too and we were the lucky winner of that," I replied.

Andrew heard our logic and laughed at how ridiculous our conversation had become. We got to our seats with a few minutes to spare. I knew what was coming and already had goosebumps. Now, Wisconsin only has a minor league hockey team, so while I'm not against the Blackhawks, I still don't root for Chicago sports teams. That said, there is no greater moment in a sports arena than the singing of the national anthem at a Blackhawks game. The crowd claps

246

the entire anthem as a gentleman belts it out which always includes a dramatic point at the flag. It's one of the most patriotic moments in sports.

I heard the announcer ask everyone to rise. I stood up, put my hand over my heart and looked up at the flag. The crowd was going wild. I had goosebumps and tears welling up in my eyes. I looked over at Tom and saw the same. We had talked with Andrew about going to a game when Tom was cancer-free, and here we were. We were still processing the last few months of our life, but this moment was one of the first that made it feel real. We had done it; we were standing at the United Center, and that meant we had beaten cancer. As the anthem wrapped up, Tom and I leaned into each other and gave each other a kiss.

"Oof, that one got me," I said as I kept my back to Andrew so he didn't see us blubbering like babies.

"Yeah, I'm so happy we are here," he replied with a huge smile.

I was happy for us; I was happy that the moment had hit me with the reality that we had beaten his cancer, but what made me happiest was the joy on Tom's face, despite the tears he was blinking away. He deserved so much happiness for the hell he had been dragged through.

On the way home from the game that night, I decided to bring up a topic we had discussed before but had put on the backburner in January.

"Can you believe we were just at the Hawks game? The national anthem got me because it made me realize we had beaten it – we said we were going to go to a Hawks game when the cancer was over," I said to him.

"Yeah, I thought the same thing. It's crazy; it's still so much to process," he replied, opening the door to where I was headed with the conversation.

"That's for sure. I know we talked about it awhile back when I was struggling, but do you think it might make sense to talk to someone?" I asked cautiously.

"Maybe," he replied, trying to put a halt to the conversation.

"I'm happy to look into finding a therapist," I suggested, knowing that the only way this was going to ever happen was if I set it up.

"Okay," he replied.

I knew he knew that he was going to need help processing everything but figured he was like me and wanted to resist the help. Particularly, for men, I think therapy is often perceived as a sign of weakness, though his giant scar would tell the opposite story.

"I know it's not quite your cup of tea, but it's helped me. If you go once and hate it then don't go back," I said, making sure he knew I would support him either way.

"I know, I'll see what you come up with," he joked, referencing my uncanny ability to find the best doctors.

A few days later I had finished my research and told Tom he had an appointment with a guy by the name of Dr. Ron. He was close by, had a great reputation and some specific expertise that I thought would be helpful through Tom's recovery. I'm sure it was one of the few moments of this cancer fight when Tom wished I wasn't such a mover and a shaker when it came to getting things done. I was eager for his first appointment scheduled the following week and hoped that he would find value in the therapy.

That same week I channeled my inner therapist and decided it was time to put away all the cards. In September, I had put out two baskets on our side table that housed the cards we had received; they were so full and had been a great reminder of all the support we had. Some nights we would grab a few and re-read them, or show some of the funny ones to visitors, but suddenly two baskets full of cards felt like a reminder of the bad, versus the support they had originally provided. I got a big plastic tub and put the cards into it, amazed by how many cards and letters we had received in the past six months. Tom walked into the kitchen as I was in mid-transfer.

"What are you doing?" he asked.

"I just thought it was time to take these out of the limelight. I'm obviously going to save them, but think it's time we put them away," I replied.

"Interesting," he replied as he grabbed a few of the cards and re-read them. "That's so many cards."

"I know. I might actually need a bigger container," I replied as I was methodically trying to fit it all in. "And it confirms that we are going to have the party," I said.

Tom and I had been going back on forth on if we should have a Cancer Survivor party in spring. I was hell bent on doing it, no matter how much work it was. I wanted to take a moment to celebrate his fight and most importantly celebrate with the friends and family who had fought so hard with us. Tom agreed that a party was a good idea as I continued wrangling all the cards into the plastic container and slid it into the closet. When I walked back to the living room, the table now looked empty, much like the emptiness of a space after putting Christmas decorations away. I cleaned up the side table as I listened to the news on the TV and rearranged the decorations that had been there. The news anchor reminded the viewers that tomorrow was leap year. I laughed to myself as I realized that the worst year of our lives would have an extra day.

March

I sped home from work as fast as I could. Tom was still on leave from work but had his first therapy session that afternoon. I was anxious to see how it had gone. I took a deep breath, dropped my rushed and frazzled state of mind at the door and acted calm, cool and collected as I walked into the kitchen.

"Hi, babe," I said as I gave him a kiss.

"Hi there," he said, as he lifted his eyebrows and let out a deep sigh.

"Oh, dear, is that a good sigh or a bad sigh? How was therapy?" I asked, nervous that he may be one and done.

"Ahh, I think…good? I don't know. It was interesting," he said, still trying to wrap his head around his first session.

"Interesting good? Interesting bad? Do you hate me?" I didn't want Tom to feel like he had to share anything with me after therapy. If that was his safe space, then so be it. He could share with me as he needed to or as he felt comfortable. However, I had put in so much effort to try to find the perfect therapist for him so I was trying to understand if this was going to work long term.

"Umm…interesting good," he said as he slid up to sit on the counter.

"That's awesome! Does this mean you may go back?" I asked.

"Yes – my next appointment is next week. He is a really nice guy and thinks he can help me deal with everything, not just with the cancer. Like we hardly talked about that today," he replied, suddenly wanting to share more.

"Seriously? I mean you explained why you were going, right?" I asked, hoping he hadn't been his typical self and tried to convince everyone around him that he was fine.

"Oh yeah; I mean I explained everything, how I ended up there, but he sort of wanted to start at the beginning and understand who I am, like with my family and our relationship and growing up, etc." he replied, seemingly on board with this approach.

"That's awesome – I'm happy for you," I replied. "You never have to tell me anything you talk about, but just know I'm more than happy to talk about it if you want to and when you want to. I know for me sometimes it takes a day to even sort out my own sessions in my mind," I said, now the expert in therapy in our family given my seven-week head start.

"I know, and I will. I feel like I keep replaying the conversation in my head. It will be interesting."

"And Dr. Crane is going to be thrilled to hear you are going back. He and I both agreed that this would be good for you," I replied with a grin on my face.

"I'm glad you and your therapist are diagnosing me," he replied, jokingly.

We hadn't necessarily diagnosed him, but my therapist was helping me cope through this strange period. I was having a hard time letting go of my caregiver role. He was about to go back to work, and I worried about his transition, and if it was too premature. My biggest fear was that he would immediately focus on everything at work and getting back to life and would stop processing the cancer. In just the few weeks of my own therapy, I felt like I was regaining control and at least understanding all my feelings, and I wanted that for him too. For now, I knew we needed to keep our therapy separate, but eventually we would need to have some sessions together as we learned more about the impact of the cancer on our ability to have a family.

I had been focusing so much on my mental health, but I knew it was time to kick physical health into high gear. I saw a coworker limping around the office and she told me she had just started a new workout program and had done so many squats she was in pain. I knew it would be exactly what I needed and told her I'd go with her as soon as possible.

When I went to the first class, I felt out of place and huge. The fitness class was a split of weights, rowing and treadmill. There is nothing I hate more than a treadmill; it's literally a machine that charts progress yet without any results. You don't move anywhere. I almost threw up twice in the first class and was ashamed of my performance. I had never been this out of shape and had to literally look at myself in the mirror and accept my reality. The treadmills in the room are up against a mirror, and as I looked at the girl staring back at me while I attempted to run I didn't quite recognize her. She was lost but knew that this was where she needed to be. It might be slow, but 2016 was going to be a better year – mind and body.

The day before Tom went back to work, we had an appointment to understand the impact of cancer to our family and what could evolve in the year ahead. We had intentionally scheduled it before he was back at work and were eager to finally meet Dr. Neiderberger. I had written his name down days after Tom's diagnosis when our fertility doctor had called back and said he had told her that we should have some hope. This appointment seemed a bit early, but we had ultimately decided to meet with him to figure out what our situation might be. We both agreed that if we waited too long and the doctor told us we could have been taking some sort of medicine, or monitoring tests for the six months prior, we would have regretted not starting the discussion sooner.

We went in with the mindset of finding out what he would recommend. We would make any decisions based on the facts he gave us, good, bad or ugly. We got up early, and the whole drive talked about what could happen.

"I'm so nervous," I said as we got on the elevator.

"I know, me too. It is weird to go talk to someone about this," Tom replied.

"Well, we are in a better spot than most people that come see him. Some guys walk into this place with no idea what could be causing problems. At least we know it's the cancer and they can focus on solutions," I replied, with my eternal optimism that often drove Tom crazy.

"That's true," he said.

As we walked into the office area, we checked in and were escorted back to a small room. A while later, our doctor's resident walked into the room and asked us a few questions before our doctor came in. We explained our situation and then he said he wanted to look at Tom, but said it as he was moving his head in the other direction. I knew that he had just asked to do an exam, but Tom interpreted what he had said as needing to give blood and began taking off his jacket.

"No, I think he wants to do an exam," I said.

"Oh…" Tom said as he looked over at the doctor.

The doctor put out both hands directly in front of him and motioned his four fingers towards him, telling Tom to come towards him. Then, he turned his hand over and motioned his hands down for Tom to drop his pants. I started laughing to myself and had to look away because I could see the look on Tom's face. He did not think the doctor was about to make him drop is pants when he had taken off his jacket.

I looked up at Tom's face and tried to avoid making eye contact with the doctor. I let out a little whimper as I tried to stifle my laughter and looked at the opposite corner of the room. I turned my head back and saw Tom looking over his shoulder at me, trying not to laugh too. It wasn't that we were immature; I just didn't ever think I'd be standing in a room, my husband's back to me, his man jewels in the face of the doctor, and the doctor looking my way. Add to the situation Tom's face when he realized he had to pull down his pants instead of taking off his jacket, and I really was about to burst at the seams.

Tom's face was slightly turned towards me and he was intentionally making faces to try to make me laugh. I wanted to laugh but instead I looked down and took a few deep breaths, trying not to look foolish in front of this doctor. After what seemed like a long time, Tom was told he could pull up his pants and that the doctor would be in shortly. I held it together until I heard the click of the door behind the resident.

I laughed out loud as I looked over at Tom. "I'm not laughing at you, but your reaction to not realizing what he had said and that you thought he wanted you to take your jacket off."

"That might be one of the most awkward things that has ever happened to me," he replied, laughing just as hard as me.

A while later, our doctor came in and discussed our particular situation. He explained so many things to us and after a few minutes I was already suffering from information overload. After his initial monologue, he looked at Tom.

"And I hate to do this to you, but today you get a two for one," he said as he motioned for Tom to get up and drop his pants again.

It took all I had to not pee my pants in that chair. Luckily, the seriousness of what the doctor had just been telling us helped temper the giggles, but I did feel terrible that Tom had to once again endure the awkwardness.

We had both thought we would find out if kids were even a possibility for our future. He actually gave us plenty of reassurance in that department. While the odds were smaller, there were things that we could attempt to help Tom's hormones bounce back. He told us that the cancer could have been what caused the fertility problems beforehand, especially considering that Tom's cancer was a form of testicular cancer.

I felt more and more optimistic as he kept talking, but then he dropped the bomb. While research is still not 100 percent on any one recommendation, it's highly encouraged to not do any testing until one to two years after the completion of chemo. I almost passed out. It had never occurred to me that we would hear today that there is a chance, be it a small one, that we could still have a family, but that we would just simply have to wait. Ultimately, Tom's DNA had changed as result of the chemo, and it wouldn't be safe to harvest or implant any sperm until we had let enough time pass.

He was glad we had come to see him when we did. We would start hormone testing and begin some medication that would, hopefully, get us on the right path. In the meantime, we could weigh our options of adoption, using a donor, or waiting. He was incredibly patient with us, answering the many questions we had, explaining it all in a way that was somewhat easy to understand.

As he wrapped up, he asked us to take care of some blood work and then schedule a follow-up appointment the next month. We thanked him profusely for his patience and time with us, and he walked out of the exam room. We had to wait for his nurse to come back with the blood orders, but I wanted nothing more than to leave that room.

"I don't even know what to say," I said as I looked over at Tom.

"Yeah, this is crazy," he replied.

I knew he was likely feeling guilt about everything we had just heard and knew that some tough conversations would be ahead. The last thing I wanted was for him to feel guilty.

I grabbed his hand and squeezed it as I looked at him. "We are going to have a family come hell or high water. I think what caught me off guard most was the timing."

"I know, me too," he said.

He wasn't saying much and quite frankly I didn't want to say much either. Thankfully, the nurse walked in, gave us all our paperwork, and we were headed home.

I worked from home the rest of the day. I had been on some calls and doing work at the kitchen table for several hours. Around lunchtime, Tom came up, pulled the chair out across from me, and looked very seriously at me.

"How are you feeling about everything?" he asked.

"I don't know...still thinking about it," I replied.

"I worry about you," he replied, still unusually serious.

"Don't worry about me. I'll figure it out," I said as I smiled at him.

"You don't have to be strong for me, babe. This is hard stuff to deal with and try to comprehend, and it impacts us both," he said.

I knew he was right, but I wasn't sure what I wanted to say. I had tried to distract myself with work all day but thoughts raced through my head. Could we afford adoption? What if we had to use a donor? What if we just weren't meant to have kids? It didn't feel right putting that all on Tom today, and I knew the same thoughts were probably going through his head anyway.

"Listen, I said it earlier and I'll say it again. The timing is what threw me off today. The whole time we were fighting this thing, I just kept envisioning certain things and being back at the hospital pregnant was one of them. I want us to be the reason the hospital plays a lullaby over the loudspeaker," I replied, trying to not cry.

We had heard a lullaby play hundreds of times during our chemo sessions. When the hospital played a lullaby, a baby had just been born. Some days it was a beautiful reminder of new life, and the good things that can happen at a hospital, but other days it was a dagger in my heart.

I looked over at Tom, who was also trying not to cry as he nodded his head. "I know, babe, and we will be," he said. "I'm glad we made this appointment now, though, so we can do everything possible to be on top of the timeline and keep things moving."

"Yup," I replied. "Why don't you enjoy your last day without work," I said, trying to divert the topic. "Trust me. It's not all it's cracked up to be."

The next morning, Tom got ready for work, a strange new dynamic in our house. I knew he was eager to get back but also nervous about seeing coworkers and being the center of attention. He hated that. I felt sick to my stomach for him and wanted to protect him. I was a mess at work that day. I couldn't focus, and I didn't want to be hounding Tom via text to see how things were going. I really wanted him to feel "normal."

At 10:30 that morning I got a text from his boss with a picture of balloons and the text, "We are so happy to have our boy back!! He has been missed...and not for the work but for WHO he is!!" I almost cried at my desk.

Moments later I got a text from Tom saying they had ordered in lunch for the team to celebrate together. I took a deep breath and realized it had been silly of me to worry. Life might be headed back in the right direction.

I was wrong. The following week, we were back at the hospital. Tom had been throwing up all morning; he couldn't keep anything down; he had an intense headache, and he was very weak. I called our oncologist and they recommended we head to the ER. I felt sick to my stomach. What if the scans had been wrong? What if it was back? We had just had almost ten days of Tom back at work and trying to rebalance our lives. I feared we might be headed back in the other direction.

They scanned Tom, ran his blood work and filled him with fluids. The diagnosis was ultimately that he was doing too much too fast. Tom was less than eight weeks out of surgery, back at work, and expending infinite amounts of energy compared to the previous months. It was simply too much. His body was going into shut-down mode to try to regain control and gave him one nasty migraine as a reminder to stop. Our ER adventure had only been a few hours, but as we headed home, we both acknowledged that we needed to tone it down a bit and remember that we still had a long road to recovery.

"I know, I just haven't been able to do anything for so long I don't want to say no to anything," he said.

"I get it, but if spacing out the fun things ensures that we can keep doing them for years then that's what we need to do," I replied.

We drove home, Tom still feeling a bit miserable, and got him settled for some rest.

"No work for you tomorrow. Email Michelle and let her know you need to work from home," I said.

"I know, I will," he said, grabbing my hand as I walked by the couch. "I love you; I'm sorry," he said.

"Please don't apologize. I just feel sick going back to that hospital. We need to take it easy. I know that's easier said than done, but we need to be smart," I said as I leaned down and gave him a kiss.

The only thing easing my mind was that Tom was seeing our oncologist a few days later. While we had finished his blood thinner shots, he remained on a blood thinner pill for a bit longer. There was already an appointment for him to meet with her and determine if we could be done with blood thinners for good, so I was happy that she was going to see all his tests from our ER visit.

I hardly slept the night before his oncologist appointment but not because I was worried about something in particular. It was the first appointment in over six months that Tom was going to attend alone. Since it was just a brief check-in appointment to confirm he could finish up the blood thinners, it was silly for me to go with him. Tom kept reminding me that I couldn't go to every appointment with him for the rest of his life. Yet it kept me up that whole night. I considered going because I worried that she might have seen something from his ER scans. I had to remind myself the ER doctors said it was fine.

Tom texted me after his appointment that morning and said he was all clear – his blood looked good, and he was able to get off the blood thinners. Also, this meant that he could have an alcoholic beverage again – perfectly timed for the day before St. Patrick's Day and his little cousin's twenty-first birthday celebration that weekend.

That night when I got home, I was eager to hear what Doctor Sobol had said. It felt strange to have to hear it secondhand.

"How was the appointment? Quick, I assume?" I asked.

"Yeah, she was surprised you weren't with me," he replied with a smile on his face, knowing that would drive me crazy.

"I would have come!"

"I know, babe, but we are getting back to normal, and I finally feel like I'm starting to remember things again. It was fine, though we did end up talking about kids…" he said, his sentence trailing off.

"What about?" I inquired.

"I don't remember how it came up, but she encouraged us to move forward and not wait too long just to find out that we can't have kids the way we had planned," he said matter-of-factly.

"Interesting. I don't disagree with her," I said.

We had been having lots of conversations over the past few weeks since our appointment about our odds of having kids, and I valued her opinion. I just couldn't understand where my feelings were at and was eager to talk with my therapist the following week.

But before that, we had a big celebration to attend. Tom's cousin Kailee turned twenty-one on St. Patrick's Day, and to celebrate, the family did a train crawl on the commuter train. We got off at selected stops and would have a drink before the next train would come. The most important part was that there were fanny packs to wear and a fun group of people. We got to the first stop, and a beer was poured for Tom. He had waited to have a drink until he was with his cousin despite being given the okay to drink a few days prior. They clinked cups and began a wonderful day. We didn't think we would be part of this day just a few months earlier. Had the cancer still been active, as they had told us, we would just be finishing up the last round of chemo and unable to partake in the festivities. It was another beautiful reminder of how much he had exceeded expectations for every timeline they had given him.

Life seemed to always crash right before my next therapy appointment, which for the time being were every two weeks. I was eager to see Dr. Crane about all the fertility stuff, but I got a hit the day before the appointment that shifted my focus yet again. My dad had called after a doctor appointment and told me that they were worried about his blood test and were sending him to see an oncologist. I was driving home from work when he told me about the issue, and it took all I had to not pull over and throw up on the side of the highway. This couldn't be happening. I had just gotten Tom through this and the thought of watching my dad potentially suffer through cancer was almost paralyzing. The worst part was that his appointment wouldn't be for another ten days, as they needed to do some blood work.

I talked with my dad and tried to get him to tell me specifics about his blood counts. Not that I was an expert, but I certainly knew more than the average person at this point. He said everything would be fine, but I knew he was a bit worried. When we hung up the phone, I burst into tears.

Later that week, I eagerly attended therapy and filled Dr. Crane in on life. We first dove into everything with my dad and he assured me that I couldn't get too lost over the next few days. He suggested I take comfort in the fact that I could be a great help to my family. That's exactly what I feared.

"What scares you most?" he asked.

"I think that I would be relied on a ton, and I want to do that for my family, and I tend to be the peacemaker in the family, so I know that would be the reality, but I just…" I paused.

"Go ahead," he said as he nodded.

"I hardly feel like I can manage my own life right now. I feel like everything in such flux that another variable terrifies me," I replied.

I didn't want to admit that I wasn't feeling in control, but I really felt lost. Tom had been back at work for almost three weeks, but he was having a challenging transition, and the hospital scare hadn't helped. I wasn't letting go of taking care of everything because I didn't want him to overdo it.

"The reality is, you won't have to do anything until you get the facts from your dad's doctor," he said.

"I know," I replied, knowing he was right but not wanting to agree.

"What can you do in the meantime?" he asked.

"I'm headed to Milwaukee on Saturday to hang out with him for the day and hopefully keep his mind off things," I replied.

"I think that's great and something that will make you feel like you're helping. There is nothing else you can do right now," he said with a nod of his head, as if I had passed a test.

Then I moved on to the fertility. As I was finishing the bulk of the details, he asked me a rather blunt question, "How are you feeling about everything?"

"I mean, I guess I just wasn't expecting to deal with the time frame, but we will figure something out. Maybe it won't happen the way we had always envisioned it, but I still want to have a family," I said.

He took a deep breath, looked up at me with a skeptical face and called me on my bull. "How do you really feel?"

I stared at him for a moment. "Sad...gypped...lost...confused..." I replied.

He nodded his head, figuring that might be my real answer.

"And sometimes angry but not at Tom," I added.

"Then angry at what?" he asked.

"I know it's probably because of our situation, but some days I feel like all I see are articles or news features on abused kids, or kids being ignored. Like today there was a woman who works on my floor who was complaining about being pregnant, and it just angered me. I'd do anything to be pregnant right now," I said as I started to spin down the anger rabbit hole.

He listened and nodded as he took in everything I was saying and started to unload the other emotions too. It was the first time I had been honest with someone about how I was really feeling about the fertility. It wasn't that I was trying to deceive anyone else, but why would I ever put that on someone?

When I left that day I felt better, but was emotionally drained. I knew that Dr. Crane had come into my life at the perfect time. I would have had a full-on breakdown by now if I hadn't started seeing him. He was helping me process, he was helping me cope, and he was helping me understand what I was feeling – something I had ignored for months.

April

April showers are supposed to bring May flowers, or so I had been told growing up. What a bunch of crock that was; how silly to imply that you know what's coming. April needed to bring some calm, and instead, it felt like everything in our lives was brewing another mess. The first weekend of April was one that Tom had been looking forward to for weeks. His dear friend, and golf buddy, Nick, was coming to Chicago for the day to try out new clubs with Tom. The item on the top of his bucket list was finally going to be purchased – his new golf clubs. In the dead of winter, on the coldest of days, on the toughest of days for him, Tom would tell me he was thinking about his new golf clubs, and being cancer-free by spring to use them.

He went to bed the night before like a little kid at Christmas. He got to spend time with Nick and get new golf clubs, something that now had an especially strong symbolic meaning to him. I, on the other hand, wasn't quite as happy. I was going to get up the next morning and drive up to Milwaukee to hang out with my dad. I loved hanging with my dad but was scared for him. The results from his blood work would be back at the beginning of the week, and I figured some quality time wouldn't hurt.

I arrived in Milwaukee early on that Saturday morning. Dad and I went for a long walk, hung out at the family's bookstore and had some lunch. While he didn't really want to talk about his health, it would randomly come up at various points in the conversation. At one point, he told me that he had a great almost seventy years of life, so what would be, would be. I almost fell apart right then and there. One, because it was as if he knew something was wrong, and two, because it felt like he was throwing in the towel.

I had just spent months with Tom, who every day made sure he told anyone who would listen that he would beat it. It felt foreign to hear someone so resigned to a diagnosis – especially one he didn't yet have. Meanwhile, I was getting videos and texts, mostly in caps with an excessive amount of exclamation points, from Tom, who was having the best day with Nick. I was so happy that he was doing this and I was excited for him. I had a great day with my dad and headed back to Chicago that evening. I still couldn't be away from Tom for the night; it was too scary. I gave my dad a hug, told him I loved him, and that I was sure everything would be fine next week. I knew I'd talk to my dad at least five more times before his actual appointment, but telling him everything would be fine in person was more powerful.

I got on the road. I had about an hour-and-twenty-minute drive and called Tom to let him know I was headed home. He told me all about his adventure and asked how the day with my dad went – I said it was fine, and told him I'd see him in a little bit – intentionally cutting off the call. I had tears welling up in my eyes and just kept thinking about my dad. I took some deep breaths and rolled down my window for some fresh air. I had music playing; I should have known better. The music, and the day, got to me, and the floodgates opened. I sobbed for the entire hour I had left in the car, and not pretty-girl sobs, more like full-on hyperventilating, probably-shouldn't-be-driving sobs. I hadn't cried this hard in months. I had hit my tipping point and I just had to let out all the emotion. As I turned down my street, I tried to pull myself together, wiped my face and took deep breaths. I walked in the garage door and Tom was sitting on the couch in the basement area.

He looked up, saw my face and jumped up. "What's wrong???"

"Nothing," I sobbed as I dropped my stuff.

"Clearly, it's nothing," he said as he grabbed me for a hug. "Are you okay? Were you in an accident? Use words."

I just sobbed into his shoulder. He stood there, holding me up and rubbing my back as I tried to take some deep breaths.

"I'm scared for my dad," I said between attempts at breathing.

"He's going to be okay, babe. You need to breathe and calm down."

I stood there, still leaning on his shoulder, and took some deep breaths. He pulled his head back a little in an attempt to see my face. I cowered more into his shoulder because I was the furthest thing from beauty.

"Look at me," he said, with a giggle since I was hiding from him.

"But I don't want to," I said, as I begrudgingly lifted my head up from his shoulder. "Dr. Crane is going to be so mad at me."

Tom laughed. "Why is that?" he asked as he wiped tears off my face.

"I got lost in the land of what-ifs on my drive back. I'm supposed to only consider facts. Otherwise, I get all upset and then I get more stressed and more worried and that's not good for anyone, as you can see," I replied.

"Oh, boy," Tom replied as he hugged me again. "It's okay. You haven't cried in a while. Maybe you just needed that."

I knew he was right. "I know, but I'm mad about the situation with my dad, and mad at myself for doing exactly what I wasn't supposed to do. Maybe I just won't bring this little snafu up to Dr. Crane," I suggested as a small grin came across my face.

As he always does, Tom managed to get me to calm down and somehow laugh. I felt so bad that I had put a black cloud in his otherwise perfect day. As I pulled myself together, he showed me his clubs and told me all about his day. He was so excited, and I hoped that he knew how happy I was for him despite my red face, bloodshot eyes and random deep breaths. As we crawled into bed that night, I was feeling bad about my earlier meltdown.

"Sorry, I was such a hot mess earlier. I don't even know how to explain what happened. I just hit a breaking point and apparently needed to cry for well over an hour," I said to Tom as we got situated in bed.

"Don't apologize, babe. How many times have I cried in the past eight months and you've gotten me back to reality?" he asked.

"A lot," I replied as I smirked, knowing he would call me out on my exaggeration.

"Hey! I wasn't nearly as bad as I could have been for having Stage 3 cancer," he quickly replied as he defended himself.

"I know, I know. I'm kidding. That's why I was laughing. I feel like there is still so much to absorb and deal with; I don't quite know how to do it all," I said.

"You and I both," he said. "We are figuring out it as best we can."

I knew he was right, and as we fell asleep that night, I tried to focus on how lucky we were to be dealing with these emotions. These were the emotions of survivorship but with that came extreme empathy for anyone that might also be headed down that path – and that is where the roads had collided earlier that day.

The next day, it was as if my prayers had been answered. I got an email from Imerman Angels that I had been matched with a caregiver, Rachel. I was excited at the opportunity to help someone; it made me feel like maybe all our heartache could have been for some reason or purpose. I had been spinning the last few weeks, trying to answer the question of why this happened, and I wanted the answer to be black and white. I knew it was ridiculous, but I wanted the "why". I wanted there to be purpose in everything that had happened.

The email provided the information on my match and I immediately began crafting a message. Yet, I wasn't quite sure what to say because this wasn't a normal email. After painstakingly wordsmithing the note, I finally hit send. I had tried to put as much information as possible without scaring her, and set a tone that implied I was here to help. After I sent it, I sat in our office and felt sick to my stomach. I got a sudden flood of the feelings that I had experienced when I was in her shoes, just a few days into a life-changing diagnosis. It almost felt like I was feeling it all for the first time yet this time my body wasn't going into shock – it had already been there. I wondered about her family and support network. Was she close to family or were they on their own? I had so many questions but would have to patiently wait until she had time to reply, which I also knew might be a while.

A few days later I received a reply, and Rachel filled me in on everything they were dealing with. The situation was similar to Tom's and I immediately replied to answer several of her questions and also give her some insight into things she wouldn't have even known to ask. I wrote pages to her, but finished the email with something I wish someone would have told me when I was in her shoes. I wrote:

"You've got this. I know right now nine weeks of chemo and the unknown seem like a never-ending road, but you will do it. I know the sick feeling in the pit of your stomach that is so confused about how life can change so fast. Take it day by day, accept the help you need and don't be afraid to ask questions and be an advocate for your husband. Some doctors and nurses can be intimidating! You've got this."

I wanted to give her every ounce of reassurance that I wish I had when we were dealing with the diagnosis. I always knew we would do it; I never doubted that, but to know that another person like us had successfully fought it would have put that extra momentum in our effort and prove that it's possible.

That week, the good news was that my dad had been cleared and everything was okay. He had some health problems, but it wasn't cancer. I excitedly told Tom, and he was thrilled to hear the news too. He chuckled, "Your dad was trying to steal my cancer thunder!"

Yet it seemed that not everything could be good at the same time, I had been feeling sick and had pain in my abdomen. I knew I couldn't be pregnant, and the pain had been getting progressively worse. I finally caved and told Tom we needed to go to the ER. I couldn't handle it, and admittedly every ache and pain now scared me. How had Tom not known there was such a massive tumor in his chest? What if there was a tumor or something that I had no clue was there? I had tried to remind myself these were ridiculous associations, but knew why I was feeling that way. We couldn't go to the ER every time we had an ache or pain for the rest of our lives, but I did finally hit my breaking point and we went to the ER.

We got checked in, were taken to a room and I could tell Tom was starting to get antsy about an hour into our visit.

"Are you okay?" I asked.

"No, I hate watching you feel so sick; this is awful. I hate this place too," he replied.

I giggled and shook my head. "Don't even go there – you're one hour into a hospital visit. Imagine doing this for the last eight months!"

"Oh, I know! I have no idea how you did this. All I want to do is fix you," he sweetly replied.

They did some scans and quickly ruled out a burst appendix, but it was enlarged and positioned the wrong way. There was literally nothing I could do about the positioning; luckily, I don't have too much vanity about my internal organs. I got a bunch of fluids, was told to take it easy, and take some pain medicine. There wasn't much else they could do but follow up with my regular doctor. I felt like such an idiot. I knew we shouldn't have gone to the ER.

"I'm sorry – I feel like we wasted our time," I said as I was getting dressed again.

"Why? It was obviously something, and now we know why you're having the pain. If we hadn't come in and it was an infected appendix, we'd be having a whole different conversation right now. Better safe than sorry," he replied.

Better safe than sorry had a whole new meaning in our household and it was one that I felt a lot of fear about. I hadn't felt safe in eight months, and wished for the day that I felt any safety again.

Five days later, I was able to get in to see my regular doctor. After examining me and reading the discharge report, he told me that the ER visit notes had signified an enlarged appendix and that I never should have been discharged from the hospital. He insisted that I immediately go see a specialist at the hospital and get a CT done. I heard what he was saying but all I could picture in my head was the day Tom was diagnosed.

Tom met me at the hospital and waited with me as I sucked down the CT drink that I had seen him drink so many times. I finished my scans and was taken to a small waiting area down the hall. It was the same waiting area that I had waited in when Tom had his biopsy. I almost threw up because all the memories came flooding back. It seemed so long ago, but when I turned that corner I felt like I was right back in that moment.

A few minutes later I was escorted to a small room with a phone where the specialist I had seen earlier in the day would discuss the results with me. The appendix was alright, but my liver was covered in cysts – I had polycystic liver disease. There isn't anything you can do about it but it explained what might be causing some of the pain I was feeling. I was relieved it was nothing, and I wasn't going to worry about it since they told me not to. I had too many other things to worry about.

Our never-ending revolving doors of doctors continued later that week when we had our follow-up appointment with Dr. Neiderberger and our fertility doctor, Dr. Feinberg. We were getting an update on Tom's baseline blood with Dr. Neiderberger, and meeting with Dr. Feinberg to discuss our options. Dr. Neiderberger's office was like déjà vu–I thought Tom might be traumatized from his previous two-time pants dropping incident, but our appointment went well. Ultimately, things were trending up, and he gave me hope that kids might still happen for us one day. He wanted to do blood work again and see us in a month. It was a simple, straightforward appointment that gave me hope.

When we walked to the car, I quickly realized that while Tom and I had sat together in the same room, we had heard two different things. I, the eternal optimist, heard that there was a chance. Tom, the guilt-ridden recovering cancer patient who didn't trust his body at all, heard that there was a very small chance that wasn't worth being hopeful about.

"That went better than I thought," I said as we approached the car.

"Interesting. I think you're trying to just hold out hope and are just setting yourself up for more disappointment," he bluntly replied. I appreciated his honesty, because he usually wouldn't have said that so forwardly. It was another sign that his therapy was helping him cope and communicate what he was feeling.

"Really? I really feel like he gave me hope," I replied.

The ride home was a quiet one. I knew we both needed to process everything and that we'd eventually talk it out. I certainly didn't want to push it though, especially because he made his opinion clear about the likelihood of a positive outcome.

Two days later we met with our general fertility doctor, who we hadn't seen since the weeks before Tom had been diagnosed. The last time we talked was two days after the diagnosis and I remember her saying that she was looking forward to seeing us when Tom was cancer-free. Back in that moment it seemed so far away, but here we were headed into an appointment with her. I was already having a tough week. I still wasn't feeling great; we hadn't had the greatest appointment with Dr. Neiderberger. To top it off, my anxiety was at an all-time high as I was preparing to leave town for the first time without Tom.

We sat down in her office and filled her in on everything that had happened. She was so thrilled to see us back in her office. She pulled up all the notes that Dr. Neiderberger had sent over and asked how our appointment had gone when Tom suddenly got quite vocal.

"It was good. We are doing some hormone testing and obviously have been told about the timelines of everything," he said.

"I left feeling hopeful that there is a chance," I started to say until Tom interrupted me.

"I think she's hanging on to a small-percentage chance and not being realistic," he said matter-of-factly.

I looked over at Tom, and then turned back to the doctor. "I'm trying to remain realistic while still being optimistic. I know we've obviously taken quite the hit here, but am I silly to hold out hope?" I asked, looking at her so Tom didn't feel the need to reply.

"I know where you're coming from, and I would do the same thing, but I really do think it's a very small chance of this working out the way you two had intended," she replied with one of those calm, bad-news doctor voices.

I felt paralyzed for a moment. I didn't want to turn back to Tom and see an "I told you so" face but I wasn't quite sure what reply was about to come out of my mouth.

"Okay…so in your opinion, understanding where we are at with Tom's timeline and the results you're seeing, what would you recommend?" I asked. I honestly didn't want to hear her answer. I wanted to go curl up in a ball somewhere. I was so angry at the cancer right now.

"I would say we should talk about alternative options, like a donor or adoption," she said.

When I heard those words come out of her mouth, I stopped listening to what she was saying and instead started analyzing her job. I knew Dr. Crane would be mad if he knew I was doing this. Rather than deal with my own emotions, I started worrying about hers.

I had no idea how she could do this for a living – be the bearer of such bad news. Now, she also probably had euphoric days when a couple she'd been working with for years could finally get pregnant. But today, I wondered how she was feeling. What must it be like for her to have to sit across from us, knowing the last eight months of our lives, and deliver a message like that? We had been taking blow after blow for months. I felt like we would get punched and then right when we were back on our feet, we'd get punched again. Hearing her tell us her thoughts on our chances was like getting punched, hitting the ground, and getting stepped on. The scariest part was the feeling of not wanting to fight back. I just wanted to lie there. I didn't want to try to convince her to tell me otherwise, or remind her that any chance is some chance. I just sat there.

Tom jumped in and started asking some questions about our different options, and the processes for those options, but I didn't say much. I peppered in a question or two, but I kept looking at her and feeling lost. Over her shoulder was a bulletin board covered in birth announcements that she had received from patients. It added a background to her face that made me resent what she was saying even more.

We wrapped up our appointment agreeing to continue to see what happened with Tom's hormones and would let her know when, and if, we were ready for any next steps. As we left, we didn't stop at the desk to schedule our next appointment, since we didn't really need one, and that added a layer of sadness on top of my frustration.

Tom grabbed me for a hug by our cars. "I love you," he said.

"I love you too," I replied.

"Only too? Are you mad at me? You only say too when you're mad at me; you're supposed to love me more," he replied, trying to keep the conversation jovial.

"I just hate cancer, and I hate that these stupid numbers and ridiculous odds keep getting thrown out," I replied. My frustration was less at him, though I was a little annoyed he had put me on blast with the doctor for being optimistic.

"They aren't ridiculous. They have to be honest with us about everything," he replied, seeing me on the verge of tears.

"Yeah, well the odds of you getting cancer were slim to none, but we managed to defy those odds. I will never say it's out of the question if there is a single percent of possibility," I replied.

"I know, babe," he said as he pulled me in for another hug.

We didn't really finish our conversation and both headed to work. I tried to distract myself by thinking about what I needed to get done that day, but I just kept wandering back to everything we had been hearing about our fertility in the past few appointments. When my mind would wander back, my eyes would fill with tears. I wasn't sure why I wasn't just letting myself cry. When it came to the fertility stuff, I felt like crying was letting it win, and now it was letting cancer win a little bit too. I rolled down my window, took some deep breaths and blinked my tears away – for the moment.

The roller coaster kept twisting as I had to focus on my upcoming trip. Katie had her baby in early March, and I was eager to meet the little guy and have some girlfriends' time down in Cincinnati. It was about a five-and-a-half-hour drive, but that seemed like an eternity away and I couldn't convince myself to fully commit to going. Luckily, I had therapy later that evening and despite wanting to talk to my therapist about everything that happened with the fertility that morning, I needed him to help me figure out what to do about my trip. Tom wanted me to go, and assured me he would be fine, yet I was terrified to leave his side. I hadn't been away from him for months and while I knew I needed to start to shed the caregiver skin, I couldn't imagine what I would do if something happened.

"What are you scared of?" Dr. Crane asked me with the voice that assured me he was about to make a point.

"What if something happens when I'm away?"

"What would happen?" he replied.

"Anything, anything could happen. Life can throw a curve ball whenever it wants to," I replied. "But I'm most nervous about leaving and something happening to him and I can't be there with him right away," I replied.

I knew what I was saying sounded ridiculous. I never thought twice about a quick weekend away before Tom was sick. I wanted to make sure Dr. Crane understood that I wasn't completely ridiculous; that I had learned something. "I know we take risks every single day when we wake up; anything could happen at any moment," I started.

"So when you get up in the morning and drive to work, why is that different?" he asked.

"I guess it's really not. I've just accepted the risks that are associated with driving a car," I replied.

Sometimes I just hated how much sense Dr. Crane made. I knew he was right; we take risks all the time. If something was going to happen, it was going to happen, and I needed to start to be okay with getting back to our "normal" lives.

"What would make you feel better about going? Is there something that would help?" he asked.

I thought about it for a moment, "Not really, just staying in contact with him, but I worry that he won't tell me if something is wrong because he wants me to go so badly."

"What do you mean?" he probed.

"I am completely aware that this trip is just as much for Tom, even though he's not actually taking the trip. For months and months, he has felt guilt, felt like he has held me back and been the reason I haven't seen family or friends. I just don't want something to happen and him hide it because he doesn't want to 'ruin' my trip," I replied.

Dr. Crane nodded as I mentioned the part about this also being very important to Tom, and we discussed strategies for how I could make this as easy a trip as possible. Ultimately, I needed to tell Tom how I was feeling, keep in contact with him, and then trust Tom. Tom already knew how I was feeling and we always talk and text so that left the one other piece back on me. I needed to trust Tom and not be scared of the cancer. I knew it was time to shed the caregiver skin, but it had been every ounce of who I was for months. I didn't need to drop it all at once. I just needed to start gradually shedding it.

Two days later I got up and was getting ready for work with Tom. I was working a half day and then would be leaving from the office to head to Cincinnati. Tom had taken my bag and put it in the car for me, and was being extra positive about my trip. I gave him a kiss goodbye and got in the car. I pulled out of the garage and headed down the street and a wave of anxiety hit me. I found myself at the stop sign at the end of the street shaking. I hadn't even realized it until I lifted my hand to turn the wheel. I panicked and wondered if I shouldn't go, if this was a sign I should stay back. I thought about what Dr. Crane had told me and took some deep breaths. I headed into work and tried to stay focused on my morning of meetings.

At noon, I wrapped up and got in the car to head to Cincinnati. I sat in my car for almost five minutes staring at my steering wheel. Then I plugged in my phone and put Cincinnati in my GPS. It said five hours and forty-one minutes based on the current traffic. When I saw the time, I started feeling anxiety again and planned my options if something happened. If there was an emergency and I could get a flight back within an hour it would be smarter to fly home and then figure out my car, but if there wasn't a flight for a while I would speed the whole way home and apologize to any cop that pulled me over. I calmed myself down and reminded myself again that this trip wasn't just about me. It was also for Tom.

I got on the road and was listening to music and suddenly ended up in Cincinnati. It was one of those drives where I had been so lost in my thoughts that I hadn't even paid attention to the trip. I managed to only cry twice in the car. The first time I cried, I was thinking about being in the car alone headed to Cincinnati and realizing that if things hadn't gone our way, this could have been my reality. I had an "aha" moment realizing that the reason I was having such a hard time leaving was because when I was alone, it was a reminder of what life might have turned out to be if he hadn't beaten this cancer. I would have had to go on without him. The thought of it made me sob, but I was happy that I had realized part of the reason this trip had been giving me so much angst.

The second time I cried was because I was worried about seeing all my girlfriends. I felt like I had been such a difficult friend to have over the past few months, and I didn't want them to feel disconnected or feel like any of our relationships had suffered. My college girls are my tribe, and I didn't like the thought that I hadn't been pulling my weight. As I pulled into Cincinnati, I decided I was pretty impressed with myself. It was just short of a 400-mile trip and I had only cried twice. Every 200 miles wasn't a terrible ratio.

I got into town and got to see old friends and enjoy dinner. The next morning, all the girls, the husbands, and the babies met at the zoo for a day of fun. It was a blast and while I kept close to my phone and was always in contact with Tom, I really was trying to live in the moment and enjoy the time with my girlfriends. We explored the zoo, I kept snuggling the babies, and relished the fact that I could be there in that moment. Afterwards, we grabbed some food and were sitting out on the patio enjoying lunch. I looked down when I saw a text from Tom, "Just got rear-ended on I-90."

I looked at my phone and blurted out, "You have got to be shitting me!" I looked up and told my friends Tom had gotten in an accident.

I quickly replied to Tom, "What!? Are you okay?!"

He replied, "I'm fine," followed by "Cars."

I quickly peppered him with three texts, "Wait, what? You're okay?"

He replied, "Cops are coming. Guy behind me is at fault."

Tom said he would call me when he was done with the cops. He was the middle car in a three-car accident and the car was likely totaled. I sat at the table and my girlfriends were trying to keep me positive. This was exactly what I had been terrified of, and I had a hard time believing Tom was okay if his car was totaled. It was almost thirty minutes later before he was able to call me. I got up from the table and walked outside the perimeter of the patio.

"Hi, babe, are you okay?"

"I'm alright. The guy behind me got the ticket for both cars. I was the middle car and he was tailing me too close. When he slammed into me, I propelled forward and hit the car in front of me, which is why both accidents are his fault."

"Are you sure you're okay?" I asked again.

"Yeah, I'm a little shaken up, but I'll be okay. The cop let me drive the car home but told me I shouldn't drive it after that."

"I feel sick to my stomach; do you want me to come back? Be honest."

"No really, I'm okay. I'm going to head home now and I'll get some food delivered tonight or something. Please don't come back. Really, I'm okay," he replied.

"Okay…I'm going to trust you," I said to him. "Do you need me to call insurance or anything?"

"No, I called them while I was waiting. I'm dropping off my car Monday and they will have a rental there for me," he said.

I was so happy to hear that he was okay, and it really did feel like he didn't need me to come home. "Alright. If you change your mind, let me know. I can be home in five and a half hours – or about four illegally," I joked.

"I know, babe, thank you. What are you doing?" he asked.

"We are eating lunch," I said.

"Awesome – well, tell everyone I said hello – and I'll text you when I get home with my clunker."

I headed back to the table and sat down and filled everyone in on what I had heard and showed them the pictures that Tom had texted me from the accident. Everyone was smiling and being positive for me but all I wanted to do was cry. I felt helpless so far away but had to trust him.

We continued texting and later that afternoon I got a text, "I need to tell you…"

"Tell me?" I replied.

I saw the dots on the screen showing that he was typing back and then it appeared. "I was starting to get so bummed about how life just keeps kicking me in the balls and it's not fair and such…but I am incredibly lucky, because I have you."

I knew he was probably feeling like he couldn't catch a break. I certainly was feeling it from afar. With everything going on with our lives, we now had to add an accident, potentially a new car, and of course all the costs of deductibles, etc. I didn't care about the money; I cared that he was safe, but I knew a bunch more was being piled on our plate. More than anything, it was a reminder of what I had feared about even leaving. Cancer or not, something can happen every minute of every day.

I replied, "You're the sweetest – I'm the luckiest to have you."

He replied, "And thank you for not driving back."

"Well…." I said.

"You better not be!" he replied.

"Just teasing!" I quickly replied.

I gave him a quick call before I headed out to dinner. We were having a girls' dinner and I wanted to catch him to see if he had heard anything else from insurance. Tom reminded me that I had so callously not asked him if his new golf clubs were okay in the accident because they were in the trunk. I could tell he was at least taking it all with a bit of humor. He sounded a bit tired to me, but I knew he had a great distraction since it was Game 6 of the first round of the NHL playoffs for his beloved Blackhawks. My sports-obsessed husband would be just fine tonight with some takeout and his hockey.

"I'll call you after dinner, or call me before you go to bed if that's first," I said. "I love you!"

"Sounds good, I love you more and GO HAWKS!"

I rolled my eyes as I got off the phone and headed to dinner. We had dinner on a little outdoor patio tucked under a big tree. The weather was beautiful and there was a guitar player playing on the sidewalk near the restaurant. I had a great glass of red wine, and even better company. It was these types of moments that I had daydreamed about during Tom's chemo treatments. We kept pouring the wine and enjoying our evening. About half way through the night, I had texted Tom, "How are you doing?" I hadn't yet heard a reply. I figured he was deep into the Blackhawks game.

When we left the restaurant an hour later, I texted him again; still no reply. I was in the passenger seat explaining to Katie that I was getting worried as we headed back to her house. I tried to call him, but after ringing it kept going to his voicemail. I was starting to feel sick to my stomach. "I'm getting worried I haven't heard from you," I texted ten minutes after I called. I was toggling on my phone between checking to see if the Blackhawks were still playing and calling him. Since the game was still on, there was no way he wouldn't be awake. I sent a series of texts over the next hour and called him repeatedly.

"Don't make me call your mom…Babe?... I'm not trying to be a crazy wife but I haven't heard from you since 6 p.m. our time… You can't be sleeping with this Hawks game going on – please answer… Babe, seriously… I'm going to throw up…I feel so panicky right now – please answer…Please, babe…Tom, this isn't funny, please answer…"

I was sitting in Katie's living room, staring at my phone. She had just put the baby down and came down to see what was happening.

"I don't want to do it, but I think I might call his mom," I said to Katie.

"I don't blame you," she replied.

"What if he hit his head in the car accident and didn't realize it, or got more shaken up than he thought?" I said.

I was struggling because I wanted to give him his space and not be a crazy caregiver, but there was no way Tom would not be watching Game 6 of a Blackhawks playoff series, and more importantly, he knew I had struggled to leave town. He wouldn't have just stopped communicating with me.

I pulled up his mom's number and hit call. It was almost midnight in Chicago. She picked up and had clearly been asleep.

"I'm so sorry to be calling," I quickly said. "Have you heard from Tom?"

"No we saw him earlier when we dropped off one of our cars for him to use. The car was pretty bad, I'm surprised he didn't get hurt," she said.

"That's why I'm calling. I haven't heard from him since six and I'm worried maybe something happened," I said.

"Do you want me to go over there?" she offered.

"I think so. I'm so sorry. It's just that I'm worried and the Blackhawks game just finished…" I started saying.

"Oh, there is no way he would have not watched that. We will get in the car and go over there," she said as I heard her wake up my father-in-law. "I'll call you in a few."

Luckily, they didn't live far from us and she knew our garage code if she needed to get in.

I tried to patiently wait for a call. The time seemed to be crawling and the longer I waited, the worse the scenario I imagined.

Finally, the phone rang; it was Tom.

"Thanks, guys, sorry…" I heard him say as his parents left.

"Are you okay?!?!?!" I tried to hold back tears.

"I'm fine, I'm so sorry. I think the accident got me more than I thought. I actually fell asleep during the Hawks game. My phone was right next to me and I didn't hear a thing," he said, though it sounded like he was still sleeping.

"Did you hear the doorbell?" I asked.

"No, my parents came in the house. I didn't even wake up when the garage opened. They came in and shook me awake on the couch. Isn't that crazy? I never sleep like that," he reminded me.

"Yeah…crazy…" I said. "Go to sleep, and I'll call you tomorrow. Sorry to send your parents over. I was just so scared and never thought you'd sleep through the game," I replied.

"I know, apparently there is a first time for everything. That reminds me," he slurred, barely awake. "Did the Hawks win?"

If I weren't so emotional, I probably would have laughed. We said our goodnights and I shot back over to my texts. I typed to my mother-in-law, "Thank you so much – if he hadn't had the accident today, I wouldn't have been so panicked. I'm sorry to wake you but thank you thank you thank you. And I promise next time I call it won't be for something bad!" My mother-in-law had recently been joking that she's scared to answer my calls because they haven't been for anything good in the past months.

"No problem. I was worried after I saw the car, but he said he was okay." The only thing I could think of to reply was that I owed them a stiff drink.

By then it was almost two in the morning and I had to get up early for a breakfast before another five-and-a-half-hour drive. I only slept about an hour. Every time I closed my eyes, I pictured the car from his accident, or my in-laws going over to our house in the middle of the night. I felt so stupid for asking them to go over, but I would have felt more stupid if they hadn't and Tom had been in danger, or sick.

The next morning as I drove home, I thought about two things. First, the blog. I never should have stopped the blog when I did. Our life now was the part of cancer very few people heard about – the struggle to get back to normal, letting go of being a caregiver, and the challenges of transiting back to "real life." Tom was having a very hard transition, and this continued onslaught of chaos wasn't helping. We had been naive to think it was "over" back in February. In reality, the only thing that was over was his treatments and surgery. I was beginning to realize that the impacts of cancer would likely never end.

When I wasn't thinking about the post-cancer struggles and wishing I had kept the blog alive, I thought about what I would tell Dr. Crane about this crazy weekend. It forced me to think through my thoughts about what had happened. By the time I got home, I felt calm. In a way, I was glad something had happened. I was so worried that something might happen when I was gone, and we got it out of the way the first time I left him, and were lucky that it wasn't something that involved him being in the hospital. The accident had validated my fears, but more than anything confirmed that we would, and could, handle anything that came our way.

May

Life was picking up pace and moving fast, perhaps too fast for us. There were so many things happening, and it felt like they were all coming at once. We were busy catching up with friends that we hadn't seen nearly enough, and adjusting to normal life. Through all the smiles and fun we were having, we were very focused on May 5. Tom was having his first post-cancer three-month checkup and we had no clue where the three months had gone.

Three days prior to our appointment, Tom completed his scans. When we saw our doctor, we'd get the results of his blood work and scans. While we assumed everything would be fine, it was challenging to get through that week. Our anxiety was building; the nights were sleepless, and the elephant in the room was if the cancer was back. Our miraculous "all clear" diagnosis was now the devil on one shoulder putting doubt in our minds that this appointment wouldn't go as we had hoped. We laid in bed the night before, restless and ready for the next morning.

"Feeling good about tomorrow?" I asked.

"Yeah. I just want it to be all good and over," he replied.

"I know. It will be good. We will go in, get the all clear, and then not worry about it for a while," I naively said.

"I hope so…" he said as he squeezed me tight in bed.

"That is what will happen and then we have the big party to celebrate!" I exclaimed, reminding him of the upcoming party.

Since early March, I had been planning Tom's Cancer Survivor Party. The party was going to be on May 21, four months to the date from when he was declared cancer-free. We had picked the date back in March when we were still in the honeymoon phase of post-cancer life and hadn't quite realized what a challenge our transition back to normal would become.

"Ha, that would be a pretty depressing party if we don't get the all clear tomorrow," he joked.

"I know, right? Can you imagine? I'll add that to my list of things to worry about tonight."

Deep down, I felt we would be okay, but the feelings didn't override the nerves. Sleep just wasn't on the agenda that night.

We got up the next morning and got ready, floating about the house both anxious and irritable. It wasn't our usual banter or goofiness. It wasn't how I wanted to start the day but knew it was where we both needed to be to make it through. We got ourselves to the doctor and sat in the depressing waiting room. As I looked around, I tried to stay positive and remember that a few months earlier we weren't sitting here for a checkup with a full head of hair; we were sitting here grasping for our lives back.

As we waited in the exam room, we hit our breaking point. We both were antsy and we wanted this to be done. More than anything, we just wanted the weight off our shoulders. Finally, our doctor walked in and immediately said, "Everything looks great!" before closing the door. Clearly, she had learned to get right to the point in her years as an oncologist. I squeezed Tom's hand and immediately felt relief. His scans looked great, his blood work was fantastic, and we sat and chatted with her as she checked Tom's vitals.

As expected, she asked how things were going with a family. We filled her in and got her valuable perspective on this topic. Ultimately, she encouraged us to move ahead with alternative options and not wait too long for any next steps. Tom and I had been tossing around the idea of just moving on, but to hear her so bluntly be an advocate caught me a little off guard. I was too exhausted and had too much on my mind to contemplate what she was saying.

Our appointment wrapped up, and we gleefully walked down the hall to the exit. I gave him a kiss as we walked down the hall, passing the rooms of people fighting this awful disease.

"I'm so glad that's done – and as we thought – you continue to kill it!" I proclaimed.

"I'm just glad it's done and that it's a great result," he replied.

As we turned the corner, we were greeted by the receptionist who quickly remarked, "Okay, so let's get you set up for three months from now…" as she clicked away in her scheduling system.

My heart broke into a million pieces. I had only been able to relax for the walk down the hallway before I was slapped in the face with the reality that this was going to be part of our new life. We were going to have this monster come in and out of our lives for months – no, years – to come. I had gotten so overjoyed with our good news that I forgot it wasn't a one-time event.

I had a lump in my throat as I softly replied, "Yes…"

I looked up at Tom who was equally jarred by our reality slap. "That just took the wind out of those sails."

Tom nodded as we pulled up our calendars to schedule our next appointment. We had until August 4th before we had to confront the monster again. Our emotions were still on high that night and into the next day, and the timing couldn't have been worse.

****

"Are you sure you're ready for this?" I asked, getting worked up about what we were about to do.

"Yeah, I think I'll be okay," he replied.

I wasn't so sure. We had been practicing and I had written a speech, but in our preparations over the past few days I knew discussing his diagnosis was bothering Tom. We were in the car and headed to a Relay for Life event, where we were the guests of honor. A family friend, Theresa, is a teacher at a high school and asked us to come speak and tell our story for their cancer awareness fundraiser. She had asked us back in March and the date had seemed far enough away that we hadn't thought twice about it at the time.

As I had been preparing our speech, there were parts that Tom couldn't describe without getting nauseous. Then, a day after the first post-cancer scans, we were going to stand up and tell our story to a bunch of strangers. We kept reminding ourselves that this was good for us, and that it was for a good cause. Because parts of the speech were challenging for Tom, I thought it was best if we went back and forth as we told our story with a slideshow. I was worried that Tom would get nauseous and that talking about it would be too much for him – not to mention the fact that he told me he was a terrible public speaker.

I don't have a problem speaking in front of a group of people. Tom, on the other hand, wasn't as comfortable, and I knew that was part of his concern. As the auditorium lights dimmed, memorial candles lit the room for people that weren't lucky enough to be standing and telling their story of survivorship. We stood at the bottom of the stairs off the stage. No one could see us as we watched the event planners introduce us. Tom and I held hands and kept whispering encouraging words to each other. After a brief intro, we were called on stage.

Tom and I walked on stage, and I put our speech down on the podium. The lights were bright and we could hardly see the faces in the audience as our eyes adjusted. We had an audience full of high school kids, parents and the faculty. I looked at Tom, he smiled and nodded, and I took a deep breath and began our speech. I introduced us and told the beginning of our story and the diagnosis before handing it off to Tom to explain what it felt like to be told you have cancer. I waited to see what his public speaking would be like. I was ready to take over if necessary.

"I'm not sure how to describe this, but being told you have cancer is the most surreal experience and still doesn't feel real most days. Of course I knew what cancer was, and have had family members not survive cancer, but it doesn't feel like it could ever touch you. I was very scared and in shock. It actually took a while for me to even cry because I couldn't believe what was happening. It was harder to watch my family as they found out and see my wife try to pick up all the pieces of our life. I didn't know what questions to ask and felt paralyzed. However, that night my wife and I decided we were going to beat cancer. I was numb and in shock but had every intention of beating it."

As Tom wrapped up his section, I was in complete awe at what an amazing job he was doing. I could tell he was nervous, but those who didn't know him well wouldn't have known. As he finished his sentence, I reached down from the podium and squeezed his hand. I was so proud of him already. I continued with my next part.

"For me, as the caregiver, being told that Tom had cancer seemed impossible. Unfortunately, cancer doesn't care who you are, what you do, how old or young you are, your personal circumstances, or your life story. As a caregiver, I had to immediately get into planning mode. I was scheduling doctor's appointments, a port surgery and chemo treatments. I was canceling our plans for the coming months including vacations, figuring out what we were going to do about our jobs and sustaining our income. I was dealing with insurance to figure out our coverage and preparing for a crazy few months. In a way, I didn't really get to process the cancer right away because I had so much on my plate. However, I was terrified. I was scared that maybe we had caught it too late and that Tom wouldn't be here; I was afraid of what it meant for our future…"

I started to get choked up. I had spent so much time making sure that Tom was going to be okay, I hadn't even considered my own feelings. When I got to the word future, I had to stop and catch my breath. I looked over at Tom and he smiled and put his hand on my back for encouragement. I took a few deep breaths, composed myself and continued before passing it back to Tom to talk about what chemo felt like.

"Chemo is hard to describe, but to put it simply it's like having the worst flu ever with a bunch of side effects. It is constant state of nausea, exhaustion and confusion. There is no way to focus on anything – I remember thinking before treatment that I would be able to read books, but I was so sick that I couldn't focus on a page – some days it was even hard to watch TV. I was completely focused on trying to not throw up or feel so sick. It consumed me. On top of that, there are terrible side effects. The most common one that people associate with cancer is hair loss, and I lost all of my hair. After my hair fell out, when I looked in the mirror, I didn't see myself anymore. That was very tough."

As Tom talked, I looked out into the audience, thinking about these kids. Some of them were only ten years younger than me. I remember being in high school and not having a care in the world. I was excited for my next part, as it got us back into the good news. I told everyone we had just had his first clear scan the day before and they began to clap and cheer as Tom started his next part.

"I am so lucky that I only had to fight this for less than a year. It was a very intense time, but many people fight cancer for years. The side effects will continue as I've had permanent hearing damage and tingling and numbness in my feet and hands. As you can see, my hair came back – though now it is curly, which is common for some cancer patients. These side effects are a small price to pay for having beat this disease and being able to continue to live my life."

I started my last part, eager for our speech to be over, and a success, without any more tears.

"We learned so much through this situation – about ourselves, about each other and about the power of the people who love us. Thinking positively and choosing to accept your situation but not let it define you is so important. When we were asked to speak tonight, they mentioned your theme this year is hope. So the obvious question is how did we keep hope, and how did we get through the hard days. I will tell you that hope isn't a selfish thing. We had hope for ourselves, but we also had to have hope on behalf of all the people who never had the chance to outlive their diagnosis and had to resign themselves to the fact that their fight would end. Moving forward, we are working hard to give hope to others by getting involved and giving back."

Tom closed the speech, and I had a smile on my face as he did. I knew he was getting energy from standing up and telling our story. I was too. The audience clapped, and we walked off stage. Tom led the way down and I followed. When he got to the bottom, he turned around and I jumped into his arms. We were on the side of the stage and no one could see us. I wrapped my arms around his neck and pulled away for a kiss.

"I can't believe you said you were a bad public speaker – you were amazing!" I whispered to him as I gave him another kiss.

"Was that okay?" he asked.

"More than okay – you did amazing. I'm the schmuck that ended up getting choked up!" I replied.

We were both beaming and stood there for a moment hugging. I could feel our hearts beating fast as we took a couple of deep breaths. I motioned for us to go take a seat in the front row as they finished the ceremony. The last part of the ceremony was a slideshow of all the people that the kids were raising money for who had lost their lives due to cancer. Tom and I slid into two seats and watched as the music played and the pictures were displayed. A few minutes in, Tom had tears coming down his face.

I squeezed his hand and leaned into him. "You okay?" I asked.

"There are too many names," he replied. He stated it perfectly. There were too many names. People who had battled cancer, but not been as lucky.

"I agree – it's reminding me how lucky we are," I replied as I put my head on his shoulder.

The ceremony ended, and the beginning of the Relay began. Teams of students would walk the entire night to symbolize that cancer never sleeps, and we joined them for the honorary lap to kick off the relay. I felt like everyone was watching us as we walked, but they were silent and respectful – I was so impressed that these high school kids felt compelled to do something to help find a cure. Once we got back into the main area, we spoke with several people who thanked us or wanted to hear more about our story. My heart was full because we had done something good from our crummy situation. At the end of the night, we got into the car to head home and both took a deep breath.

"Hard to believe those kids will be walking all night," I said to Tom. "I'm glad it's over for the sake of my nerves, but I felt really good about doing it."

"Me too – it's just strange to talk about it in the past tense since it feels like we are still very much in the fight," he replied.

"I know, I was thinking the same thing. I know we both got into conversations with different people, but I met some really nice people who had some very positive things to say."

"Did you talk to that guy with the plaid shirt on?" he asked.

"Briefly. What a story," I replied.

"He came up to me, shook my hand, and told me how inspired he was. He's been fighting cancer for eight years. Eight years," Tom said as he shook his head.

"Oh gosh, he didn't tell me all those details. He shook my hand, wished us the best, and mentioned he had talked with you for a while," I replied.

"I don't feel like a survivor," Tom said.

I almost drove off the road. "Are you serious? Why would you say that? You're a survivor!"

"I only had cancer for one hundred twenty days. I feel like I cheated. You meet people like him and it makes you realize how easy we had it," he replied.

"That blows my mind. We did not have it easy. You had one of the most intense chemo treatments, and had it twenty times in twelve weeks. Twenty times. Sure, your active cancer time may have been short, but I don't think we got off easy," I replied.

"I know. I just can't imagine someone dealing with this for years. I mean, I know I'm a survivor..." Tom trailed off.

"I'm so proud of you," I said as I leaned in and gave him a kiss.

We talked together the whole way home and were happy that we had agreed to do the speaking event. It was the first time that we told our story out loud, and it felt like we owned the story, like we had taken our own narrative back. For months, cancer had been telling our story. Cancer had been dictating what we did, but that night we stood up and told our story and more importantly told it as if we had a choice. While cancer had determined the fate of our story for a while, we never gave it the right to decide how we had handled it.

The next morning I was sitting in the salon chair staring into the mirror.

"Are you ready?" she asked as she looked at me through the mirror.

"Yup – let's get it donated!" I exclaimed.

In less than three seconds nine inches of hair was chopped and donated for cancer wigs. I hadn't done much with my hair in the last year other than let it grow out and once Tom was diagnosed, I was determined to donate it.

The only problem with my plan was that I wasn't good at relaxing or being pampered. I was getting highlights because one of the symptoms of Tom's cancer was gray hair for me. I couldn't sit still this long and I texted Tom, "I'm so bad at taking care of myself and relaxing...but get ready for a wife with short hair again!"

"Try to enjoy a few minutes with just your thoughts. You are so amazing, donating hair and beating cancer with me, just think about all the laughter we get to share for the rest of our lives." He was so darn sweet sometimes.

I managed to suffer through an hour and a half in the chair and then headed home. I got in the car, looked at my hair and loved it. I ran my fingers through it and looked at it for a minute before bursting into tears. These weren't the kind of tears that you felt coming either – they came out of nowhere. I felt so light. I never thought my haircut would be such an emotional moment, but it felt like I was saying goodbye to that chapter. I felt like I had just cut those bad memories away. It was refreshing.

I had felt this feeling a week earlier, too, when we got a new car after Tom's accident. I was so glad to see his old car gone. It felt like we were starting things fresh. I never thought a material object or my hair being gone would provide such a sense of relief, but they did. In my perfect world, we would sell the house too because lately that hadn't been full of many great memories. It was an intense desire to start everything over, to start fresh, as if it would somehow erase what had happened.

I knew Dr. Crane would tell me this was normal, or at least I hoped. When I saw him the following week, we discussed how our speaking event went, the scans and the chaos of our lives for the past two weeks as we recovered from Tom's accident. He could hardly believe how crazy things had become but assured me that everything we were feeling was normal.

"I feel like I'm having a hard time with what we hear versus what we feel," I told him.

"What do you mean?" he probed.

"I feel like when we told our story, I started to realize the magnitude of what happened. It's really crazy when you think about it. And Tom made an interesting comment about talking about it in the past tense...I don't know, I guess I'm just having a hard time reconciling what everyone is telling us like 'you guys are amazing role models,' 'you are doing so well,' 'his hair is back,' and matching that to what we feel. It doesn't match up," I replied. Before I let him speak again I continued, "It's like everyone says all these nice things, and they all truly mean the world to us, but then I just want to look at them and tell them that's not how we feel – you have no idea what our lives are like right now. His job is the perfect example. Someone comments, 'I can't believe you're back at work and back in the swing of things so soon,' when the reality Tom is struggling at work. He's not sure what he wants to do, where he wants to do it, and is starting to flounder a bit."

I had just word vomited quite a lot to him, and he patiently helped me work through it all. In a way, we had created a happy exterior to keep everyone around us from worrying, but behind the scenes, things were rough.

Things only got rougher when we had our first real argument in months. Tom was supposed to do blood work for a fertility appointment, and it had to be within a certain time frame so they could track progress accordingly. He had told me he had done the blood work and would schedule the follow-up. I eventually asked enough questions and found out that he hadn't done the blood work, had missed the window, and had lied to me about it all.

I was so upset and I shut down. For months, I had done every single thing in my power to make things as easy as possible for him, taking care of everything, and making sure that everything stayed in order. I never asked for a thing in return and I never wanted anything in return. However, the one thing that he knew meant more to me than anything was that we kept on top of the fertility testing so that we could keep making progress. His lying and lack of follow-through felt deceitful. I doubted everything he had said to me about wanting a family, about fighting this for us and for our future. I was crushed. I did the only thing I could do and grabbed my keys and left.

I drove around for a while, furious, crying, and sad. I had the windows down, the music playing and kept driving. I tried to get myself under control and then did what I always tried to do when we had an argument – tried to put myself in Tom's shoes. Why would he have done that? Why did he feel like he had to lie? I was more upset about the blatant lying than him not doing the blood work. Once I had some time away, I pulled back into the garage. Tom was in the kitchen as I walked up the stairs.

"Hi," he said, very somber.

"Hi," I replied, with a lack of happiness in my voice.

"I'm sorry," he replied with tears in his eyes.

"Why did you lie? I'm honestly more upset that you lied. Are you scared to tell me something? Have I been anything but understanding for the last seven months? Why did you lie?"

"I just…" he started to say but stopped himself.

"Just what?"

"I just…" his cliffhanger approach to this was making me even angrier.

"You asked and I just said yes for some reason, and I just…"

I looked at him and stared. I wasn't going to play games, or dance around the truth. I just stared.

"I just don't want to know the truth. I'm scared. You deserve better than this. You should go marry someone you can have kids with. I know we need to do this, but I also know that every appointment gives us more information that is hard for you to hear, and I feel so much guilt about all of this…"

I stood in the kitchen, looking at him trying to hold back tears, and my anger transformed into sympathy. He didn't want to deal with our reality, so he avoided it. It wasn't my favorite approach, but I certainly understood why he had done what he had done and could at least believe that he didn't do it as an insult to me.

"I understand, but you can just tell me that? Please don't lie. We still have a long way to go, and we can't add lying into the mix or we might not make it out on the other side together with our sanity. I love you so much. I'm not going anywhere, but you have to know how much that just hurt."

While I felt sympathy for him, I also wanted him to know that it wasn't easy for me to swallow, and that he had hurt me. This was a hard transition because for months I had kept my own emotions on the back burner. I had tried to keep my feelings out of the spotlight so people didn't worry about me, especially Tom. I didn't want him to worry about me, but as I was trying to deal with everything now, I was realizing that it wasn't the best approach to have taken because rather than keep them out of the spotlight I had buried them, and now, I felt like I hadn't had a voice for months.

We had survived our first argument since he had cancer, and were eager for our first big adventure later that week. I had to be in Dallas for a conference for work from Monday to Wednesday, so we were flying out to Dallas on Friday for a long weekend. We needed this time away more than ever, but for me it was going to be especially challenging. I had barely survived my first weekend away from Tom a month earlier, and this was the first time I was going to be a plane ride away. Tom was going to be flying back Sunday night, and I wouldn't be home until Wednesday. I was having so much anxiety and hoping we didn't have another incident like the previous month. On top of everything else, the Saturday after I returned was the big Cancer Survivor party that I was throwing for Tom. To say it was going to be crazy was an understatement.

We arrived in Dallas early Friday morning, immediately started our sightseeing, and had so much fun exploring a new city. As we crawled into the hotel bed that night, we both realized what a difference a change of scenery made. A hotel room and a different bed was a treat. It felt like old times, a weekend getaway. I had missed going on adventures with him.

Saturday was another chock-full day, which included the baseball game that night. We had hit the pavement pretty hard which was evident Sunday when Tom asked to go back to the hotel before his flight. He had run out of gas. It was the slap-in-the-face reminder that while we had been able to get away briefly, we were still far away from the "way it was." The timing was terrible because he was boarding a plane that night. I felt sick to my stomach and considered going back with him so he wasn't alone.

"I'm sorry," he said as he looked at me from the bed.

"Don't apologize, it's okay," I replied. I wasn't mad at him, just frustrated with cancer.

"I'll be fine at home. I don't want you to worry," he said as he fell asleep.

I knew he would be fine; I knew I needed to just power through the next few days so we could continue to make progress together, but it still scared me. He woke up a while later, and I walked him out to the rental car that he was driving back to the airport. I was worried about him, and he was worried about me, but I eventually stopped hugging him and he left, feeling a bit better than he had that afternoon.

I headed back to the hotel room and pulled out my computer to start looking over my list of things that needed to get done before the party. We had invited so many people and were shocked by the response; we were expecting close to 140 people at our house. Some family were flying in, and many were driving in from Michigan, Ohio, Kentucky, and Wisconsin. I had already ordered a tent, tables, and chairs to be delivered for the backyard. I had a plan for all the food and drinks, Tom's mom was taking care of the cake, and I had recruited Tom's aunt to help with centerpieces and décor. I had all the tablecloths, tableware, and anything else that I could get done ahead of time. The last place I needed to be for four days before this party was in Dallas because there were so many things that needed to be done. The kicker was that a last-minute work trip to Houston had been added to my schedule the Monday following the party. I was already running on empty, and knew the week ahead was going to be especially draining.

I survived the conference and returned home on Wednesday. Tom eagerly picked me up from the airport and it was like our old days of dating long distance. Given the last nine months of our life, three nights away had felt like an eternity. For the next few days I cranked out work during the day and then worked on the party details late into the night.

The day of the party I was nervous. I suddenly had doubts about throwing the party and wanted everything to go smoothly. There were going to be many people we hadn't seen since Tom had been sick, and I was worried about all of the emotions that would be floating around. With the help of family, we had all the last touches on the party ready to go in time for the guests to arrive. We had set up corn hole and games in one area of the backyard and had tons of food and drinks around too, along with a giant frame on an easel. In the frame was a piece of board that read "In Memory of Those Who Didn't Get Their Cancer Survivor Party." I wanted to have a place where everyone could take a moment to remember someone who didn't get their survivor party. I felt that it was important. We weren't just having this party for Tom but for many others too.

One of Tom's favorite things was the cake and cake pops – his mom wanted to do the cakes and Tom had requested a cake that looked like a torso with his scar so that he could cut into his scar. He even got an upgrade because the cake had six-pack abs. In addition, my mother-in-law had cake pops made in the shape of different sports balls including footballs, baseballs and golf balls, with a sign that said, "It Takes Balls to Beat Cancer," which not only was true but a perfect pun for someone who had beat a form of testicular cancer.

One of the most important people to show up that day was Mother Nature; we got a perfect day. Our friends and family weaved in and out over hours of fun, and it felt like a dream. In a way, it was like having a second wedding. Tom and I divided and conquered to make sure that we were able to thank everyone for coming but about halfway through the party, I gave a quick speech. I felt that it was important to thank everyone, and have a toast to Tom and all the people who were listed on the poster board that didn't get their parties. As I looked out, I saw a sea of faces and it stopped me dead in my tracks. I felt overwhelmed with the love. They had come from near and far because they wanted to celebrate with us; they wanted to remember someone they loved and they wanted to be at a party like this, and it was a party of joy.

We partied late into the evening and our hearts were full. As the final guests left, we crawled into bed, completely exhausted from the day. I curled up into Tom with my eyes barely open.

"What a day," I said.

"What an overwhelming day," he replied.

At the time, I thought overwhelming was a good thing, but I soon learned it would take us down an incredibly dark path.

The Monday after the party I was on a flight to Houston. I only had to be gone for one night, but I was quite uneasy. The party had worn us both out, and Sunday had been a strange day, as Tom had pretty much been down for the count. Not only was the party a very long day, it was an emotional one too. We had expected it to be emotional and had expected to be worn out afterward, but our emotional exhaustion far exceeded what we had imagined. On the plane that morning I looked out of the window, exhausted, but unable to sleep. I was nervous. The anxiety of being away was building and the plane started to feel very small. I tried to channel Dr. Crane and took some deep breaths. I tried to shift my focus back to work.

As I walked into the hotel room later that day, a text popped up. It read: Hey, Honore – would you have any time to talk on the phone this evening? Having a pretty hard day – it's totally okay if you're busy. It was Rachel – the caregiver I was mentoring. I dropped my bags and immediately called her. We had been exchanging tons of emails, but hadn't yet chatted on the phone.

After a few rings I heard her pick up the phone, and her voice was exactly what I had expected. It was a strange moment because I felt so close with her given all our communication back and forth. She unloaded to me that she was having an especially tough day because test results came back less than ideal. It was almost the exact situation that had happened to us on Christmas Eve. I felt for a moment that I was back on that day as she explained her feelings. I tried to comfort her by explaining how the same thing had happened to us, but the tests had been wrong. We talked for almost an hour, and with each passing minute I felt stronger. I felt like my ability to help her was helping me work through our own situation too. It made me feel like a pro instead of an amateur, and with so much emotion in the past few days, I had barely felt like an amateur. More than anything, it made me hear myself say out loud that we had beaten it, and that they would beat it too. My heart was the happiest it had been in a while because I had been able to pay it forward.

As we finished chatting, I realized I was an external processor. I felt more content than I had in weeks because I had talked with someone who understood my situation. In my efforts to help her, I was helping myself too, and it was fulfilling. I walked downstairs and headed to the bar to meet up with my coworkers. We had a long meal and I kept catching my mind wandering. No one knew how heavy my mind was, how much I wanted to call Tom and fill him in on my conversation with Rachel, how much I just wanted to hug him and thank him again for how hard he fought. Yet I had become a professional at smiling and getting through, so that's exactly what I did.

The next afternoon I was back on that plane, almost home to Tom, and eager to see how he was doing. He hadn't sounded great on the phone, so I was getting a little worried. I knew I was struggling with my own emotions after the party, so I imagined he was too. On top of everything, he was having a hard time at work. His transition was less than smooth and the pile-on effect of so many things happening at once worried me.

At work the next day I got a text from Tom that his boss's mother-in-law was diagnosed with cancer and that he had made it through talking to her but then cried in his office. I picked up the phone and called him. I could tell he was still upset.

"I'm sorry, babe – are you okay?" I asked. Michelle was his boss, and he didn't know her mother-in-law, but I knew this was likely striking a chord with him, as she was one of the first people to be diagnosed since he had been sick.

"I just can't stop thinking about Day One, going to random doctors to hear more shitty news," he said. "If I close my eyes, I think I'm back in the hospital – it's just so scary," he replied.

I could hear the sadness on the phone. I wanted to help him, but deep down I knew there was nothing I could do other than support him. He was going to have to work through those emotions.

Later that evening, I sat in Dr. Crane's office, on the verge of tears.

As usual, he started with, "How are you doing?"

I usually tried to start slow, but I couldn't. "Tom is really struggling at work. I'm having a hard time processing everything that happened with the party. Tom called me from his office today practically paralyzed upon hearing about someone else's diagnosis, and I miss our old life," I answered.

"Tell me about the party. Did something bad happen?" he asked.

I wasn't quite sure where to start with the party so I rambled, "The party was amazing. We were surrounded by 140-plus people, the weather was amazing. Everyone was so happy, but I have not felt good about it since we had it," I replied.

"Not good?" he asked.

"I can't really put my finger on it, other than to say I'm not sure what we were celebrating. I mean I know what we were celebrating, but I'm also not sure. It was weird to see the reactions of people whom we haven't seen, and everyone's comments made me realize the magnitude of what we have been through. Some days we took it hour by hour, but I guess as I step back and realize everything we did, it really is pretty crazy. I don't know. I just feel so emotional about it all."

"That's normal; it was a big day for you both. Talk to me more about what you were celebrating..." he asked very slowly and deliberately.

"I'm scared that I don't know what we are celebrating yet," I bluntly replied. I hadn't even thought of that reply it came out of my mouth and surprised me as much as I'm sure it surprised him.

"Scared?" he probed.

"How can we celebrate something that we don't even understand yet? I thought we understood it all, but it's clear we didn't. Tom didn't beat cancer; he beat his diagnosis. Cancer is still around, it's still haunting us, and it's still terrorizing our ability to make decisions or sleep well at night. What if we can't have kids – did we just have a big damn party to be happy about that? Were we stupid to just spend well over a thousand bucks on a party and not just donate it on his behalf to help with research? Maybe I'm overthinking it; I'm probably overthinking it. I don't know. During the party I just felt so surrounded by love and support. We were on cloud nine, but if I had anticipated this aftermath, I'm not sure I would have still had the party. I just feel lost. Lost is the right word – maybe not scared but lost."

"Explain more about the lost feeling," he asked.

He was good at making me talk things out to have my own revelations. I hated it some days and loved it other days.

"I thought that we would have this party, four months after he was declared cancer-free; we could celebrate with friends and family, thank everyone for the support and then have some closure. Yet there was no closure at all. Instead the party was a smack in the face – this was our reality, this was what happened. I distinctly remember looking around at one point and wondering if it was a dream. Was I really twenty-eight years old, having a Cancer Survivor party at my house for my thirty-one-year-old husband? It felt foreign, almost like I was watching from the outside. It was a strange moment to feel so lost, surrounded by 100-plus of our closest friends and family." I started choking up, but was determined to not cry in therapy. I had managed to not cry for this long and was determined to keep my streak going.

He talked me through some of the different things I was feeling and helped me organize the feelings. In reality, I hadn't yet accepted Tom's diagnosis. I hadn't avoided it intentionally but it wasn't a priority at the time. I had to immediately get into "run mode" when he was diagnosed; I was able to avoid acceptance with the hundreds of things that needed to get done. As we wrapped up our session, I felt calmer. I was so grateful that I had made the decision to get therapy a few months earlier, and I thought I would be able to start winding down the sessions soon as we closed the cancer chapter. In reality, the chapter hadn't even started, nor did it have a title.

A few days later, I got a text from Tom at work. "I hate today; I want to crawl in a hole and never leave." I quickly replied, "What's wrong?" He replied, "Everything but I'll be fine." I had a rough time after the party, but it was hitting Tom twice as hard. I would venture to say he didn't even know he had cancer until after that party and after his boss's mother-in-law was diagnosed. I was worried about him and so thankful he was seeing a therapist but was not sure how else to help.

I tried to help him via text but really wanted to just go give him a hug at work. Three quick texts popped up on my screen.

"I just want to be happy, babe; I just don't know what to do to make that happen…Life is too complex. I don't have cancer, so I should be happy, but I'm not…I love you, and you are amazing, but everything else sucks."

I saw those three texts and stared at them for a moment. I didn't know how to reply. He was really struggling, and I knew the fact that he was admitting it meant it was really bad. I hurried home that night and we talked for an hour in the kitchen. He had been crying on and off at work all day and was feeling like he was spiraling a bit. He kept saying he would be fine, which I knew was just him trying to convince himself. We were supposed to be headed to Milwaukee for my little cousin's graduation the next day, and I offered to cancel our trip. He was adamant that we still go, and I knew that was mostly because he didn't want more guilt. My gut was telling me to cancel, but I didn't listen.

The next day we met at home after work and headed up to Milwaukee. Tom was worse than the day before and had another rough day at work. He kept crying on our drive up to Milwaukee, and I almost turned the car around twice. Again, I should have listened to my gut. He kept insisting that we go. He had never struggled so much in his life, and he wasn't changing his decision-making, despite his altered mental state. I was struggling to let go of my role as caregiver, but it was hard to let go when I felt like I needed to help him make decisions because he wasn't in the clearest of minds.

Fast forward to the next afternoon, and I was standing in the bathroom at my aunt's house, handing Tom a Kleenex as he heaved into the toilet. He had overdone it. There was too much going on mentally and physically, and he had shut down. As he cleaned up, I slinked out of the bathroom to let my parents know we were going to sneak out and head back to Chicago. I assumed his sickness wasn't anything major but felt better being close to our doctors in case this didn't clear up quickly. I told my parents that we needed to go. I could tell my parents were concerned, and I tried to reassure them that he was likely fine, but that it made the most sense to head back. Deep down, I just wanted to curl up in a ball and cry. I wanted our old life back where we hung out with family all day and made memories.

We left the party as discreetly as possible and headed back to Chicago. Tom got in the car, put his seat back and closed his eyes for the ride back. I drove and tears streamed down my face. I tried to stay as silent as possible so he could sleep. I kept looking over at him to make sure he was okay. About halfway through the drive, he woke up briefly and turned on his side in the seat.

"I'm sorry. I love you," he softly said as he reached out for my hand.

I took one hand off the wheel and squeezed his hand. "Don't apologize, it's alright…"

I wasn't mad at him. I was mad at what cancer had done to our lives and that our new normal wasn't yet recognizable.

Part 3 – Take 2
June

We were back at square one. The end of May had been a plane crash, and I felt like we were surrounded by fire, yet no one could see it but us. From the outside looking in, I'm sure things didn't seem as tough as they did to us, but I felt like we were falling down a dark hole. The only thing keeping my mind clear was working out, specifically running. In hindsight, the blog had helped me cope through Tom's diagnosis, so I found myself looking for an outlet again to help process and tell our story.

I pulled up my laptop and started a new blog. I was going to attempt to run twenty 5k races for a variety of great causes to bring awareness to how hard the post-cancer transition can be. I wrote my first post and published it but decided to wait to tell anyone about the site until I made sure I was able to make this a reality. I looked at the stock photo of a girl running at the top and scrolled down to read what I had just posted.

"Let me make sure one thing is known before I type anything else on this blog – I hate running. There are very few things I hate in the world, but one of them is running. Another thing on my hate list is cancer, which is where these two worlds collide.

In September of 2015, my amazing husband was diagnosed with a rare cancer and was turning the corner towards late Stage 3 by the time we found it. September was when a bomb exploded in our life, and we were left to pick up the pieces. I don't know how to describe this other than with a puzzle analogy. Remember as a kid when you would get a fresh puzzle? I would always dump out all the pieces and then prop the cover of the puzzle into the bottom of the box so I could see what it was supposed to look like. The next logical step was to separate the pieces into groups based on color, edges, etc. It wasn't much, but it still provided a guide and a way to sort of figure out how to get to the end. Our cancer puzzle has no edges, and the box doesn't have a picture on the front. The pieces of our life were everywhere – and we had no clue what our new picture was supposed to look like, so how the hell were we supposed to put our life back together?

Do you want to know what the craziest part is? This putting our life back together phase has been the harder part of this whole adventure. Things have been rough. It's taken a lot of time, effort, energy, therapy, patience, crying, laughing, confusion, frustration, humor, and gratitude to get this far, but we are just at the beginning, and the road ahead continues to be a puzzling one.

So that's what this all about. I watched my husband go through twenty chemo treatments and there aren't words to describe how proud I am of him - he did it with such wit, humor and determination. It inspired me, to say the least, to challenge myself, to not back down from something because it's hard, to rebalance my life again and remember what's important, and most

importantly try to make him feel for one moment how proud I was, and
continue to be, of him. That's when this crazy idea popped in my head. I hate
running (but I love a free t-shirt), so what if I worked hard and ran twenty 5K
races, one for each of his chemo treatments? I'm not talking world-record pace
by any stretch of the imagination, and my flat feet aren't really thrilled with
this whole idea, but I know it's something that will provide me with a new
perspective, create some discipline, and maybe provide some insight to others
on how life after a cancer-free diagnosis is just the beginning. So let's see how
this goes…"

I finished reading it and immediately hit the New Post button on the
screen. I felt like I should make sure everyone knew how I felt about running.

Running hasn't ever been my thing. There are several reasons that
running and I haven't had the strongest relationship. First, I have always been
more of a short distance runner: I played basketball for many years, so I mostly
was doing short circuit sprint-type running. Second, I have completely flat feet.
I can't sneak up on anyone on a pool deck; I sound like a duck with my flat feet
flopping around. That makes for challenges with my feet/knees as a result.
Traditionally, if you've seen me running, it's probably to a cupcake or glass of
wine. It usually has not been by choice. But, alas, that will change…I think.
People often talk about these amazing running highs, and I think that's crazy.
There is nothing euphoric about my legs cramping, my back hurting and
running from Point A to Point B. Regardless of all my hate for running – Tom
did something he hated twenty times over. I run a 5K, and I'm done, maybe
sore the day after. He got chemo, and was sick for weeks as a result and has
side effects for the rest of his life as a result. I can deal with this, right?

I hit post, and tried to figure out what my plan of attack would be for
getting this out there. My first 5K was about a week and a half way, so I
decided I would get through that first before deciding to share the new blog.

Things kept spiraling, and it seemed like the run might not even happen
because things were so out of control at home. Tom was at the lowest point I
had seen to date, and I was worried that this was no longer something that just
therapy could help with. I came home from work and Tom was sitting on the
kitchen counter with his head down.

"Hi, babe, you okay?" I asked as I walked over to him.

"Uh uh," he grunted as he grabbed me, hugged me, and started to cry.

"What's wrong?" I asked, not letting go.

"I wish it had taken me. It's so messed up, but I wish the cancer had just
won. I don't know if I can do this; I can't handle it all. Maybe it would have
been easier if I had just died," he said as he cried.

I quickly pulled back and looked into his eyes. I was hoping I had
misheard what he just said. I could tell by his expression that it was exactly

what I had heard. I started to spin. Should I take him into the hospital? Was he just having a tough moment? Should I tell someone? Should I leave him alone? I swallowed hard.

"You don't believe that, do you? You fought to be here. I know this isn't easy, but you belong here," I said to him as I wiped tears away from his face.

"I am really overwhelmed," he said with his head down. "I don't feel in control of my mind."

I had so much to think about, but I kept my mind clear and calmed him down for a long time in that kitchen. The tears eventually stopped, the conversation shifted to a plan, and eventually I got him to laugh. I knew it was a temporary moment, but I was happy that I could get him to a better place. Luckily, he had therapy the next day and would be able to talk with his therapist about everything he was feeling.

The next day, he came home and seemed a little bit lighter, but his therapist acknowledged that he was dealing with PTSD and depression. I don't think it shocked either of us, but there was something about it that angered me. Why hadn't anyone warned us that this could happen? I researched it that night, and it's very common in cancer survivors and even more common in cases of men that were diagnosed as abruptly as Tom. No one had warned us, no one had mentioned it could happen, and perhaps that was because they were always telling us how well we were handling things. However, despite how well we handled the treatment, that didn't mean that his brain wouldn't eventually catch up and create the mental turmoil that he was struggling with now.

I felt better that his therapist had given a label to what we were dealing with, but the logical next question was what do you do? One option was an antidepressant, but Tom was pretty adamant that he didn't want to start there. He had a bad perception of antidepressants. He wanted to go with the option that got him something he had wanted for ten years, a dog. Dogs have been proven to be remarkable companions for people struggling with PTSD. Given the dark place we were in, I was actually considering it. I wasn't against a dog, but, in a way, I had my own PTSD. I had handled everything for so many months that when he mentioned a dog, all I heard was one more thing on my plate that I would need to manage. He had secretly snuck a dog on his post-cancer bucket list too one night, so while I knew it was likely imminent, I wanted him to continue working through everything with his therapist before we made such a big commitment.

Tom relentlessly reminded me that having a dog would be great. Meanwhile, the ups and downs of his emotions were brutal. Later that week I walked in the house to find him crying in bed. We were supposed to be at my niece's birthday party in ten minutes, and he was in a heap on the bed. I didn't rush him and most importantly didn't assume I knew why he was upset. That was something that I learned that I will take with me in how I handle these situations in the future. There were many reasons he could be crying, but I wanted him to tell me what it was.

"What's going on?" I asked.

"I heard a song lyric on the way home," he said.

It wasn't quite what I had expected him to say, but clearly this was part of his PTSD. "What song?" I asked.

He knew I wouldn't know it so he grabbed his phone and pulled it up. It was "Spirits" by the Strumbellas. He started to softly mouth the words as we listened to the song.

> I been looking at the stars tonight
> And I think oh, how I miss that bright sun
> I'll be a dreamer 'til the day I die
> But they say oh, how the good die young
> But we're all strange
> And maybe we don't wanna change."

He started to cry again at the end of the verse. I gave him a hug and laid my head on his shoulder as we kept listening to the song.

> I got guns in my head and they won't go
> Spirits in my head and they won't go
> I got guns in my head and they won't go
> Spirits in my head and they won't go
> But the gun still rattles
> The gun still rattles, oh
> I got guns in my head and they won't go
> Spirits in my head and they won't go.

He cried, rolled into me and squeezed me tight. I didn't know what to say to him, so I wrapped my arms around him and let him cry. He gradually calmed down. I asked him if he wanted me to call his family and let them know we wouldn't be coming to the party but he insisted we go and that he would be fine in a few minutes. I knew he didn't want to raise suspicion by not going, but I worried about what the "pretend like everything is okay" approach was doing to his recovery and his mental health. I knew it wasn't the time to argue, but I asked him one more time to be sure.

Fifteen minutes later we were at the party, mingling and smiling with friends and family. He wasn't his complete self, but he was putting on quite a good show. I felt like a fraud but was happy to be around the good energy of family. We didn't stay long. Once the gift opening was over, we grabbed our things and headed out. Nobody really questioned it, but it would have otherwise been unusual for us to leave so quickly.

The reality of our situation was wearing on me, and I liked to think I wasn't showing it, but I clearly was failing. One day at work, a coworker asked me if everything was okay. I told her about Tom but was mostly surprised that she had picked up on it. A few days later, my boss asked me the same thing. I took a deep breath and told her that Tom was having a hard time and that there was a lot going on. I wasn't sure why I had been so hesitant to tell her. Why when it was cancer did I have no problem telling her what was happening? I wasn't ashamed but I didn't feel like people quite understood PTSD and depression. When I was at work, I was worried about Tom and if he was having an okay day. I didn't think Tom would ever commit suicide, but some of his comments had me worried. I wasn't entirely sure about what Tom, struggling with PTSD and depression, might be capable of doing. I was starting to spiral myself because I had the weight of the world on my shoulders and very few people knew what was happening. On top of it all, I really didn't tell him how I was feeling because I didn't want to add more to his already full plate of mental health challenges.

I would lie awake at night and wonder what went wrong, what should we have done differently, or what we could change to make it better. One thing for sure was that Tom had gone back to work way too soon. He was back full-time within eight weeks of his surgery, before having a chance to fully comprehend his cancer. At the time, it seemed like a good idea. It made him feel like himself again and that he was getting back to life. For every potential cause for our current situation, there was an argument that it was a reason that we had made it as far as we had. It was a vicious cycle.

I tried to keep Tom's spirits up and both of us busy so that he didn't have too much time to dwell on his reality. Perhaps that wasn't the best approach, but it was all I could do. I had my first 5K the following weekend and while we'd had an especially trying week, I hoped that this would be a fun morning adventure for us. We got downtown, and I lined up for the race. It was intense, and I knew I wasn't in peak shape just yet, but hoped I'd be able to hold my own. As I crossed the finish line I almost cried, and I wasn't sure why.

I felt very accomplished when I was done. It hadn't been pretty, and my time wasn't great, but I did it. In March, when I first started running, I could hardly make it a quarter of a mile. Progress was progress, no matter what the clock or my aching body said. As I posted my blog post about the most recent run, I still wasn't sure if I would continue down this path and tell people about the site. Tom had cheered me on and seemed happy to be there, but it was clear that he wasn't having the strongest of days. I woke up every morning hoping that the day would be better than the one before, but this extensive string of terrible days was really challenging to navigate.

The following week I was at the office and had a gut feeling that Tom hadn't gone into work. I'm not sure how I knew. I called his office and he didn't answer. I quickly got a text that said, "I'm not at my desk. What's up?" His company has their phones hooked into email so voicemails send email notifications. I knew he was lying. I waited an hour or so and then called again but didn't let it go to voicemail this time, so he didn't get a notification. I figured he would see the missed call and call me back. He never did. I waited until early afternoon and sent him a text asking if he was working from home. I saw him typing back and trying to figure out what to say as the "in progress" dots showed. He texted back that he had ended up working from home that afternoon because he wasn't feeling great. I knew he was lying. He hadn't gone in at all, and for some reason he didn't want to tell me.

I got home that night and after discussing it for a while, he finally admitted that he hadn't gone in. Getting out of bed in the morning was so overwhelming for him right now. I understood what he was feeling, but not why he felt the need to lie to me about it. It came down to the fact that he was embarrassed and ashamed. The worst part was, he had lied about going to work a few other times too. What he didn't get was that I only wanted to know what was happening so I could support him and also keep my mind clear. When he was unable to go into work, I was sitting at work uncertain where his head would be when I got home. It made me sick to my stomach.

Later that week, we both got home within minutes of each other. He had gone to work that day, and I walked into the bedroom to see him crying again. It had been a tough day for him and we were supposed to be at a dance recital for our niece that evening. My heart broke for him. He had been struggling to get up and go to work in the morning and he couldn't really articulate what specifically was bothering him, which confirmed that this really was a deep struggle with the PTSD and depression. What terrified me most was the unpredictability of mental health challenges.

The night before this meltdown I had been at therapy and as I stood in the bedroom trying to support him and get us to the dance recital, I tried to think of everything I had discussed the night before. One of the things we focused on was my inability to measure progress. His cancer treatment had been a straight trajectory; we made progress, we moved on to the next thing, and continued on that path until we had completed all the chemo treatments and surgery. In many ways, it was easy because it was predictable and measurable. However, this sudden change in our life wasn't so simple. A good day didn't signify progress anymore - it just signified a good day. There was no predicting if the next day would be another good day or a bad one, and it left me feeling helpless and that I lacked the ability to care for Tom and help get him better.

In addition to the abrupt ups and downs, I had been sick to my stomach about him skipping work, the lying, and the comments he had made about wishing the cancer had taken him. Dr. Crane and I started discussing how that conversation had impacted me.

"I can't imagine that is easy to hear. How did you react?" he asked.

"You know, honestly, the immediate reaction was shock, and then I wanted to make sure I really grasped what he was saying and whether he needed help immediately. After that, I was paralyzed for a minute and had a flashback that caught me off guard," I replied.

"What was the flashback?"

"I…" I wasn't sure I wanted to talk about it because I never really had. I paused and took a deep breath. "In college, I was the student manager of our student center. It was a 24/7 facility, led by two university staff members and two student managers. Jim was the main boss. He had been there for years. He was a great guy, always personable, and so kind to all the students. One afternoon when I was working the front desk, he came out of his office and told me what a great job I was doing as a manager and that the scheduling had been so much easier since I took it over. We chatted and joked for a minute, and I thanked him for the compliment. Then he said he was going to run to the bank and would be back in a bit if anyone needed him. He was beaming from ear to ear. He seemed so happy that day, euphoric almost."

"That's an interesting flashback…" he replied with a pause, assuming my story was likely not done.

"My shift ended, and I headed out. I worked the early morning shift the next day, and when I arrived I saw Jim's wife and two daughters behind the desk near his office with our other boss. Jim hadn't come home the night before and no one had been able to get a hold of him. They asked me when I had seen him last, and it became clear that I had been the last one to see him at the student center. I told them that he said he was going to the bank and that it wasn't anything out of the ordinary. They left the building with the campus police to go look for his car as I sat down for my shift, feeling uneasy at what could have happened. Later that afternoon they found Jim. He had killed himself. And I guess, in hindsight, he was a bubbly guy four out of every five days, but the off days were very off. And it scares me, because right now Tom isn't himself most days. I never would have believed Jim would kill himself, but he did, so I don't treat it as an empty threat. When Tom said that, I saw Jim's daughters crying at the funeral; I saw all the people who loved him, and I felt as sick to my stomach as I did at his funeral. But more than anything, I remember how happy Jim was that day, and he killed himself hours later."

Dr. Crane nodded at me and didn't say anything at first. He stared at me as I sorted my thoughts – it wasn't something I talked about often.

As we talked, we worked through everything I had just said. We wandered back to the topic of how these types of challenges made it hard to measure progress. I spun in circles as I tried to come up with different ways to measure progress.

As we were wrapping up, he made a suggestion. "For progress, I would consider thinking about it in three buckets. Frequency, duration and intensity.

How often are the bad moments or days happening, for how long are they happening, and how intense is it," he remarked.

"Wait, you've had the answer all along?! That would have been helpful fifteen minutes ago," I joked.

When he said it that way, it suddenly clicked. Our progress post-cancer wasn't a straight line on an axis of time and progress. Instead it was the ups and downs with the frequency, duration and intensity determining how many of those twists and turns were happening.

As I stood in our bedroom thinking through everything we had discussed in that session, we were able to pull ourselves together and get to the dance recital. We sat up in the balcony area and watched as these sweet kids danced all around the stage. One of the special dances each year was when the dads danced with their daughters. This year, it was my niece's turn, so my brother-in-law was in the dance number with her. The sappy music started and I watched as these little girls danced with their dads. I could tell Tom was reacting to this, as I was. It had been a tough week with Father's Day reminding him that we still don't have the family we so desired – as well as the work issues and his general struggle with mental health.

The hardest thing about it all for me was that I, foolishly, tried to be happy for two people. I couldn't double my happiness in an attempt to make him feel better. Yet at the time it didn't occur to me how stupid that was, and I tried relentlessly to make him as happy as possible, often at the expense of what would make me happy. I would get overexcited about something that made him happy because I hoped that it would keep him happier longer, and it wore me down fast. It's hard enough to be happy all the time for yourself, much less for two people.

As summer approached, I felt that we had hit rock bottom. But I thought we had already hit it a few times before, so as we sat on the bottom with our world falling apart around us, I prayed that this rock bottom didn't have another trap door.

July

It was birthday month, but it didn't feel like it. June had taken us to a whole new low, and the pressure to be happy for my birthday wasn't helping. I knew Tom wanted to make it a special day, but I also knew he didn't have much in him right now to make it happen. We skipped the family 4th of July celebration and instead just vegged all day, out of our norm. It was becoming too hard to smile through the sadness, and there was such pressure to do so at family events. While I had watched Tom spiral down into this dark place, it wasn't until my birthday week that I realized that I too had gone to a bad place. I had been fooling myself to think that I was powering along without any problems. I knew I didn't feel well but wasn't quite sure how bad it was until I met again with Dr. Crane.

Days before my birthday, I was at therapy. As I was talking, I wasn't even sure what I was saying; instead I was asking myself how this had become normal. Days before my twenty-ninth birthday I was talking to my shrink, trying to figure out what was wrong with me. The toughest ten months of my life had just happened, and twenty-eight had proven to be a year filled with challenges. I never felt like a "grown up" before, but as I approached twenty-nine I felt I had experienced more grown-up things than many fifty- or sixty-year-old people.

"How are you feeling?" he asked.

"Rough," I bluntly replied, seemingly catching him off guard.

I usually tried to start on a more positive note, but I couldn't that day. As I explained everything that was happening and all the ups and downs that continued to occur between our two-week sessions, he smacked me with a dose of reality.

"Do you notice when I ask how you're doing, you tend to tell me how Tom is feeling and focus on him?" he asked.

There was no denying what he was saying was true, but right now how Tom was doing heavily impacted how I was feeling. Or was I using that to avoid my own feelings?

"I guess I agree, but how can it not be about Tom at some level?" I asked, but then continued before he could answer. "I'm struggling with everything, and I feel like as we unpack the magnitude, it's harder to handle some of the day to day. It's like his car accident. After a car accident, you're jumpy for the next few days because you just had a wreck. In a way, I feel very jumpy about all this aftermath." As I talked it all out, it was starting to make sense to me. "I feel like this all changed me at some level, and that can be a bit scary."

"How so?" he asked.

"Oh goodness, so many ways. The biggest one I think is that while we are navigating back to this new normal, I struggle to make decisions. Before all this, I could make relatively sound decisions because I knew what our normal was; I could at some level "predict" the outcome of decisions. I can't do that anymore. I can force myself to get used to the new normal, but I can't seem to make decisions; it's too dangerous. I still can't trust our life. It's terrifying," I replied.

"What else?" he asked.

I could have gone on for days, but tried to focus. "Another big one is my career. I was always so career-focused, wanting to climb as fast as possible. Yet since everything happened, I've wondered what exactly I was climbing to. Was it a title or a certain amount of money? I just had a great performance review and usually that would have lit a fire in me to keep going, keep climbing. Instead I just stared at my boss. I was proud of myself, don't get me wrong, but I no longer value career in the same way. That's a big change for me, and a bit scary because now I'm not sure where my 'place' is, or my purpose."

As I talked through these components, it was starting to make more sense to me. "Trust is another one," I quickly blurted out. I'm nervous about trusting my gut, trusting how Tom is feeling, trusting the day, trusting the moments of happiness, trusting that the bad days are temporary, trusting that we aren't going to have another ball come out of left field," I continued. The puzzle pieces started to click together.

"I'm missing closure; I'm not sure how to get closure from this all when I feel like it has fundamentally changed me. I can't have closure if my daily anxiety reminds me that it happened or that I can't make decisions."

"What do you think will help you with closure?" he asked.

"I suppose it's just time, but I'm not sure I can have closure until I have all the answers," I replied.

"Answers in regard to what?" he asked, nudging me to acknowledge what I didn't want to talk about.

"If we can have a family. I guess I can't get closure until I know the final impact. Which, even as I say that, I know it is ridiculous. We may never know the full impact of his cancer. It could have taken years off his life, and we will never know. But I'm sure you get what I mean; I feel like I can't cope with this all until I know the immediate impacts. And while all of that is swirling in my head, I'm trying to deal with these nuances that have changed me. It's exhausting." I stopped for a moment and stared at him. I wondered if he had heard this a million times or if I was unique in my ability to handle this situation.

With such patience he talked me through what I had just word-vomited and assured me that none of it was unusual. In a sense, if the cancer hadn't changed me, it would have been even stranger. It should have changed me, and it did. I had to decide what control I gave it, though, and that was the tricky part. I heard what he was saying, but still wondered to myself if I had actually changed, or whether it was my perspective that changed. I wanted so badly for everything to be black and white, when in reality we were going to be in murky gray waters for a while as we figured it all out.

"I wouldn't say I'm feeling depressed because I don't think that's what this is," I remarked as we were talking about these gray waters. "I think I'm just feeling the diagnosis for the first time and feeling the sadness of it all. It may have taken away so many things from us. It's sad. The emotions are harder to deal with now than when he was dealing with the actual cancer."

I wasn't sure how to explain it to him, but perhaps it was the shock wearing off and the aftermath setting in. I'm not sure which one released the emotions, but they were coming with a vengeance. I still had not cried during one of my therapy appointments, but I felt I was on the edge of tears. In fact, I hadn't cried in quite a while. I had pushed the emotions so far away to stay strong for Tom that they hadn't had a chance to even manifest as tears.

As my birthday arrived, there was little fanfare. Tom had repeatedly asked what I wanted to do, and I had decided a drive home to have brunch with my family was what I wanted. I was eager to see them and we walked on the lakefront, one of my favorite places in the world. It didn't feel like my birthday, and I wanted to feel that excitement for a minute of the day. I coasted through the day, enjoying all the birthday messages and love but as we drove back to Chicago that afternoon, I couldn't turn off my mind. I was thankful that I had a birthday, because this was the first time in my twenty-nine years that I had so closely witnessed someone having to fight hard for his next birthday.

The following weekend, we had a BBQ at Aunt Paula and Uncle Rick's for a belated birthday celebration. Tom and his cousin were joining us after the Cubs game. They arrived and walked into the backyard, and I knew immediately he wasn't feeling well. I could see it in his eyes and his color. He went around giving hugs to everyone and when he got to me tucked his head down into my shoulder. I discreetly asked him if he was okay and he softly shook his head no. I told him to sit down and that I'd grab him some water. It had been a hot day at the game, and he hadn't had a single drink, so there really wasn't a logical explanation for him feeling this way. We began to eat and I watched as Tom pushed his food around his plate. A few moments later, he got up and went into the house. I knew he was either throwing up or needed to cool down in the air conditioning for a minute. I waited a few minutes and then walked into the house to find Tom lying on the couch and looking terrible.

I sat on the edge of the couch near his hip. "Are you okay?" I asked.

"I just threw up; I feel terrible," he replied.

"Why don't we head home," I quickly offered.

"No, it's your little birthday gathering, I want to stay. I'm going to rest my eyes for a bit and hopefully feel better," he insisted.

I returned to the backyard to continue visiting. His family asked if everything was okay, and I assured them he was fine but just needed to rest for a few minutes. A few minutes turned into over an hour, and every twenty minutes or so I would go in to check on him. On one of my checks, Tom tried to sit up. He had his head in his hands, and I heard the patio door open. My sister-in-law Staci was heading out and was going to say goodbye. I turned over my shoulder and just waved, and she waved back with a concerned face. As I sat rubbing Tom's back in silence, I wondered what she must be thinking. His family hadn't seen many of these moments since he had been so sick, and I hoped it wasn't causing any additional worry for them.

Tom's parents started packing up, and I knew we would be right behind them. Tom got up to say goodbye, and then came in the backyard to chat with the rest of the family. He had color again; he looked great, and we ended up sitting outside chatting for almost an hour. He was making jokes, laughing and happy as could be. Yet two hours earlier he could hardly function. It created a tough dynamic as I tried to shed my role as caregiver.

As I rolled into therapy the following week, I felt panicky. I hadn't made much progress and almost felt like I was in a worse place. Dr. Crane immediately asked me how I was doing and how my birthday had been.

"My birthday was different, and that's okay, but it was just different and made me think way too much," I replied as a grin came across my face. Dr. Crane always told me I had to try to live in the moment so that I didn't get too caught up in my worry. My admission of over-thinking was my acknowledgment that perhaps I hadn't done well with that the last few weeks.

"Thinking about what?" he inquired.

"We were driving back from Milwaukee and I don't know how to describe the feeling other than to say that I'm lost. I don't know who I am right now. There are so many different "versions" of me: I'm a wife, a caregiver, a daughter, a sister, a professional, a friend, a goofball, and yet in all those versions of me, I sort of just long to be a kid right now, when times were simple. I have this nagging feeling that a piece of me is missing, and I don't know what it is," I said.

"Describe that," he pushed.

"It's big, joyous, fulfilling and an 'a-ha'," I said matter-of-factly.

"Tell me more," he pushed again.

"I'm not sure I have all the answers, but I do know things like mentoring other caregivers seems to fulfill me," I replied. I was continuing to mentor and felt very happy when I was able to provide some guidance or perspective.

"What else?" he asked.

"Writing has been very therapeutic. I know I've told you before I'm working on a book, and that has been good. It's funny, though, because some days I can write, and other days it's too terrifying to get my mind back into that darkness. But lately, when I work on the book, I black out a bit," I replied

"Black out?" he inquired.

"Yeah. If I write about a specific situation or topic, I sometimes will just feel out of control, like I don't even know what I'm typing and then I'll go back and read the few pages I wrote and have no recollection of what I wrote. It's as if I'm reading it for the first time," I explained.

"It's a coping mechanism called disassociation," he replied.

"You know, it's funny you say that, because I was thinking about that the other day. The blog ended up being a story for me. I told the story of our lives and by telling what was happening I was able to pretend it wasn't happening to me. I was just telling a story. Maybe that's why I'm having such a hard time accessing the emotions," I hypothesized.

Dr. Crane nodded his head, I had obviously nailed it. It was all starting to make sense. While still challenging to deal with, understanding what I was doing, and why, helped me feel a little more normal and that it could be worked through. I told him what had happened with Tom at his aunt's house and that it had scared me a bit and as a result I had turned off the emotions again.

"Why did the emotions turn off?" he asked.

"I was finally feeling everything. You saw me last week, and I was a mess. Then I had to snap back into caregiver mode, and that turned it all off. I can't get to the emotions anymore, and I know I need to. Plus, we are heading up to our family reunion this weekend, and I'm starting to get worried about that too, so that keeps emotions away. It's just a lot to balance."

"How are you balancing everything?" he asked.

It was such a simple question that it caught me off guard. I took a deep breath and answered honestly, "I'm not; I don't even know what to balance anymore. It's too much." I wasn't trying to avoid his question. During Tom's cancer treatment there was also a lot to balance, but it had been easy in retrospect because the magnitude of the emotions hadn't hit yet.

One thing I was hoping would help rebalance us was a trip the following weekend to the Upper Peninsula, or UP, of Michigan. My dad was born and raised there. It's a tranquil place; until only a few years ago they hardly had cell reception. It's a slower pace and a great place to relax. Our extended family gathers there each year for a family reunion at McClain park and as we started our seven-hour drive, I had a nagging thought that I had to get off my chest.

"Are you excited for the trip?" I asked.

"Always. I love the UP, and I get to hang out with Rookie for a few days. That's a win-win," he replied.

"Yeah…are you nervous about seeing people?" I asked. We were still in this weird phase of seeing lots of family and friends who hadn't seen us since he had been sick. Usually, that meant there were a lot of questions or conversations around the topic. We were used to it, but sometimes it made us a little nervous because we didn't want to be the center of attention.

"Not really. It will be nice to see everyone," he replied. The family had called and sent so many care packages and cards that it felt like they supported us through it all.

I knew I needed to bring up what was making my stomach churn but was trying to avoid it. I was doing my common coping strategy of not telling Tom how I was feeling to avoid making him upset.

"I have to be honest, it might be a strange to be back at McClain," I stated.

"Oh yeah?" he asked, not yet making the connection.

"Yeah, I'm just glad you're with me in person to go, instead of going there to spread your ashes. I still am haunted by the conversation we had to have that night in the hospital about spreading your ashes," I stated in a matter-of-fact tone to avoid tears. It seemed so strange to be going to a place that was so special to both of us and had been part of Tom's last wishes if something happened. I hoped it wouldn't bother me too much, but it was a strange to say the least. We drove on and never really talked about it again until we pulled into the ranger station a few days later to pay for our day pass into the park. We had already had a great few days of vacation but were taking it easy for Tom. As we drove into the park, I got goosebumps. I tried to not think about it, but it was all that I could think about. Tom looked over at me and smiled, and I leaned in and gave him a kiss.

"I love you," I said.

"I love you more," he replied.

We had said everything we wanted to say with our eyes and our "I love you". I didn't want to dwell; I wanted to be happy about our return here. We unpacked our coolers, games, and beach stuff and headed to our normal spot. The food was laid out, the games started, and a day full of fun began. Our picnic spot is on the top of a bluff overlooking Lake Superior. You can get down to the beach level, but from the top there is a tremendous view. In the afternoon Tom and I had walked down the cliff a bit to look out and sat in two chairs that faced where the sun sets each night.

It was beautiful, the sun was shining, and the temperature was perfect. I looked over at Tom as he looked out to the water.

He looked over at me and smiled. "I'm glad I'm still here – times like these make me glad I'm here and didn't give up," he said.

"Me too," I replied as I reached over and grabbed his hand. "I know it hasn't been easy, babe, but thank you."

"Thank you?" he asked.

"Thank you for being you and trying to keep me happy while our lives are falling apart. You could have taken the easy way and been mad and difficult, but you didn't. I know this has been tough, especially these past few weeks."

"It's been so hard. Thanks for taking care of me. I feel like I've been living in either anticipation or anxiety. I went back to work too soon. I never thought these emotions would take me down like this," he replied.

"Yeah, these emotions have gotten so sneaky! I almost wanted to throw up when we pulled in earlier," I admitted.

"Me too," he said as he turned his head back out to look at the water.

We sat and watched the waves and kept squeezing each other's hand. We had a few hours until sunset. One of my favorite things in the world is a sunset, and the ones in the UP are some of the best you can find. We headed back to the hotel to get cleaned up and planned to grab a to-go pizza before heading back to the park for the sunset like we had done previous years. As we pulled back into the park, I didn't have the same reaction I had felt earlier. We grabbed our food and headed to a gazebo on the cliff that provided a perfect view of the sunset. This time last year we were about eight weeks away from our world falling apart. It was hard to believe we managed to be back now with our health somehow intact. We ate our dinner and walked out from the gazebo down to the beach. I dipped my feet in the cold Superior water, and Tom and I watched as the most glorious orange and red sunset lit up the sky. As we walked down the beach, we passed two women who were also watching the sunset, and I asked them to take a photo of us.

As we headed back to the car, I showed Tom the photo.

"Cute shot, right?" I asked.

"Great shot. That was an awesome sunset tonight," he replied.

"Great ending to a great day…thanks for being here with me," I replied.

Tom nodded his head and we got in the car and headed back to our hotel. It occurred to me that regardless of what happened in the last year, Tom did want his ashes spread there one day. As much as it had paralyzed me to get out of the car and acknowledge the reality of what could have been, I knew that nights like tonight and spending time with our family was the reason it meant as much to him as it did to me. We both had some peace in this little part of the world and memories and watching sunsets there. I had taken back the ownership of the park – it didn't scare me anymore. Instead, it reminded me of all the great memories. We were lucky to have a place like that.

August

A week after vacation might be the worst time to run a 5K. I was continuing to run but had abandoned the idea of the blog. It felt too complicated to put all our dirty laundry out there this time; there were too many emotions. However, it didn't stop me from running. To think in March I could hardly run a minute and now I was able to run three miles without stopping was a great reminder that while it didn't feel like it every day, I was making progress. Running had become an escape, a way to process what I was feeling, and I was continuing to have epiphanies about myself when I was running. I tried to think through things while I ran and "leave it behind" at the end of my run. It worked sometimes, but other times it didn't work at all.

The first week of August began with Tom's second checkup. The fact that another three months had passed seemed impossible. When we had been at the first checkup, things were great but so much had happened since then. The scans quite frankly had been the least of my worries in the past two months because so many other things were falling apart. Tom went to his scans on his own before work, and our results and meeting with the oncologist would be a few days later. He called when he was done and said it was fast and easy. I felt relieved and carried on with my day, eager to get the results.

About an hour later, I got a text from Tom that he had thrown up and was leaving. I called him to see what was going on.

"Are you okay?" I asked as he picked up the phone.

"Yeah, I don't know what's wrong. Maybe it was nerves, but I'm just going to head home," he replied.

"Do you want me to come home?" I asked.

"No, I'm going to probably throw up again and then sleep. Please stay at work," he requested.

I heard Dr. Crane in my mind telling me that this is the perfect opportunity to continue to shed the caregiver layer and trust that Tom was being honest.

"If you want me to stay at work, I'll stay at work. Can we just make a deal that if you need anything or start to feel worse you'll let me know and I'll come home?" I said.

"Promise," he said.

I had to trust that he was being honest with me. I wondered if some of his reaction was nerves about the scans in addition to all the changes that were happening. Tom was in the process of interviewing for a new job and knew he needed a fresh start. He had been interviewing before he got diagnosed, but there was so much going on his head already that adding a new job was daunting. He loved his coworkers and enjoyed his job, but he wanted to take on more and he had maxed out his opportunities at his medium-sized company.

I hung up the phone at work and stared at my computer. My body filled with anxiety. All I wanted to do was get in the car and drive home to make sure he was okay, but that wasn't going to be reasonable for the rest of our lives. Plus, it would forever prevent us from making the shift back to husband and wife versus caregiver and patient. I stayed at work, but I couldn't focus at all. I was going through the motions and was puzzled as to how I had done this for so many months in the winter during the "off weeks" of his treatment. I felt helpless.

The next night, I was explaining my feat to Dr. Crane.

"Aren't you proud of me? I stayed at work!" I exclaimed.

He laughed and nodded. "How are you feeling about the oncology appointment tomorrow?"

"I mean, it gets to the point that regardless of what they tell you, you just want it to be done either way. That's where I'm at. I want it to be 9:45 a.m. tomorrow so that it's done for another three months," I said, "but I'm exhausted. I hardly sleep for these few days beforehand. I just want to feel relaxed for a minute."

"That's understandable. What makes you relax?" he asked.

It was a fair question, and I spun in circles, unable to answer it. "It's funny; this weekend marks the ten-year anniversary of when Tom and I started dating. I'm surprising him with a float in a sensory deprivation salt tank and was considering doing it myself, but I don't think it would relax me."

"I don't think you belong in a sensory deprivation tank," he bluntly replied.

I laughed out loud at the frankness of his comment. "Right? I agree!" I exclaimed.

Tom had been eager to try a sensory deprivation tank. You float in water with extreme salt content, in silence and darkness. As a result, your mind goes to different places because it doesn't have to process sounds, colors, smells, gravity, etc. None of your senses have to be engaged.

"Well, he's wanted to do it, and it's apparently great for people who have PTSD as they can clearly think about and process what happened. But yeah, that doesn't sound relaxing to me at all," I said.

"From what I can gather from the months we've been talking, you need to channel, not turn off, to relax," he said.

It was a very interesting point, and he was right. I was more relaxed when I was writing and working on the book than when I was staring at the TV. In fact, for years Tom made fun of me for my inability to just sit and watch a show. I always needed to be doing something else to make the TV watching "productive." It was an "aha" moment for sure. If I turn off my mind to relax, I started having problems because I would get depressed. Relaxation takes many forms, and not all of them are the traditional ones. I felt validated in a strange way and hoped for some relaxation on the other side of the scans.

As we wrapped up the session, Dr. Crane told me to call him if I needed anything. I hoped he wasn't offering that because he thought something would go wrong with the oncologist, but there was comfort in knowing I could call him if I started to unravel.

The next morning, we got up and headed in for Tom's appointment. My hopes that this would become easier quickly disappeared. We felt the same feelings we had three months earlier. Others who have done this before us and our therapists promised that this would get better with time, so I was disappointed that I was feeling so anxious. Clearly, more time needed to pass, but in the moment it felt like we weren't healing fast enough.

"Hello!" she proclaimed as she walked in the room. I couldn't help but smile. While our experiences with her are associated with a lot of anguish and despair, she's also a huge part of the reason Tom had such a great treatment and outcome. Thankfulness is the overwhelming feeling that still hit me like a truck every time I saw her.

"Hello!" Tom and I both said as she shut the door behind her.

"You know, we really do miss you, but also are really glad we aren't seeing you every day anymore!" I said as she sat down and pulled up to her computer.

She smiled and agreed. I always wondered how she managed her own emotions since her range of conversations in a day were extreme. When she walks into our consultation, she can celebrate with us. Yet one room over could be a conversation about a terminal diagnosis with no treatment option. I often thought about how emotionally tough the job must be for these oncologists. That said, we were happy to be patients that remind her that all her hard work could yield such great results.

She let us know that Tom's scans and blood work looked great and that she was pleased with all of his levels. It was another moment of euphoric relief. We started to fill her in on the chaos that had occurred since we had last seen her. Tom explained how bad things had gotten and that he was struggling with PTSD and depression. As expected, she echoed that everything that was happening was normal, and while difficult, was something we could beat, just as we had with the cancer. I distinctly remember her saying that if any couple could deal with these challenges, we could. These words of encouragement from her felt very sincere, and I was once again reminded how lucky I was that Tom and I had a solid relationship before this all happened. I knew that if we hadn't, one of us would have cracked by now.

As we danced through our conversation, we again talked about our quest for a family. We were in a bit of a holding pattern until Tom hit one-year without cancer. We had been tossing around the idea of just moving forward with a donor, but I ultimately had pulled the plug on that idea. I wanted to wait until we had all the facts. As we continued talking, she looked over at Tom as she reviewed the numbers from his vitals.

"I'm a little worried about your heart rate," she said.

"Heart?" Tom asked.

"Your resting heart rate is a little low. It's common for it to be low after a surgery, but based on your record, yours recovered and has started to decline again. That is likely a result of the chemotherapy, but we will need to keep an eye on it for the next few months. Be careful with cardio. If you have any dizziness or feel light-headed, you need to go right to the ER," she replied.

As she explained her concerns, my mind shot back to our original office visit with her after Tom was diagnosed. I remember her mentioning that the chemotherapy drugs could cause long-term damage to the kidney, heart or liver. At the time I was more worried about everything else that came with the diagnosis, especially as it related to our ability to have a family. While none of this sounded foreign to me, I hadn't paid much attention back then.

"So that's normal then?" Tom asked.

"This is lower than normal, but we will keep an eye on it," she replied.

As we finished up our appointment, I started to feel really anxious. I hadn't prepared for this shot out of left field. I was only planning to hear about the blood and scans. I got angry at myself for being so naïve to not expect something unusual in one of these appointments. We thanked her, made the dreaded next appointment for November and headed downstiars to get an EKG.

"Well that was interesting," I said to Tom as he grabbed my hand.

"Yeah, how about that?" he replied.

"I remember her mentioning organ damage as a potential side effect, but were we not going to do chemotherapy?"

"Exactly what I was thinking," he replied.

Tom quickly completed his EKG, and I sat in the waiting room puzzled as to how our life continued to take turns.

We didn't say much and climbed into the car to head home. The emotions after these appointments still took time to process. As we drove down the street, Tom finally piped up again.

"I feel like this is the first time I've had to think about cancer taking some years off of my life."

"I know, but the alternative was that it would have taken a lot more years," I tried to rationalize.

"True, but still shitty."

I wasn't feeling my usual relief. Instead, I was worried about what we had just heard about his heart. I was feeling myself inch back to caregiver, and I was desperately trying not to as we were working so hard to get back to husband and wife. I was feeling sick to my stomach, but not wanting him to know how worried I was. The heart was such an ominous thing to worry about because there weren't direct symptoms, but it's obviously critical. The more I thought about it, the more I worried, and that couldn't have been good for my heart either.

Two days later, we walked into the float studio. It was ten years ago to the date that Tom and I had started dating and we had a fun day planned. Tom was so excited to try the tank, but I hoped he wasn't setting the bar too high and thinking that sixty minutes in a sensory deprivation tank would make everything better. We got him checked in, and I walked to Michigan Avenue while he had his float experience. Part of me was jealous that he was doing it, but I knew it was a badplace for me to be with the way my mind operates.

It was such a hot day. I walked in and out of stores, keeping an eye on the clock to make sure I didn't wander too far. I wondered what was popping into his mind during his float. Maybe this would turn the tide, move us back to happier times. The rollercoaster we were riding was already tough, and the heart news wasn't helping shift us back to a more positive headspace. A short while later, I eagerly walked back into the studio right as Tom was saying thank you to the owner.

"How was it?!" I asked as we walked out of the studio. We were headed to lunch and I was eager to get the details during our walk.

"So cool, but yeah, you would go nuts in there. My skin is so soft from the salt too," he said to me as he rubbed his arm on me.

"Did you have any visions?" I asked.

"I think you definitely need to do it a few times. Apparently, that's common. It does take a little while to get used to the sensation. At first I was floating into the sides of the tank, but once I got the hang of it, I liked it," he said.

"I'm so glad you liked it! Did you get any clarity?" I asked, not sure what I meant by my own question.

"I was thinking about my job and career and what I really want to do and what I want to be when I grow up, and I thought to myself, what do I want with my life…" he said as he looked over at me.

"Please don't tell me you're enrolling in Clown College," I replied as we walked into a restaurant for lunch.

"No, but it was so weird; I saw a shadow of your profile," he replied.

"Whoa, really?" I said.

"Yeah. I couldn't even tell if my eyes were open or closed, but I saw in my mind your profile," he said.

"What do you think that means?" I asked.

"That no matter what I do with my life, there is nothing I want more than to spend it with you and have a family," he said.

"Well, geez…" I replied, not expecting such a sweet reply.

We sat on the patio at the restaurant and he continued to fill me in on the details of his float. The more he explained, the more curious I got, and I convinced myself that I should try it too. I kept asking questions as the drinks arrived at the table. I grabbed my prosecco. "Happy Tenth Year," I said as raised my glass.

"I can't believe we've been together ten years. Even my subconscious knows how much I love you," he joked.

"This last year makes me feel like we should add some extra years. We packed a lot into year ten if I do say so myself," I said.

Later that evening, when we were back at home, I grabbed my surprise for Tom and handed him a wrapped gift.

"Wait, I thought we weren't doing gifts!"

"I know, this is more of a peace offering than anything else," I replied.

He unwrapped the box and smiled as he pulled a leather collar out of the box.

"It's even engraved," I said.

I had a dog collar engraved with the name "Doc" for Tom. It was my official peace offering that I could get on board with a dog. At this point, it was beyond the bucket list and was more about the positive impacts that dogs can have on people struggling with PTSD. We had stopped at a few shelters randomly over the past few months, but until now they had been just visits.

"Since you don't like my other name, I think Doc is the right fit. Hopefully, a dog will help with the PTSD and provide some much needed therapy as we navigate all this crap and be your last cancer Doc," I said.

"Your name was so dumb," he reinforced as he leaned over for a kiss.

I had thought naming the dog Peeve would be fun, so that I could have an actual pet peeve.

The following week, I had to stop by the hospital to pick up medical records so I could see a specialist to deal with my appendix scare in April. I hadn't been in the actual hospital part of the medical buildings since we had been released from Tom's surgery. As I turned the corner to head down the hall, the smell and feelings hit me like a truck. I stood in the hall for a moment and looked around and observed. I walked over to the desk and proceeded to pick up everything I needed. Within minutes, I was set to be on my way, but I couldn't leave. I walked across the hallway into a waiting area, sat down, and watched everyone going by. For the first time in months I was content. I couldn't explain it. I tried to understand it as I sat there, but it was a feeling of safety that I hadn't felt in so long. When Tom was so sick, these sounds, smells, and people helped make him better. At some level, we "lived" here for a while. Now, as we managed through the mental health pieces, I didn't feel like we had that same comfort of support. We were navigating on our own. Yes, we had the help of our therapists, but it was different. I sat in the waiting area for almost twenty minutes because with that feeling of safety came a few moments of peace. It was eleven months after the day of his diagnosis and it started to scare me that I found such comfort in this part of the hospital. I got up and headed back to the car, my mind racing. It was the beginning of my own realization, beyond my trouble with leaving Tom for weekends, that I was having some of my own PTSD reactions.

The next day, I headed to see my specialist. My appointment was at 12:30. At 1:15 pm, the nurse finally called me back. I was getting annoyed because I had come over on my lunch break and didn't have too much time. The nurse took my records, asked me a few questions and said the doctor would be in shortly. I was feeling more and more anxious as the time ticked by. I had spent too much time in doctors' offices in the past year, and the fact that this one was about me was especially irritating. I started to pace at 2 p.m., when the doctor had still not come into the examination room. At 2:15, I lost my cool, grabbed my things and headed down the hall. The nurse looked up from her computer station and asked where I was going, and that's when I snapped.

"I have to go. I have to get back to work and it's almost a full two hours after my original appointment time. I think I've been more than patient, but this is flat-out insulting," I said to her in as nice of a tone as possible, which wasn't very nice.

"I'm sorry, ma'am. I can get the doctor now," she replied as she stood up.

"Are you serious? So not only am I sitting in that room waiting, he's available right now and was just choosing to have a patient sit and wait almost two hours? No, I'm good. I'll see a different doctor who has a little more focus on patient care," I replied as I headed towards the waiting room.

The nurse ran down the hall after me and repeatedly apologized. I couldn't look at her I was so mad. She followed me out the door to the waiting room before once again asking me to stay and see the doctor.

I'm not even sure what I said. I know I didn't yell, but I do know that based on the faces of the people who were in the waiting room, it wasn't one of my prouder moments. The last thing I said as I turned and walked away was that I think the core need of any person, doctor or not, is respect, and the complete lack of respect for my situation and my time was unacceptable. As I walked out of the waiting area to the elevators, a woman looked at me, smiled and said, "You go, girl!"

I took the elevator down and tried not to cry. I was so irrationally upset about this appointment. I darted to my car, got in, and sobbed. I hadn't felt so upset in a long time, and I knew my reaction wasn't just about this appointment. It was the buildup of the hundreds of appointments over the past year. It was the recent developments around Tom's heart, and because I meant what I said about respect. But more than anything, I was exhausted. This appointment had been the final straw.

The following week, we found the dog. We had been shelter-hopping a bit and were looking for a dog that was good with kids and not a puppy. I was still managing so much and while I was eager to get a dog to hopefully help Tom's recovery, I knew we were taking on quite a bit considering our lives had been falling apart for months. He was a beagle mix, and his name was Trevor. Obviously, we would rename him Doc, as I just couldn't get on board with a "human" name for a dog. This dog was very much for Tom, his bucket list and the PTSD, but I knew Doc might help with my own therapy too, given my meltdown at the doctor days earlier.

We took him for a walk at the shelter and then to a dog park area. Tom and I sat and watched him sniff around.

"You think he's the one?" I asked.

"I think so. I like that they take him to adoption events. That means he's good with people and kids, and he's not too much to handle," Tom said.

"Alright, well, if he's the one, then let's do it…"

"Are you sure? I know this is a lot for you because you didn't grow up with dogs," he said.

"Yup, I'm good," I replied, only partially believing myself.

We headed back into the main visitation area with the dog and told the volunteer we would move ahead with adoption. We filled out some paperwork and planned to pick him up in a week after he got snipped. It seemed too easy.

The week before we officially got Doc, things continued to spiral. Tom had made a final decision to leave his company and pursue a new opportunity. His current boss had helped mentor him through the interviewing process and was happy for him to start a new role. Tom knew it was the right thing to do, but it was going to be a big change. As Tom gave notice and officially accepted his new role, I worried about what all this change would do to us and wished that we already had the dog for him.

"Are you feeling good about everything?" I asked as I was making dinner.

"I think so. I know this is the right move. I was looking for a job before I got sick, but I know I'll never have such great coworkers again," he replied.

"Yeah, they are pretty great," I agreed.

"You know what I'm most excited for?" he asked.

"A challenge? More money? Discounted products?" I started to fire off guesses.

"I'm excited to not be cancer boy," he bluntly replied.

It caught me off guard for a minute, but then I understood this whole additional layer of "new" that he had been searching for. His current company was fantastic, and due to his job in payroll, he knew most people in the 500-person company. After five years, he had relationships across most of the business. As a result, when he got sick, they all followed along and cheered him on. In fact, they were some of the top blog readers throughout his treatment. Yet when he went back to work, he felt like things were different. Everyone was so happy to see him, but he felt like he couldn't kick the "that's the guy who got cancer" shadow that followed him.

For the time being, he was excited about the new job and some positive change, and I hoped it would last. The following Monday, Tom picked up the dog on his way home from work and suddenly we were dog owners. He walked in with the dog, and I wasn't sure what to do. Doc sniffed around, we let him outside in the yard to explore, and I paced around.

"You okay?" Tom asked, as we watched him in the yard from the deck.

"Yeah, I just don't know what to do," I replied.

"To do?" he asked.

"Yeah, like, do you entertain him or what?" I asked.

"No, babe, he's a dog. He sleeps most of the time or runs outside."

I wasn't convinced it would be that easy. The whole evening we followed the dog around the house to see what he would do. I'm sure if dogs could talk he would have had a few choice words for his helicopter owners. The next day, we went to work and Tom assured me that if we put up a gate and made Doc stay in the basement all day he would be fine. Apparently, we had to gradually give him more space in the house so he couldn't run free in the house right away. Tom set up the iPad in the basement and downloaded an app that allowed him to see the dog at random times throughout the day. I figured nothing too bad could happen.

After work, I headed to my workout as a text popped up from Tom. It was a picture of all the blinds in the basement, which Doc had ripped down and chewed. I put the phone down, and walked into my workout. I couldn't comprehend what I had just seen on my phone. My greatest fear had happened within twenty-four hours of having the dog. Luckily, working out and running had become a critical place for me to clear my mind. By the end of my workout, I was much calmer and had a clear mind about it all. I took care of a few problem-solving things on the way home, but when I walked into the house, Tom looked terrible.

"Do you hate me? Do you want to give him back? Maybe a dog was too much for us right now?" he said.

"Babe…" I started to reply.

"You're mad at me, aren't you? How effective is a therapy dog if it makes me feel worse?" he quipped.

"Stop. Listen. I think you and I had very different expectations. Mine are much lower than yours. This poor dog has been in shelters and is getting used to a new house. We should have gotten him a crate to start. I texted your aunt and she said we can borrow hers. Kailee is bringing it over shortly. Something like this was bound to happen. It happened; it's fine, and we will deal with it. I'm really not mad. I stopped and got paper blinds to put up now and I'll reorder the custom ones. Really, it's okay," I said.

Tom just stared at me. I don't think he had expected me to be so calm when he knew that I had come a long way to even get the dog in the first place. He walked over and grabbed me for a hug.

"We're good," I said as he hugged me.

"I'm so glad I married you," he replied.

As we were hugging in the kitchen, Doc sat by our feet and looked up. I looked down at him… "You, on the other hand...we aren't good yet. Listen, we make enough money to buy you food, so let's not eat the blinds."

A few days later, I headed in to see Dr. Crane. He had been on vacation, so I hadn't seen him since the day before Tom's scans at the beginning of the month. My anxiety had started to build in his absence, and I was eager to see him.

"How are you doing?" he asked.

"Well…that's a loaded question. I've missed you! Let's see. Tom's scans were all clear, but now there is some concern with his heart. We got a dog. Tom is taking a new job. I sat paralyzed in the hospital for over twenty minutes because I felt comfortable there and things just still feel…. messy…" I replied, not sure how to comprehend the last month as I said it out loud.

"Wow…" he started to reply. He knew that the dog had been a struggle for me because I was worried about that responsibility falling on my plate, but I was curious where he would want to dive in first. "What happened with the heart?" he asked.

I filled him in on all the medical updates.

"So how are you feeling about that?" he asked.

"You know, I've had time to process it all, and I'm still not sure I can answer your question. Part of me was angry, part of me was heartbroken. When Tom had the realization that cancer, regardless if he beat it, cancer may have taken years off his life, but more than anything I think I felt panicky. I feel like it's created a strange shift," I replied.

"A shift?" he asked.

"I mean…for example…for the last few months, we've had this post-cancer bucket list. Every time we've knocked one off the list, it's been celebratory. But suddenly, I feel less joyous about those. I feel like we need to get it all done in case this is just short term. And I know realistically it isn't, but the heart stuff and the slap in the face of the damage from chemo has shifted my feelings. I'm scared. I don't want to beat cancer temporarily; I want to beat it forever. I guess I have to let go of the concept that we beat the initial diagnosis, but we didn't beat cancer. It's still lingering, and it might always linger. I hope less and less over time, but we didn't beat cancer, he beat his specific cancer diagnosis."

He nodded as I explained my logic. We weaved and bobbed through all the other chaos that had happened and as we started to wrap up the session, he asked me the question I hated most.

"How are you doing with everything?" he asked.

"I'm scared; I'm tired, and I have no idea what September is going to bring, especially with the anniversary of his diagnosis. I'm just blah. For as much as August has been a mess, I'm scared that it's just a preview of what September will be," I replied.

I hoped I was wrong, but I knew deep down that as we approached the one-year mark, we had a high likelihood of additional challenges. My only comfort was that I had somehow figured out how to navigate everything that had been thrown our way so far.

September

The following week, I was back at Dr. Crane's. I had scheduled an appointment so soon because I knew I was in desperate need of guidance. We had one hell of a month ahead, with the most daunting being the arrival of September 16th. I was deep in conversation when Dr. Crane asked me a very raw question.

"Who have you told you're scared?" he asked. We had been talking about how I had been feeling scared lately. Scared of the month ahead, of Tom's progress taking another turn, of the anniversary.

"No one, really. I mean if you're asking if I've directly said to someone, 'I'm scared,' then no," I replied.

"Why not?" he asked.

I knew that would be his question, and I didn't have an answer. I fumbled.

"I can see you're uncomfortable," he said.

"I just don't know what telling someone I'm scared does. It doesn't solve the problem, and it makes people worry. I genuinely don't think I've intentionally not told people I'm scared. It's just sort of a random thing to bring up," I said. "Plus, the scared feeling has some layers of anger in it too that hadn't been there until recently," I admitted.

"Anger?" he asked.

"Yeah. It's almost the anniversary of his diagnosis. Obviously, it's not a day to celebrate, but I'm treating it more like we are taking back the day. I want to fill the day with good memories so it doesn't have power. Yet each day that we are closer to the 16th, I get angrier. I'm not sure why it hasn't hit me until now, but I'm angry at cancer. I'm angry at what it took from us. I'm mad. I'm mad at the cancer; I'm mad that the day has power, and I never thought it would be such a significant day," I replied.

"That's not unusual," he replied.

"Well, that's good…and I know I need to feel all these feelings, but I don't want to…" I replied, hesitating to see what his reaction would be.

"I think you're afraid to give a little and let yourself feel because you're afraid you're going to feel all of the feelings you tucked away in the last year," he replied.

"Yes…" I replied, pausing to look at him. He hit the nail on the head. "I think you're right. I hate the feeling of not knowing what's coming next, and I think that just as easily applies to the emotions," I said.

"So it's mostly anger and sadness right now?" he asked.

"Loss. Loss is another one that I haven't felt until these last few days, and I know that's one that Tom is dealing with too. And that's what makes this much more complicated. I'm suddenly feeling all of this, and I'm still trying to be strong for Tom and make sure he is okay too, because I can't imagine this is any easier for him. In fact I know it isn't," I replied.

"Of course," he replied as he nodded. "Tell me more about the loss."

"You know, for the most part, I've stayed as positive as possible, and while I wish none of this had happened, lots of good came from a really crappy situation. But as we approach this one-year mark, I'm feeling the loss. The loss of time, the loss of a "normal" life, the potential loss of a family, the potential loss of years from Tom's life. I can't comprehend that it's almost a year. I know we didn't "lose" the year; in fact some of our favorite memories are from the past year. But I can't help but feel this overwhelming sense of loss," I replied as my voice wavered. Acknowledging the loss out loud forced me to process it.

Dr. Crane patiently listened as I continued to discuss what loss felt like.

"So what are you going to do on the 16th?" he asked.

"Back in May, Tom and I were at a Cubs game and he mentioned that it might be fun to go to a Cubs game on the one-year anniversary. We checked the schedule and realized that it was a Friday game, Cubs versus the Brewers, and knew immediately that our two teams playing that day was too good to be true. So we are going to the game with his parents and his aunt, uncle and cousins. But the Monday of that week is his last day at his job, and then Tuesday to Thursday my best friend and her family are in town to have a golf extravaganza. I'm hoping it will be a great week for him," I explained.

"That sounds fantastic," he replied.

"I'm also surprising him – his name will be up on the scoreboard congratulating him on his win against cancer," I said as a smile came across my face. "He's going to be so pumped to see that, and there is a chance with the way these last few weeks are going that it could be the playoff clinch game," I explained. As I talked about it, I got more excited. "It feels strange to be excited for an anniversary that isn't a good thing, but I'm trying to think about it as a celebration of how far we have come in a year," I said.

"An anniversary is in the past for a reason," he said.

That struck the perfect chord with me. He was right. We were going to take back the day and then this anniversary would stay in the past. It signified a day, but we weren't going to let the trauma of last year own the day.

"You're right," I replied. "It's such a blur. I think back and I don't feel like I'm part of the memory."

"What do you mean?" he asked.

"You know how when you think of a memory, it's from your viewpoint? You visualize it the way it happened for you?" I asked.

"Yes," he replied.

"For some of the past year, I don't visualize it in that way; I see the memory as a third party. I see myself sitting on the couch in the hospital. It's like I'm looking in on the memory and seeing myself. Does that make any sense?" I asked, starting to think I might be sounding crazy.

"Absolutely. It's called depersonalization," he remarked.

After explaining the psychology behind what he was describing, he acknowledged that I had been describing a lot of situations that occurred with PTSD.

"You know, I've thought that for a while. Being afraid to leave Tom was part of that, my freak out at the doctor and other things made me realize it too. It's normal though, right? This is just us navigating back to our life?"

He assured me it was all normal, but the world "normal" felt like such a strange word to describe our world right now.

Later that night, I got home and talked with Tom about everything I had discussed in therapy. We sat at the table for a few hours chatting about how this looming date was bothering us both and that it felt strange and hard to describe. After dinner, he went into the basement to watch a game and I was upstairs working on the book. A few hours went by and I realized that I hadn't heard from Tom in a while. Usually he'll pop upstairs and see what's going on or grab a drink from the fridge. I started to walk downstairs and called out his name. I peered into the basement and saw him lying on the couch with his eyes closed. Tom is such a light sleeper so I just yelled to him to wake him up so he could go to bed. He didn't move. I froze. I pictured everything the doctor had said about his heart. I quickly darted down the stairs and took the few steps towards him while continually saying his name. I reached out and shook his shoulder.

"Babe, wake up. Tom....Tom..." I said as the seconds went by like minutes.

He finally woke up and looked up at me, confused. "Whoa, I must have been tired," he remarked.

"I seriously thought you had a heart attack," I replied as I turned to walk upstairs, as if it hadn't bothered me at all.

I walked right into the bathroom and put my hands on the edge of the sink, letting my head drop. I let out a deep breath and took in a deep breath. My hands were shaking and I couldn't get the voice of the doctor out of my mind. I knew it was unreasonable to freak out every time he didn't respond, but it was so unusual for him, and it was the first time anything like this had happened since we had heard about his heart. I heard Tom walk by the bathroom a few minutes later and snapped back to reality. I lifted up my head and looked into the mirror. The woman having a freak out looking back at me wasn't me; I didn't want her to be a part of me. I wanted to live our carefree life again.

The next week, Tom wrapped up his job and was ready to celebrate a few days off. He had three days of golf lined up and was eager to play some amazing courses. He was playing with my best friend's dad and brother, and they had been talking for months about this week of golf. During the day, they golfed and I hung out with Katie, her baby and her mom. It was a refreshing change of pace to take some time away from work and have them visit from Cincinnati. Each night when we went to bed, Tom would fill me in on how much fun he had. He lit up. We had talked for months about celebrating his being cancer-free with this golf adventure, so for it to actually happen was another very tangible sign of progress for him. We were both so grateful to have had these few days before the official anniversary.

On the last night, we had dinner and had to say our goodbyes. As we drove home, Tom seemed a little quiet, but I figured it was exhaustion. Three straight days of golf was still a lot for Tom physically, and I hoped he was feeling okay. I resisted being a caregiver and asking directly but was keeping a close eye on him. Later that evening, I walked downstairs and sat across from him to talk about the plan for tomorrow morning.

"Are you alright? Ready for tomorrow?" I asked.

"Yeah, it's just weird," he started to reply. I knew he was struggling to put words to what he was feeling too.

"You okay?" I asked. "If I didn't know any better, I would think you might have been crying," I suggested. I did know better, and I knew he had been crying.

"I just...I had the best time with Joe and Mark these last few days. But there was one point during golf that I was just jealous."

"Jealous of what?" I asked.

"Mark. He's got an amazing dad that he has these amazing memories with," he remarked.

I was surprised to hear this, but it made sense. Through therapy, other issues had surfaced that Tom had avoided for years, like the relationship with his biological father.

"I just want to have a family so I can have that with my son, and I'm scared to find out about what cancer may have done to our hopes for a family, and I worry I'm not going to be a good dad," he replied as he started to tear up again.

"Don't be ridiculous, you are going to be the best dad in the world. It's one of the reasons I love you so much," I said.

"You're just saying that. Denny was the best stepdad, and I know I'm more like him than I am my biological father, but sometimes I worry about the genes and that I won't have the connection with my kid," he said.

I looked across at him, unsure what to say. "The fact that you're worried about being a great dad proves you will be a great one. You and I want a family more than anything in the world and I think we will be great parents. We will figure it out in our own goofy way. It will be fun. Then you can play baseball with your son and golf with him. You are going to be a great dad..." I said.

"I hope so..."

"Did you know how to be a husband before we got married?" I asked.

"Well, no, but that's different."

"How so? Same exact thing. You didn't know how to "be" a husband, but you were surrounded by great examples and figured it out. Same thing with being a dad. You've got great people around you: Denny, Uncle Rick, my dad, your brothers-in-law, Katie's dad...the list goes on..." I replied.

"I know. I think it's everything with this week. I miss the days where I didn't feel my emotions!" he joked. Prior to his diagnosis, Tom could compartmentalize things, tuck them away and not actually deal with them. However, that had changed after his treatment.

"I think it's so sweet that you care so much, and I'm excited for tomorrow," I said, lightening the mood.

"Me, too, especially if they clinch."

With unbelievable luck, there was a chance we would see the Cubs clinch a playoff bid. However, it depended on how the games shook out that evening and if the Cubs and Cardinals won or lost. There were several scenarios that could play out. The first was that the Cardinals won, and Tom could see the Cubs clinch by winning the game we were attending. The second scenario was that the Cubs clinched the night before the game because of a Cardinals loss. For the second scenario, if they did clinch because of the Cardinals game then the game we were attending would be the first game since the clinch, and it was expected that they would celebrate during the game. We were hopeful that regardless of how it happened, Tom would be part of some celebration.

The next morning, I rolled over and curled into Tom, who was already awake.

"I love you," I said as I did most mornings.

"I love you more," he replied.

It felt strange. It felt like something, but I wasn't sure what. It had a similar feeling to a birthday or other important day when you feel a difference, but it wasn't the most joyous of reasons to feel that way. Surprisingly, Tom seemed to be in a really good place and was very excited for the game. The second scenario had played out and the Cubs had clinched as a result of the Cardinals game the night before, so he was hoping to see a celebration.

As we started our day of fun, no one directly mentioned the anniversary. Once we sat down for breakfast we did a "Cheers" to what a difference a year made and how perfectly it had played out that this game was a Brewers and Cubs game. I was rocking my Brewers jersey while everyone else was decked out in Cubs gear. We got into the bleachers and grabbed seats that ensured we would see the jumbotron. Everyone but Tom knew that the scoreboard surprise was happening, and I was anxiously awaiting the middle of the 5th inning to see his reaction. As we looked up to the sky and checked the radar on our phones, it was evident that we were about to get poured on. About an hour of hard rain was showing as starting exactly at game time. It was a beautiful metaphor for the storm that hit us a year ago. About ten minutes before the game was supposed to start, it misted, then disappeared out over Lake Michigan, and the sun came out. An even better metaphor.

The game was a blast, but I couldn't pay attention because I was so excited for him to see his name up on the board. The stadium was electric because of the events that had played out the night before. Towards the end of the fourth inning, Tom suggested grabbing some food and I immediately shot him down. I needed him to stay in his seat and not miss his shout out. A few minutes later, he asked if I needed sunscreen and that he could run buy one. Nope, I'll burn. Stay put. The top of the fifth inning ended and they started to show the shout outs on the jumbotron. Everyone was looking at the board when his popped up. "Congratulations, Tom Nolting – You got your "W" against cancer!" The Cubs organization has a white flag with a giant blue "W" on it that flies when they win. In fact, there had been one at my house all season because Tom was gifted one at his survivor party. I turned and looked at him as he smiled, with tears in his eyes, and leaned in to give me a kiss.

We all clapped and celebrated, and he admitted he had a sneaking suspicion that something was likely happening when I repeatedly denied wanting anything and when everyone pulled out their phones in the middle of the inning. I smiled and took a deep breath now that the surprise part was over. I squeezed his hand and looked up at him.

"I hate that I feel my emotions!!" he whispered into my ear.

"I'm so proud of you; I love you so much. The world should know you got your W against cancer. You fought hard," I said back.

The game was electric, and I was thrilled my Brewers were winning. However, in true Cubs fashion, Tom's team came from behind in the 9th inning to push it into extra innings. The Cubs ended up winning on a walk-off home run in the 10th inning. I've never heard a place so loud. As they won the game, the NL Championship celebrations began and the shirts, hats, and champagne came out. Tom's face exuded joy. A lifelong Cubs fan and baseball fanatic ended up being at the Cubs come-from-behind win to celebrate the NL Central Championship. A game where his name was on the scoreboard to celebrate his progress, on what had previously been the worst day of our lives. It was poetic, it was symbolic, and it was pure joy.

When we got home that night, we both crashed. I was crying; he was crying; we were talking about how the day felt like something, but not anything we had ever experienced before. No one understood this but the two of us. It was comforting and terrifying at the same time. I couldn't process the flood of emotions we were experiencing, so I tried to just be in the moment. I was realizing that by staying in the moment, I was giving myself a break later on.

A few days later, I was trying to describe the anniversary to Dr. Crane.

"It was strange. In a weird way I felt disconnected from the day a bit. I'm wondering if that's because I wrote through the whole thing. It forced me to explain what was happening and then maybe move on?" I questioned. "I was emotional all day, but I still can't figure out what exactly the emotion was, other than that nagging sense of loss," I explained.

"What else did you feel that day? It sounds like it was a perfect day," he remarked.

"It really was. I'm not sure you could write a movie plot that perfect. You know, there was a point in the day where I looked over at Tom and he had just pure joy on his face. In fact, I snapped a picture of it on my phone. But later I was thinking about that, and while we've obviously made tremendous progress, I started to doubt the progress," I commented.

"I mean, physically he's obviously progressed beyond everyone's wildest expectations. He beat it, had massive surgery, and is recovering. Last year he was lying in a hospital bed. So that's easy to say A to Z was progress. Yet, from the mental aftermath, I'm not sure what progress has been made. At some level, cancer still owns us…"

"Owns you?" he immediately asked.

"I guess owns isn't the right descriptor, but yes, we are still treated differently in some situations. I am still struggling to let go of the caregiving thing. Comments and questions still come up, which I know is normal, but cancer is still very present in our everyday life. I'm eager for it to just be an occasional visitor. Cancer has overstayed its welcome," I joked.

"I'm sure it has," he said, smiling back at me.

"How was your urge to be a caregiver last week?" he asked.

"You know, I did pretty well. I was a little nervous about how much physical activity Tom was doing, but he kept up pretty well. We both crashed hard the day after the game, but I think that was because of the emotions. I'm trying so hard to let it go, I really am."

"What's holding you back?" he asked.

"I think I know, but I'm not sure I want to admit it," I said.

"Really?" he asked.

"I don't want to get back to normal and then have the feeling of upheaval again," I bluntly replied.

"Upheaval how?" he asked.

"His heart…or it coming back…" I replied. I never liked to say that out loud; I didn't want to put it out in the universe.

He nodded his head at me. I was sure that he was waiting for me to figure that one out on my own. I really am very aware of myself and why I do things. It doesn't mean I can easily change things, but I've always been very proud of my ability to step outside my own thoughts and check myself.

"The sick feeling I get when I think about how fast our lives changed, how much I had to learn, and how much I had to juggle. I don't even know why I'm saying all of those in past tense. Perhaps staying in this in-between is my defense against something bad happening again, because if something bad happens and I haven't been able to enjoy the "normal" life again, then it won't hurt so much."

"You keep going back to this concept of "normal," he challenged.

"I know, and maybe that's part of the issue. I need to accept the fact that we aren't going back to life as we knew it. I'll be floundering for the rest of my life if I keep looking for that. It's going to be gradual, I know…"

I didn't want him to think I was a complete idiot. I knew I was still trying to divorce myself from the idea that some of the worst parts of our life, like scans every three months, were going to be part of our normal whether I wanted them or not.

"All of this is good; these are all signs of coping," he reassured me.

I believed him, for the most part, but desperately wanted to cope faster. Meanwhile, Tom was in his first week of his new job. It seemed like he had made the right move and he was eager to take on the new role. Most of all, he was eager to not have a backstory. I felt his excitement gradually rise, and I was hopeful that I had been wrong about how hard this part of the year might be.

His first week of work wrapped up, and I had a 5K on Sunday morning. It was a beautiful day, and I was once again proud of myself and the progress I had made with my running. The run was early, and we watched the sunrise as I headed off for my race. That afternoon, Tom headed to the driving range and I worked on the book on the back patio. I sat at our patio table, watching the dog in the backyard, with my laptop on my lap, writing about the past few weeks. The temperature was perfect, and the leaves were starting to fall. I stopped writing several times and just looked at the world around me. I didn't get to experience much of the seasons changing this time last year, and fall was my favorite season. I sat outside for a few hours and kept catching myself smiling as I wrote. Last year at this time we were about to start Tom's chemo and had just finished a whirlwind week of appointments and chaos.

I was startled when I heard Tom come out onto the patio. "Oh goodness, I didn't realize you were back," I said as I looked up at him. He had his guitar in his hand as he sat down near me.

"How's writing going?" he asked.

"Pretty good. I'm pretty sure writing and running are the only reason I haven't completely fallen apart," I joked.

"And my unconditional love?" he asked with a serious face.

"Of course! Are you going to play for me?" I asked.

"Maybe…" he said as he strummed the guitar.

I kept writing as he played random chords and parts of songs that he could remember off the top of his head. I watched him play for a while and my heart felt full. We were sitting at our house, which we still owned – a genuine fear of mine with all the bills when he was first diagnosed – he had a smile on his face as he played his guitar, the weather was beautiful, I had run a 5K, and I was working on a book that I was hoping would help someone else who had to deal with cancer. Most importantly, while these days were tough, we still had our relationship intact.

Tom started making up goofy words to a song he was playing and I laughed as he mumbled ridiculous phrases and tried to add in my own goofy lines. What I was most proud of in that moment was that despite everything that had happened in the last year, we hadn't lost "us." Our "us" had evolved a bit differently than expected, but as I sat there I felt peace knowing we were still "us," and if I was being honest, we were a stronger "us."

October

I woke up and rolled over, wondering where Tom was as he walked back into our bedroom. He had a few pairs of my underwear hanging off his hand.

"Why are you holding my underwear?" I asked.

"Doc seems to like your underwear. These were out on the living room floor," he replied.

"I was foolish to think we would ever have a normal dog, wasn't I?" I asked. While he wasn't normal, he had stolen my heart quickly and I was becoming more of a dog person every day.

"Yup, we don't do normal; we needed a dog as crazy as us," he replied as he crawled back into bed with me.

"Ha, isn't that the truth. Are you all packed?" I asked.

"Yup – you?"

"Nope, I should probably do that," I replied.

We were heading to Milwaukee to celebrate my dad's 70th birthday. It was a milestone birthday and I was eager to celebrate with him. What I wasn't eager about was another room of what I now called "newbies." I affectionately referred to people that we hadn't seen since his diagnosis as "newbies" since the conversations usually ended up being lots of questions about what had happened. I wasn't opposed to filling people in on everything, but what that meant was that the cancer became a topic that wouldn't go away.

As folks filed into the party, I noticed a strange yet familiar nagging feeling. In these types of situations, it always seemed like all eyes were on us, our interactions, our comments, etc. If someone asked me a question about Tom's treatment, it often quieted a room because others wanted to hear the answer. I thought the blog would help minimize this in our life, but it did the reverse because our openness meant people felt comfortable asking questions. It didn't anger me; in fact, it filled my heart that so many people cared, but it was pressure. I didn't want the day to be about us. I wanted it to be about my dad's birthday – and it absolutely was – but when the party ended and it felt like all I had done was talk about the chaos of our life, it seemed like we had been the focus, even if we hadn't been.

I couldn't kick the uneasy feeling. It gnawed at me. For two nights after his party, I couldn't sleep. I would overthink our lives, the answers I had given, and how I could have deflected the conversation to another topic sooner. Yet in reality, I was reliving something in the past, something I would never be able to change. I knew that, but it didn't seem to stop my mind from spinning. Luckily, a few days after the party I had an appointment with Dr. Crane. I was eager to see him and started talking the minute I sat down in his office. I didn't wait for him to ask me how I was doing.

"I'm spinning a bit. I know I'm supposed to stay in the moment, but I've been spinning since my dad's birthday party. I don't know why I've been so irrationally emotional about everything – but I think the things that bother me most are people's questions," I immediately said.

"Why questions?" he asked.

"I hate not having answers. I hate that I sometimes can't give the real answer. I hate that it's socially unacceptable to tell someone to stick it where the sun doesn't shine when they ask an inappropriate question," I replied, getting worked up.

At this point, I had become a pro at deflecting. I was shocked by how many people, especially people outside of my inner circle, would ask such personal questions. Normally, people wouldn't flat out ask me if we can have children – so I couldn't understand why cancer gave them that right. It shouldn't, it didn't, and it put salt on an already large wound.

Dr. Crane could tell I was having a tough day and that I was already exhausted, and yet this was just the beginning of all the anxiety I was feeling. As we were talking he made a point that made me really think. After all of this, he acknowledged that I needed to allow myself to accept the emotions.

"I don't think I can do that because the acceptance of the emotions makes everything behind the emotion real and that is too dangerous a place for my mind," I bluntly replied. I wasn't even sure what emotions I hadn't accepted. Maybe the anger, maybe the sadness. Yet, I knew why I couldn't accept the emotions.

"How can I accept something when I don't know its full impact yet?" I asked, though we had discussed this before.

"What don't you know?" he asked.

"I've been thinking about this a bit, and as much as I want to move on from cancer, I need to accept that at some level it will never go away. I can wrap my head around that; it's like when you lose a loved one. You can't change that reality, it never goes away, but with time it gets easier and doesn't feel so fresh."

"I would agree," he said as he nodded for me to continue.

"See, I don't even have closure yet – the death of this cancer hasn't happened yet, and I don't think it will until I know the outcome of what it did to our ability to have a family. How can we move on? How can I accept the emotions of all of this if I know I might not have experienced the worst ones yet? How can I put it in the past when it still has such a hold on our future?" I almost cried just saying the words out loud.

We were starting to turn the corner towards the one-year anniversary of his chemo, which was when we would have the ability to do some testing and see if we had a chance to have a family. That date was only about eight weeks away, and it was floating in our minds all the time. I knew that the was part of the reason my anxiety was building.

I took a deep breath. "And you know what, I've never said this to anyone, but I'm going to say it to you; the scariest part of this whole thing, beyond the ability to have kids…What scares me most is if we can, and we do, and then the cancer comes back, and we aren't as lucky the second time around. And I know that's irrational. Would I ever doubt starting a family if cancer hadn't happened? Of course not. Yet, in theory, that same risk would exist. I could get pregnant tomorrow and Tom could get in a car accident. I know it's ridiculous, but I love him, and want a family with him."

As Dr. Crane and I continued to talk, I wondered where I would be if I hadn't started seeing him ten months earlier. Being able to talk to him, no judgment, as a third-party that didn't have relationships with the people in my life, was the only reason that I was still sitting there with my wits about me. I'm not ashamed to admit that, if I hadn't started therapy, I don't know what condition I would have been in. I was grateful for Dr. Crane, and especially grateful for the conversation that night. As I walked out to my car, I felt a little weight off my shoulders because I had talked through some of what had been spinning in my head. It wasn't gone, but I had helped myself organize it in a way that didn't give me such anxiety. It's like Dr. Crane was a professional organizer of my thoughts – a messy job indeed.

A few short days later, I was waiting on a random street corner in Chicago to meet up with my girlfriend Maggie who was running the Chicago Marathon. She was inspired to run a full marathon, and had asked Tom and I if she could raise money for a charity that meant a lot to us on behalf of Tom's cancer fight. We had selected Imerman Angels, and she had raised thousands for them. I figured the least I could do was run a few miles with her during the race, especially because running and I had become such good friends. She arrived at our planned meeting point right after the mile 18 marker and I ran alongside her. I was planning to run about three miles with her. Tom, my girlfriend Jenna and her husband, Andrew, were meeting us at that location. From there, Maggie was going to finish the last four miles and we would see her at the finish line. I started running next to her, and I couldn't believe she had already run eighteen – as I ran next to her I was thankful that I was as tall as I was and that she was a bit shorter because the difference in our stride was the only reason I was able to keep up with her.

She wanted to slow her pace to get ready for her final few miles and we chatted as we trotted along. We talked about our careers, about Tom & I wanting a family, and how appreciative I was that she was doing this for Imerman Angels. This was a physical demonstration of how many people had helped us, and for us it was one of the good things to come from cancer. If our story helped her decide to run, and totally crush, her first marathon, then we chalked that up as something "good" that came from cancer. While cancer was the hardest thing in the world for us to deal with, I truly believe that if we had kept tally, more good, in many shapes and forms, came from it than bad. My heart was full that night as I went to sleep. I was so proud of Maggie and I was also proud of myself. A year ago I wouldn't have been able to run half a mile, much less feel confident enough to run three with Maggie. It was a reminder that for all the anxiety I was feeling, for all of the tough days we were having, there was still progress.

A few days after the marathon, we got the text that my sister-in-law, Christina, had delivered her new baby boy. We were excited to meet him and while he was a little earlier than expected, everyone was healthy and doing fine. My sister-in-law and I chatted and planned that we'd see the baby the following night. I wanted nothing more than to hold the little peanut, but part of me was anxious about going into the hospital. She had delivered at the same hospital where Tom had completed treatment, and it would be the first time we would be in a patient room since we left after his surgery.

We had a day to prepare our minds, but I found myself getting anxious as the day went on. I worried about Tom too, but had learned my lesson with our speech back in May and was trying to focus on my own emotions. When we both got home from work, we agreed we were both okay to go and that we would power through – we wanted to go to the hospital for a positive reason so we could start associating better feelings with the place.

It was strange to park in the same parking structure and walk through the same hallways where I had carried our things back and forth to the car for chemo, but nothing struck a chord quite like the smell. It's that sterile, clean, hospital smell that hit my nostrils and sent a wave of emotion through my body. It was different from when I had picked up the medical records, and I wasn't sure why. I grabbed Tom's hand and we both squeezed. We quickly made our way to the elevator to her room. Surprisingly, Tom was doing better than I was as I almost threw up. I felt relief when the door shut behind us. The room was filled with familiar faces, my sister-in-law, Staci, and her family, and so much love that I was able to calm down.

As we visited with them and I snuggled the baby, I felt at peace knowing that while I struggled with the hospital itself, the concept of all the love within hospitals remained the same. When people came to see us they didn't have the joy of a newborn, but there was still so much love. We had conquered the first official hospital visit, and it was another thing we could check off the list of our recovery – for the best reason ever – baby Jonathan.

Despite all the excitement, my nights were sleepless again as I was flying out to Washington DC for a friend's wedding. Tom wasn't coming because we were taking another trip the following weekend, and a back-to-back weekend was still a lot for him to handle. That meant that I was leaving him alone and would be a flight away. Given how emotional he had been lately, how much he was struggling, and of course just the fear of something happening, I almost canceled my trip multiple times that week.

"I don't know if I can get on the plane tomorrow," I said as I was packing in the bedroom.

"You're going. Your sister and the baby are out there, you have family to see out there, you're going," he said.

"I know you are right, but it's still hard. Can you just stay in the house in bubble wrap?" I asked as I smiled at him.

"No, I need to go out and get sushi because you're away," he joked.

I knew he was trying to understand where I was coming from, but he would never completely understand. I think his mindset was more go, get back to life, and don't hold back, while mine was still struggling to break from my caregiver shell. I still felt like such a protector. He had only been in his new job for about three weeks, and the time of year was impacting both of us.

I got on the flight that Friday night and arrived in DC. I headed to my aunt's house and saw my cousins, sister, brother-in-law, and nephew who were also attending the wedding. It was late, and I was feeling so much anxiety about being away. I crawled into bed, but it felt empty. I once again realized how accustomed I had become to being with Tom all the time. I couldn't even enjoy the solitude. Instead, it just felt wrong.

The next day, I tried to focus on spending time with my family and being in the moment with them. My sister started the day by telling me that she was going to make me an aunt again and that she was pregnant. I was excited for her, but these milestones put our own timing in perspective. Tom and I had been trying to have a family before my sister had her first child and now she was pregnant with her second. I was so happy for her, and our whole family, but these types of events put the spotlight on how fast time was moving and how long our lives continued to be without a family - which at times could be very overwhelming.

Tom and I texted back and forth all day, and he assured me that he was fine and that he wasn't going to crash the car while I was away this time. In the afternoon we headed out to the wedding, which was being held at a vineyard outside of the city. The setting was beautiful and the ceremony started just before sunset. It was a small intimate wedding and a perfect day. As I sat there watching them recite their vows, I found myself becoming more cynical, which quickly shifted to anger. I remembered my own wedding. I remember saying the same words they were saying, but having no clue, and perhaps being too naïve to really think about what they would mean over the years. Some couples deal with the trials of richer and others deal with the poorer. Some couples deal with sickness while others can avoid it for years. These words were hitting me to the core; they felt like punches to the gut. So much had already manifested in my own marriage in just a few years. And yet, during their engagement, he and his fiancé had dealt with challenges as they both lost their fathers in the months leading up to their wedding. I knew they would be okay, and my anger turned to protective feelings. I wanted them to never, in their entire lifetimes, feel a moment of the pain we had experienced in the last year.

I did what any normal person would do in this situation when the emotions are unexpected and strong. I headed to the open bar. It was those moments that were always toughest, the ones that caught me off guard. I didn't think I would have that reaction to being at a wedding, but I had, and it wasn't easy to deal with alone. Yet as I looked around the room, other than my family and the bride and groom, I was anonymous, and it was refreshing. No one knew my story. No one in that room could feel bad for me, and no one in the room would ask inappropriate questions. It was oddly delightful.

The next morning, my aunt and I ran to a few of my favorite places from all my years of visiting. She had asked if I would stop by and see my uncle's grave. My uncle had passed away a few years earlier after a years-long fight with cancer. She had crafted a beautiful headstone and she wanted to show me how it had all come together. I happily agreed to stop with her, and we pulled up to a beautiful cemetery. We got out of the car and she led the way to the stone. We got to the stone, I looked down, and I immediately felt like sobbing. I took a step away and couldn't look back at the stone. I sort of danced around by the other graves and continued my conversation with her.

That could have been me. I could have been the widow standing at my husband's grave. I was mad at myself for my reaction. How dare I wimp out on acknowledging his beautiful gravesite. How dare I tell her that it was affecting me. My aunt had lost her husband; my cousins lost their father. They probably often wonder what life would have been like if their dad had beat cancer. Regardless, in my mind my uncle had beat cancer because of how beautifully he fought it. The weekend had smacked me with so many unexpected emotions, and I was eager to get back to Tom. We wouldn't be home long, as Tom and I were leaving the next weekend to head to Las Vegas with my dad. We were taking him to Vegas for his 70th birthday and it had been on our post-cancer bucket list, so we were excited for a few days away.

While we were in Vegas, the World Series was in full swing. Tom was so excited that the Cubs were making a run for the World Series and more than anything it was providing a great distraction for these few weeks, as there was so much energy and excitement. On our first night there, the Cubs won the NL Pennant and were headed to the World Series.

The next day, I woke up in the hotel room to the symphony of Tom throwing up. It had become strangely normal for me to not react to this, and hope it was temporary, yet to my dad I'm sure it was strange. Tom eventually came out of the bathroom and flopped on the bed again to rest. The day of traveling and the Cubs game had been too much for him. My dad headed off to play a tournament, and Tom slept. I was feeling very sad and wasn't sure what to do. We were in the hotel room, and I felt like everything I did was keeping Tom awake, so I decided to go for a walk so that Tom could sleep.

I walked down the Las Vegas strip and people-watched. If ever someone needs a prime people-watching opportunity, it's a Sunday morning in Las Vegas. I could only hope that some of the walks of shame were headed to church. My mind was racing, wondering if Tom would be down for the whole day, if he was okay, and if this trip was a bad idea. We had yet to take a trip where he didn't get sick, and I missed the days of our spontaneous adventures. I went back to the room to find Tom awake and feeling a bit better. It was a tricky dance we would have when he wouldn't feel well; we had to take it slow and hope that he would rebound. Luckily, he came around and we spent three fun days with my dad gambling, eating food and enjoying the best people watching in the world.

We returned home the day before our anniversary, and I already knew that our anniversary plans were going to change.

"So, I was thinking…maybe we can postpone our anniversary dinner until this weekend…" Tom said with a smirk.

"Could that have something to do with game two of the World Series?" I asked with a smile on my face.

"Perhaps…" Tom said as he came over and gave me a hug.

"That's fine, babe – it doesn't bother me at all. You unintentionally set the bar so low last year," I joked.

"What do you mean?" he asked, confused.

"Last year our anniversary was our first day home from chemo, you had to get a shot, were nauseous, and sleeping most of the day. The bar was so low last year that if eating takeout and watching the Cubs game is our anniversary celebration it's still one hundred times better. Plus, this year you are cancer-free so you already gave me a gift!" I explained.

"You're the best," he replied as he gave me another hug.

"I'm confused about how we are celebrating this weekend. There are games on Friday, Saturday and Sunday night," I said.

I saw the look on Tom's face as he realized that I was right. "I mean…maybe we could go to an early dinner one night or something?"

"Let's just do it sometime after the World Series. It doesn't bother me in the least," I replied.

It truly didn't. He was cancer-free. Our relationship was intact, and I knew our vows were stronger than ever. Even if I hadn't heard the line in our vows about how important World Series Cubs games would be.

The last weekend of October was the first weekend that I had been home the entire month. I was exhausted and had been traveling so much. However, those same months last year I was desperate to get out of the hospital and travel. We had come such a long way.

Since I was finally home, I was outside raking and getting ready for winter, which was quickly approaching. It was a gorgeous fall day, the temperature was crisp, and the leaves were falling. I cleaned up my flowerbeds before I grabbed the rake and started to drag all the leaves to the curb. About ten minutes into raking, I burst into tears. Last year, I hadn't had the opportunity to rake. Family had all pitched in and helped take care of the yard while we were in and out of chemo. I didn't realize how much I had missed it until I stood there raking. October was my favorite month – it's one of the reasons it was the month we got married. Yet now, here I was crying like a baby because I was raking.

It was the feeling of loss again – we had lost all the time last year and didn't even realize it until we got it back. It has been said you don't know what you have until it's gone, but I think it's also fair to say you don't know what you lost until you get it back.

November

"Breathe, please!!!" I yelled at Tom from the couch.

"I am!" he said, not taking his eyes off the TV.

It was game seven of the World Series. The Cubs had come back from being down 3-1 in the series, and this game had gone back and forth. They were up, then they were tied, then a rain delay, then extra innings. It was exhausting, and watching Tom watch the game was painful.

"Okay – you have a weak heart – you've come too far to have something happen during game seven!" I joked.

It was just Tom and I at home watching the game. I was kind of surprised that he hadn't wanted to go out, or head downtown to Wrigleyville and watch it there. However, Tom wasn't necessarily someone who could sit still and watch a Cubs game. He needed to pace around the house, throw his hat and do a myriad of superstitious activities during the game.

It was fun to watch the game with him, though nerve-wracking. As a Brewers fan, I didn't have much at stake, but I did want this for Tom. In fact, so many friends of ours, who usually support other teams, had been texting and telling us they were rooting for the Cubs for Tom. As I watched him watch the game, I couldn't help but think of last year. The Cubs had just missed the chance to be in the World Series, and that loss occurred during our third round of chemo. I was thinking back to that night when they lost the game. His morale was already down because of a chemo week, but after the game his outlook had been surprisingly positive. He had said that maybe it was a good thing – and predicted they would win next year when he would be able to celebrate.

How right he was. A little later he was screaming at the TV as the Cubs, after 108 years, won the World Series. Fireworks were going off outside, neighbors were out banging pots and pans, and Tom jumped down the stairs and out the front door to hang the Cubs "W" flag with pride. He was beaming. I had wanted this for him so bad. He didn't crawl into bed that night until almost 4 a.m.; he had been too excited to sleep.

That was the peak. Then it all crashed again. Two days later, I came home from work, which happened to be the day of the Cubs parade, and Tom was crying. I knew it could only be one of two things – either he had watched a replay of game seven, or something was wrong. He was a mess, emotionally all over the place, and very much wandering back to the dark side of the depression and PTSD.

"What's wrong? Are you okay?" I asked.

"Yeah, I don't know. I'm fine," he said.

"Well, obviously not," I replied.

I sat up on the kitchen counter as he moved around the kitchen. I had a feeling I knew what was happening, but wanted to see if he had figured it out too.

"Can I tell you something and you not get mad?" he asked.

"You say that like I'm a monster – of course – fire away," I replied.

"I should have gone to Wrigley to watch the game. I'm regretting that I wasn't down there for the game. I wanted this for so long and I should have just gone," he said.

"I begged you to go downtown – you insisted on staying at home!" I replied.

"I know, and here's the part where I don't want you to get mad, and I love you, but it felt like last year," he replied.

"Last year?" I questioned.

"Last year, it was just you and I stuck in this house. It just felt strange that it was just you and me – I kept thinking it was last year," he said. "And I love spending time with you, and I had fun watching it with you, but it was just weird."

"I get that, babe, I wish you had gone down there," I replied. "I worry about you though – I think maybe the Cubs were a bit of a distraction," I said, hoping he wasn't going to get defensive.

It had occurred to me that the Cubs had been distracting us since the one-year anniversary of his diagnosis. I was having a hard time with these fall months myself, and it had surprised me that it wasn't affecting him more. He certainly had several rough days in late September and October, but I think he pulled himself together by always having a game to look forward to. Now that may sound crazy, but Tom is an obsessed Cubs fan; it truly would have been the light in an otherwise tough day.

"I know. I agree. I think I used it all as a distraction," he replied.

I was a little shocked he was so agreeable to my observation, but I was glad that he was able to recognize it.

"Well, I have an idea!" I proclaimed. "How about this. We never got our anniversary dinner, so why don't we go downtown this weekend and have our anniversary dinner and then at least go to Wrigley? It's all still covered in the chalk, and we can get your picture with the marquee. I know it's not the same, but it's only been forty-eight hours, so I'm sure it's still electric."

"I didn't tell you this to solve the problem, I just wanted to tell you how I'm feeling," he said.

"I'm not trying to solve the problem, but we were planning to have our anniversary dinner anyway so why not stop at Wrigley? It's your call, but I'm up for it if you want. You decide."

It's how my personality works; I take facts and create solutions. I wasn't trying to fix the emotion, but rather try to find a middle ground that helped him not feel like he had completely "missed" everything since the parade had just happened and there was plenty of electricity still flowing around the city. It broke my heart that he felt like he had missed out, especially because last year he had such optimism about the win happening this year.

The next night, we had our anniversary dinner and headed over to Wrigley. It was still buzzing and it was amazing to see all the hustle and bustle around the stadium. Once the Cubs had made the World Series, fans had gone down to Wrigley and written messages with chalk on the brick stadium. It was filled with inspirational messages and memorials; it gave me goosebumps. We walked around the stadium on that late fall night, and I hoped that this was helping Tom and that this little dip was only temporary.

Unfortunately, it wasn't. He was really having some tough days. We had planned to head to Cincinnati for the weekend to meet up with friends, but I ended up canceling the trip at the beginning of the week. It was too much for us at the time, and I didn't want to force Tom to be in social situations all weekend when he wasn't feeling well. I was learning how to navigate all the post-cancer challenges and putting on a happy face and smiling though those situations became too exhausting for us.

I was curious what Dr. Crane would think about me cancelling the trip. To date we had always managed to power through on plans, no matter how tough. When we talked that week, I had to be honest about how I was feeling.

"I canceled our trip this week, and for some reason I worried I was being judged," I said.

"By whom?" he asked.

"I sent a note to all my girlfriends and was honest that things just haven't been great, and I worry they think I'm crazy because they don't understand it. It's like what I imagine it's like for someone who is a new mom, and she says that she can't make it somewhere, or are very late or something, and she gets judged for it by someone without kids. I mean, how does a person without kids throw judgment? They shouldn't. Yet no one understands this situation. Obviously, I'm happy none of them have the experience – I wouldn't wish this upon anyone – but I just don't ever want them to doubt how much I love them. Am I even making sense?"

"Yes," he replied as he nodded.

"And these last few weeks, Tom has just been having a really tough go of it, and I keep trying to balance my role of wife and caregiver, but he's all over the place, so I feel out of control. I feel like I'm letting people down and that they don't understand how challenging our life is right now," I said as I tried to organize my thoughts. "Plus, to add insult to injury, we have the next round of scans next week so the sleepless nights are beginning again. I just want everything to be okay. Even if we get great news from our doctor, our reality is actually the opposite. How's that for irony?' I remarked.

Dr. Crane did what he did best and helped me make a plan to deal with my reality. It was terrifying how radically my reality could change in the days between sessions. I left his office that night, thinking I had a plan of attack for the week, but just a few hours later I felt terrified again. Tom and I were sitting on the couch and could hardly believe our eyes.

"Is this really happening?" I asked.

"We are so screwed if it is," he replied.

We were watching the news coverage on election night and at that point, it was clear that Trump was going to be elected. It hadn't even crossed our minds that it could happen. It was terrifying. Among so many concerns we had about him being elected, repealing the Affordable Care Act would have a massive impact on our future. We headed to bed in hopes that all the predictions were wrong.

The next morning I rolled over and checked my phone. It wasn't a nightmare. A few moments later Tom walked into the bedroom.

"I'm sorry I got cancer," he said, holding back tears.

"Don't you dare – you didn't do this on purpose – and we just need to hope that something comes out that proves this isn't true, or that he doesn't repeal it" I said, trying to make him feel better.

It was depressing to think that Tom felt the need to apologize to me for getting cancer because of the president-elect. Regardless of party, what upset us most was the uneasy feeling of not knowing what the alternative would be. Never once in Trump's campaign did he specifically explain what he was going to do to change the Affordable Care Act. The uncertainty of potential changes ahead created an empty feeling for both of us.

There were two components of the Affordable Care Act that had huge impacts on us. The first was that there are no lifetime maximums – meaning that the insurance company couldn't dump us once we got too expensive. To this point, we had billed almost two million, yes million, dollars for Tom. Prior to the Affordable Care Act, Tom would never have been able to be insured again. The second was coverage for pre-existing conditions was in jeopardy. Previously, if you had a pre-existing condition, like cancer, the insurance company could deny coverage. Those two components alone could dramatically change the projection of our future. Paying for medical expenses out-of-pocket for the rest of our lives would mean drastically different and possibly very dangerous choices. What frustrated me most was that there were people in our lives who didn't understand why we were so upset. In reality, they didn't understand how insurance and the Affordable Care Act worked, which was even more frightening.

We were both upset and scared. I was happier than ever that I had cancelled the trip to Cincinnati because of where we were at, trying to cope with the election and headed into a checkup week.

You would think at some point we would start to catch a break, but in almost poetic form, the opposite occurred. Monday of checkup week, my grandmother was put into hospice care and wasn't likely to make it through the week. She had been in a nursing home for a while, and for years had longed to be with my grandpa, who had passed away years earlier. Now in her 90's, she had lived a full life, but it didn't make it any easier.

On Wednesday we got the all-clear on Tom's scans. It was a relief, and the doctor was eager to hear about how things were going in our recovery. It felt like we would always tell her the same update. In a way, we were in a holding pattern; we needed time to pass to have any sort of meaningful changes to report. The sense of relief we had when walking to the car felt like a huge weight off our shoulders. Each successful checkup made me a little more hopeful for the next one, which would hopefully make them less daunting each time.

Usually the night after the checkup I would sleep hard, having more peace of mind. But this time was different; my grandmother was still in hospice. I hadn't focused too much on Tom's checkup with my family because I knew everyone had so much else going on, but I was glad that our good results had been a moment of happiness for the family. My grandmother passed away peacefully the day after the checkup. The priest had been in the room with her and prayed a Hail Mary. As he said the last line, "…now and at the hour of our death…Amen," she took her last breath and passed away. In my wildest dreams I couldn't have prayed for a better ending for her. It was peaceful, dignified, and she was surrounded by so much love.

Her death was another first that caught me off guard. She was the first person who died since Tom's diagnosis, and wrapping my head around her death was harder than I had imagined. Usually, when someone died I could rationalize, understand and even accept the reality of the situation. For some reason, I couldn't do that as well this time around. The only solace was knowing that she was with my grandpa. He had passed over fifteen years earlier, and she missed him so much. She always said she was ready to go be with my grandpa, and now she was at peace and with him.

In less than fifteen days, the Cubs had won the World Series, Tom was in the lowest place he had been in months, Trump was elected, we had checkups, and my grandmother passed away. Emotionally, I felt broken. I was trying to keep it all together for Tom, but I was starting to slip myself. Tom was continuing to see his therapist and had come to the realization that last year he had put all of his effort into his physical fight. This year, he was experiencing it all emotionally. The loss, the guilt, the impact, the magnitude – it was like an avalanche picking up speed.

I rolled over one morning and heard him sobbing in the bathroom. I jumped out of bed and knocked on the door to see if he was okay. It was 5 a.m. and I was worried something had happened.

"What's wrong?" I asked as I grabbed him for a hug. His eyes were bloodshot, his face covered with tears.

"I don't even know, I am so overwhelmed," he replied. I stood there, half asleep, and squeezed him so tight.

"I'm sorry, babe..." I softly said as I rubbed his back. "I love you so much."

We stood there for several minutes, not saying a word as he composed himself.

"It's cold out here – come back to our warm bed..." I said with a smile as I pulled away from our hug.

We crawled back into bed and I curled into him.

"I don't know why I woke up and got so overwhelmed," he said.

"You don't owe me an explanation, babe, I get it..."

It was these moments that actually kept me from falling apart because I knew that I needed to stay strong for us.

Days later, we sat at the Thanksgiving table, and despite the complete mess that our lives were, we had so much to be thankful for. It was our year to spend Thanksgiving in Milwaukee, and I was eager to be with family. My grandmother's wishes were to donate her body to science, which meant that a funeral wouldn't happen for up to eighteen months. While I was so happy that she chose to help people even after she was gone, it left me without closure for the time being.

On our way to Milwaukee, Tom started feeling a bit nauseous, as he was thinking back to the holidays last year. I was surprised that this trip was sparking this kind of reaction in him, because we had been to Milwaukee several times since his surgery and it didn't bother him. However, it was the fact that it was the holidays, given how challenging those had been last year, that was making him flash back.

"Do you want to stay home?" I asked.

"No, I'll be fine. I just need to be sad for a minute," he replied as he squeezed my hand.

As we sat at the Thanksgiving table, I was so happy that despite how we felt, we were surrounded by so much love and had so much to be thankful for. As we went around the table, saying what we were thankful for, I had so much to say but had one thing in particular that I wanted to make sure I said before I burst into tears. I almost immediately began to cry but somehow managed to blubber out some words. What I was most thankful for was Tom. In the absolute worst year of our life, he had tried with all his might to cope with a smile, while trying to make me laugh. I was so proud of him for working through all the post-cancer challenges and having the strength to say that he needed help. Tom always said he felt so weak – but all I saw from him in the last year was strength. Beyond everything, Tom was full of gratitude all year. I never did something for him that he didn't thank me for and acknowledge. Even on the toughest days, he would roll over and kiss me on the forehead and thank me for being so strong. He had gratitude all year long, something that would have been easy to forget, but he didn't, and I was more thankful than ever for that.

We got home from Milwaukee on Friday and I crashed. It had been very emotional to be home without my grandma at the Thanksgiving table in addition to the chaos that had ensued the previous three weeks. I did something I rarely do; I curled up in a ball and didn't leave my bed for the rest of the day. I even skipped a holiday event with Tom. I had hit a bit of an emotional rock bottom, and I knew that I needed to let my mind and body recover for a few hours. I was foolish to think a few hours would be all I needed, but I was proud of myself for prioritizing what I needed in that moment. It was the first time I had done that in months.

December

I woke up every day hopeful that life might feel a little more normal, but as time passed, it felt like the reverse was happening. Life felt so disjointed. It felt like we had missed a year of our lives and with other milestone anniversaries upon us, I was nervous as to how things would transpire. It was hard to believe that we were approaching the one-year anniversary of Tom's chemo ending, which would continue to be memorialized with his birthday. However, we had a fun celebration planned. A dear friend of mine from college was getting married in his hometown in Colorado, and Tom and I had been planning to attend. We had extended our trip for four days to go skiing.

Skiing had been on the post-cancer bucket list and it seemed like a great opportunity to make the most of a plane ticket and celebrate how far we had come in a year. It seemed impossible that chemo had finished a year ago – that creeping feeling of loss reared its ugly head. The days felt slow, in fact some dragged on, but the year as a whole had flown by. We hadn't had many breaks, a few quick weekends here and there, but I really needed to get away.

The wedding was beautiful, and it was so good for us to be surrounded by friends. The morning after the wedding, we woke up and Tom was down for the count. He hadn't had a single drop to drink the night before at the wedding, and still it had been too much for him. Another trip, another day down. It was in these moments that I got really mad at cancer. Before cancer, I never would have had to worry about Tom not feeling well on vacation – we would get up and explore and not have to think twice about energy and being able to keep up with a full day of fun. I hated watching him be miserable, and I especially hated how bad he felt about being miserable. It was a vicious cycle.

What worried me was that while he was already feeling terrible, we were about to drive to an even higher altitude. We rested that morning and I hoped he would start to feel better, so we could enjoy these few days of celebration. I knew he wasn't feeling well physically, but I worried that the pending chemo anniversary was also making him not feel well mentally. After some fluids and a bite to eat, he started to turn the corner and we headed up to the mountains for some skiing. We drove through beautiful, snowcapped mountains and I was eager to see the ski towns all decorated for Christmas. As we traveled the windy road, we chatted about the days ahead.

"So really, on a scale of one to ten are we worried that I've never skied and have only watched YouTube videos to teach myself?" I joked with Tom.

"I hope this ends well…" he said as he laughed with me.

"It seems easy enough. If you want to go forward, you make your skis look like French fries; if you want to stop you make your skis look like a slice of pizza. That seems like the important stuff," I said with confidence.

I knew it was driving Tom nuts that I hadn't been able to take a class, but I have always been more a baptism-by-fire kind of girl anyway.

We pulled into beautiful Beaver Creek, toured the cute town and got acquainted with where we would go the next day to ski. Our hotel was unbelievable, with a fireplace in the room. It was a ski in/ski out resort, and it was enchanting. Later that evening, after we had explored the surrounding towns a bit, we walked over to the downtown area of Beaver Creek. There was an ice rink in the middle surrounded by sitting areas and fireplaces. We were already bundled up and we curled up together next to a fire pit where we watched the few people on the ice rink. Everywhere you looked there were Christmas decorations and, thanks to the time of year, the town was practically empty. It was magical. It felt like we were at the North Pole, and more than anything, I was so happy to be on this getaway with Tom.

"I know it's a long time away, but I want to bring our kids here someday. This is such a cool town, and it would be so fun to do a family vacation here," I said. I hoped he would take my comment simply, versus think about all the question marks surrounding our pending family.

"Me too – I want to ski with my kids here, but before they are too cool to ski with me," he joked.

We sat there chatting about your future and it gave me hope. A year ago the only future we could talk about was his upcoming surgery; anything after that seemed so tentative. It was late and getting colder, so we headed back to our hotel and decided to jump into the hot tub. It was outdoors, but there was something so fun being in a hot tub, surrounded by snow. It felt like we were in a snow globe. No matter where I looked it was like an image on a postcard. We floated in the hot tub and for the first time in weeks, things felt calm.

The calm quickly passed the next morning when I was standing at the top of the bunny hill with Tom, about to click into my skis for the first time. Tom had skied previously, but it had been years, so he wanted to go down the bunny hill a few times to get his "ski legs" back. We were standing in the area next to the gondola, and Tom told me how to pop into my skis.

"I wouldn't put your boot in your ski that way. You need to be perpendicular to the hill or you'll start sliding down the hill," he said.

"Oh, I see," I replied. I turned 180 degrees and put my skis down and started to put my boot in the ski again as I heard Tom laugh out loud.

"You just turned the other way, but you're still going down the hill. You need to put on your skis perpendicular to the hill," he said between laughs.

"I don't remember this part in the YouTube video," I said, laughing.

I knew this might be a disaster, but I was already having fun, even if my ability to snap the boot into the ski wasn't going well. I got all secured and then needed to figure out how to actually ski. The videos must have worked, because I sort of just figured it out. I pushed myself forward, got adjusted to the skis and then began to work my way down the bunny hill. I made it down, slowly, and can always say I didn't wipe out on my first hill experience. Tom looked like a natural and we decided to do the bunny hill again. At the bottom of the bunny hill you can turn and start going down a "real" hill.

"You picked this up way better than I anticipated," he said.

"I'm almost a pro!" I exclaimed as I struggled to stop on my skis.

"What do you want to do?" he asked as he looked downhill.

"I'm game. Let's give it a shot!" I said as I pushed myself towards the first part of the hill.

Luckily for Tom, he married a lady who isn't afraid to throw caution to the wind and give it a shot. What was the worst that could happen? Tom led the way, and while it was a little more challenging than the bunny hill I was able to make my way down the hill. It zigged and zagged until we hit the final part of the hill, which was the "real" part of the hill. It looked very steep. Up to this point, the pizza and French fry moves had been effective. So I did what any idiot would do who had only been on skis for thirty minutes - I turned onto the hill and faced my skis downward.

I tried to "pizza" myself to safety and failed miserably. What I hadn't seen in the YouTube videos was that, once you are on a real hill, you have to stay perpendicular. I quickly picked up speed and couldn't figure out how to stop. I got closer and closer to an edge that would cause me even more problems, so I wiped out. The minute I landed, I knew I had really hurt my tailbone. It was so bad I couldn't even get up from the ground while snapped into my skis.

A moment later Tom caught up to me and was kind enough to tell me that you have to stay perpendicular to the hill. I managed to make my way back down the hill without falling and I was in so much pain, but there wasn't a snowball's chance in hell that I wasn't going to power through the day so that we could have our day of skiing. We went up and down the hills for hours and I started to get better at skiing, while biting my tongue in pain. I took a break and sat by the fire as I waited for Tom to come down one of the harder hills. I watched all the people coming down and kept my eye out for Tom. I eventually saw him making his way down and couldn't help but get emotional.

It was exactly one year ago that he took his last bag of chemo, and here he was skiing down a mountain. He had been tethered to an IV pole last year with no freedom, and there he was gliding down the hill. The analogies were abundant, but I just sat there with tears in my eyes and was full of gratitude.

We had the most wonderful trip, and when we got home I felt so thankful that, despite the year we had, we were able to take a trip. I had worried so much that we would have to sell our house or deplete our savings to make it financially. We certainly took quite a hit, but so far, we were making it.

For every high, I had been conditioned to be ready for a low and it was strangely natural at this point to be ready for a low. It was a coping mechanism, but after the trip I had hoped we might start having fewer lows. The next week I woke up to hear Tom throwing up in the bathroom.

"Throwing up?" I asked when he came back into the room.

"Not even, I just kept dry heaving," he replied.

He powered through, but I felt helpless. I left for work and he was dressed and right behind me. I knew he wasn't going to go into work, but I didn't want to doubt him. He had been having an intense sequence of bad days, and I knew he was slipping back into the dark times we had experienced in summer. It was scary, but I tried to talk myself out of it. I got to my office and was texting back and forth with him all morning.

"How are you feeling?" I asked.

"Not great, but alright."

"Did you go into work?"

"Yeah."

I knew he wasn't at work but I gave it a little more time before saying anything. Then it occurred to me that I had a way to see if I was right. We had installed a smart thermostat the week prior, which is synced to our smart phones. The thermostat learns our patterns and helps lower energy and heating costs while allowing us to control the temperature from our phones while both home and away. I clicked on the app to see if it had us as "away." It would only be in that mode if both phones were out of the house. I waited for the app to load and my stomach dropped when I saw that it had us as "home."

I grabbed my phone and texted him calmly "Did you really go into work? Please don't lie if you didn't, just be honest."

"Alright, I'm sorry. I couldn't take it today. I'm working from home. So there you go; you're always right."

"I'm not trying to be right; I just want you to be honest."

"It's hard to tell you I'm struggling sometimes because I don't want you to go into caregiver mode."

"I understand that, but the deception actually pushes me further into the caregiver mode. Knowing what's going on helps me deal with facts. The guessing makes me assume the worst, which makes me be a caregiver."

"I love you…I just want to be strong for you, and it's hard to admit I'm struggling sometimes. I want to feel like myself again."

"I know, babe. Trust me; you are already strong in my book. The struggle is real; I have it too, and there is nothing wrong with dealing with that."

I tried to be calm, but I was really hurt that we were once again dealing with his struggling and his wanting to hide it from me. I don't think he made the connection that it was his behavior that drove how I reacted. When he wasn't being honest, and trying to hide how he was feeling, it forced me to jump into caregiver mode.

I was feeling defeated, and I acknowledged why our situation was bothering me so much. I felt like I had lost my voice. I wasn't speaking up on certain topics because I worried about him and how he would react. I didn't want him to interpret my worries as guilt, because he was already carrying too much of that. Earlier that week he had insisted that he snow blow during a storm because he "owed" me from being unable to do any shoveling last winter. Words like that were like nails on a chalkboard. He owed me nothing; we were a team, and while I had taken on a lot the year prior, it didn't mean he owed me anything in return.

The other thing that was bugging me was that a part of me felt like Tom wanted me to be madder. I think at some level, whether he knew it or not, he wanted me to tell him I was mad about our situation so that I could validate his guilt. It's just not who I am. Cancer was out of his control, but his actions now were in his control and that was a fine line that I was trying to understand. While I knew he was coping with a lot, I also feared that he might stay in this state for too long. To me, everything he was feeling was natural, especially the fact that he was experiencing all these emotions for the first time, but I also needed to balance that with progress. My greatest fear was that we'd be in the same emotional turmoil next year because we didn't force ourselves to move on. I wasn't going to allow a pity party; we had never had one to this point, and we certainly were not going to start.

We took each day one by one, especially as we approached the holidays. He continued to wake up and throw up or dry heave in the morning, but was finding a way to go into work most days. We had an early Christmas with my family and then settled in to celebrate Christmas in Chicago. While I was sad to not be with my family, I was happy that we didn't need to travel for the Christmas weekend. I knew it might be emotional and was happy we would be able to lay low and try to relax.

On Christmas Eve, I went to mass before we headed over to his parents' house. Tom had offered to come with me, but I let him off the hook for several reasons. I walked into church and it was packed. I found a space on the back wall to stand for the mass and immediately regretted my shoe choice for an hour of standing. Mass was at 3 p.m.; it was the kids mass, the only one I was able to attend before the Christmas Eve festivities. As I stood in the back, I looked around at all the families and kids who had the magic of Christmas in their eyes. The music was beautiful and I started to feel overwhelmed. This was precisely the reason that I had thought it was a bad idea for Tom to come too.

I wanted nothing more than to be celebrating Christmas with a little one. I wanted the joy that these families were experiencing as they patiently sat through mass knowing that Santa would be coming soon. I made it twenty-five minutes before a tear rolled down my face. I quickly wiped away my tears and took a deep breath. I didn't want to feel so sad on Christmas Eve, but this kind of day made the absence of children front and center in our lives, which in turn put cancer at the front and center again.

We had a wonderful Christmas and it helped us acknowledge how far we had come. Yet I would be lying if I had said we weren't drained. We had such a busy month and Tom's emotional state had made it even tougher. As we wrapped up the holidays, we approached New Year's Eve exhausted.

"What do you want to do for New Year's?" I asked Tom.

"I don't know. What do you want to do?" he asked.

"If I'm being honest, I want to order take out, be in bed before midnight and give 2016 the middle finger," I replied.

Tom laughed and agreed to my romantic plans.

"Except, I was thinking I'd run another 5K on New Year's Eve morning if you're up for cheering me on," I replied.

Tom agreed and a few days later I was once again standing at a starting line for a 5K. I was already freezing cold, but I was starting my seventh 5K of the year. The freezing temperatures helped me move quickly and as I ran the race I felt an overwhelming sense of pride. I never thought I would be much of a runner, and I wasn't running the fastest time, but I was running and making progress in my own way. As usual, I saw Tom cheering me on at the finish line, and I was so happy that he had been so supportive of my running. As we crawled into bed that night we were ready to say goodbye to the year.

"It's weird, because as hard as this year has been, I've had some pretty great days too," he remarked.

"I know, I think that's why this all feels so weird. I want this year to be done, but it had some great moments. We were able to take some trips, I've been running, we've both been seeing therapists…" I started to say.

"The Cubs won the World Series…" Tom interrupted.

"Yes, I know, the Cubs won the World Series…" I replied.

As we lay in bed chatting about the chaos of 2016, I knew there was more to us than the previous year, but it had certainly defined us, and refined us, in many ways. Many of our friends and family had been shocked to hear that we had so much dislike for 2016. In their opinion, the logical response was that we had beat cancer this past year and how could we not have loved that? While that was true, it wasn't the whole story. In 2015, we had nine great months before his diagnosis. In 2016 we had to deal with the aftermath from a few months in 2015 and it was one hundred times harder. It had been brutal; it had been isolating in a way we had been secretive about it, but those 366 days, thanks to the leap year, had been the hardest of our life.

January

I started the New Year with a kiss on my shoulder and a whisper in my ear, "Happy New Year, babe, it's going to be a great year."

I smiled as I started to wake up. It was a great way to start the year. I was cautiously optimistic that we were going to have a much better year, and I was determined to do everything in our power to make it a true statement.

With the New Year came the opportunity for Tom to take the fertility tests that he needed before seeing the specialist again. He had been able to take them a few weeks earlier, but we had waited until the New Year because of where we were at with insurance and out-of-pocket costs. It may sound crazy, but it was the difference of thousands of dollars.

There was something so delightfully fresh about a New Year, but the struggles of 2016 were still with us. Tom was still not in the best place, and he was continuing to have these random throwing-up episodes. I started to wonder if this wasn't his anxiety and depression manifesting but rather a sign of a bigger problem. I was scared that maybe problems were brewing, and that these were early symptoms. Tom came out of the bathroom one morning looking completely defeated.

"I can't wait for the day when I can feel sick and not immediately be terrified that it's cancer," he remarked.

I knew what he meant because it was the same fear I was having. On top of that, we were constantly reminded in the news that there would be dramatic changes to the Affordable Care Act, which would significantly impact us.

Tom completed all the tests in the first few days of the New Year and we were able to schedule the big appointment where we would find out about the future of our family. Our doctor usually took several weeks to see, so I called to make the appointment, figuring we wouldn't be able to get in until the end of March at the earliest. I started talking to the receptionist and she informed me that she had just had a cancellation on her previous call and if we could make it she would be able to get us in on January 20th. My stomach dropped, as that was much sooner than I anticipated. I quickly grabbed the appointment and was happy that it was aligning on the same day as other appointments. I hung up the phone and immediately called Tom.

"Hey, babe…. I just got off the phone with the doctor's office and you're not going to believe when we can get in to see him," I said.

"Let me guess, April?" he said.

"Not quite…next Friday," I said, hopeful he would be able to make it work with his schedule.

"Holy crap!" he replied.

"That's going to be a crazy few days. We've got this huge appointment a day before the one-year celebration of you being cancer-free…" I said.

"That's crazy…" he said.

I wished I could have told him in person, but since it was only a few days away I wanted to tell him as soon as possible so he could talk to his manager. I was hopeful that he was alright with these two days now being even more emotionally charged. I wasn't sure how I felt about it. Part of me felt like it was almost destiny that we were able to see the doctor the day before the one-year anniversary. I wanted nothing more than to get answers so we could move on, and this might provide the opportunity.

Two days later, Tom told me that the doctor had called and that they wanted him to go back to take another blood test. This was a result of his original blood work and it made me sick to my stomach. I Googled the test and found that its sole purpose was check for prostate cancer. My heart sank. I had no idea why the doctor would suddenly need to test for this and made the poor decision to continue reading articles online. I finally had to put it away because I was making myself worry even more. I tried to be calm to not scare Tom, but I had real concerns. The worst part was we were going to do the test on Saturday and still had six more days until our appointment.

I wasn't sleeping well as we started into our big week. I was starting a crazy week at work with the launch of a project I had been working on for months, and we had our fertility appointment followed by the one-year cancer-free anniversary. My panic about the blood work, along with the fertility news, was consuming my thoughts. I was eager to see Dr. Crane and see if he could help me gain control for a few days leading up to this appointment. I filled him in on everything that had transpired in the first few days of the New Year.

"You know, I'm bracing for the worst, but hoping for the best this weekend. More than anything – good, bad, or ugly – I just want some answers on Friday. I think that will heavily dictate how well Saturday goes," I said.

"What are you planning for Saturday?" he asked.

"We are going to a fancy seafood restaurant so Tom can eat some crab. It's the only thing he wants to do. I asked him if he wanted to get away for the night and he insisted that he wanted to be at home that night, in our bed. It's funny because we were invited to a wedding on Saturday in Indiana and my best friend's thirtieth birthday party in Cincinnati, but we aren't doing anything. We are going to see how the day evolves, but based on how these other milestone days have gone, we aren't planning too much," I replied.

We started focusing on what was really bothering me, which was the fertility appointment.

"I feel a little lost in the fertility stuff," I said.

"How so?" he asked, seeming to be surprised by my comment.

"It's like there is the cancer, and the impact of the cancer to our family, and I've sort of just become this side thing. And I don't mean that like someone is doing that intentionally, but obviously I have a huge part in this. This is the biggest thing that has happened as a result of cancer, and we both feel it deeply. I'm not just a caregiver for this one; I'm a directly impacted party," I said.

"Very much so," he said.

"My anxiety has been out of control. I'm not really sleeping, work is insane, but I do have this ability to compartmentalize. I'm sure that's not what my therapist wants to hear, but while it might be a bad thing right now, I will say it's probably the only reason that I survived the past year," I rationalized. "I just need to figure out how to deal with this anxiety."

Dr. Crane started discussing different strategies with me, and I had the epiphany that the issue was that my emotions weren't matching my intellect. It didn't make sense at first, but as he was describing it I had my "aha" moment. I had been suppressing the emotions and trying to be so tough that my mind wasn't able to reconcile my intellectual understanding with what I was feeling.

"It's funny you say that, though, because I think it's my ability to compartmentalize that helps me avoid the emotion," I concluded. "I've been coming here for a year, and I think about all the conversations we've had, and how rock bottom I've been, yet I've never cried in front of you."

He looked at me as if that couldn't be true, and after a few moments realized that I was right. I wasn't necessarily proud of it, but it did demonstrate exactly what he was telling me I was doing with my emotions and intellect. I knew that no matter what happened on Friday at the appointment, I needed to feel whatever it was that I was going to feel. I looked up at Dr. Crane as we wrapped up the session. "This sucks," I said.

He paused and looked back at me while he nodded his head. "For now..." he said.

I knew he was right; I knew this peak anxiety and nerves were only temporary. Yet, in my sleepless and emotionally exhausted state, it was exactly the reminder that I needed in that moment. What I wanted to know more than anything was how long "for now" would last. We needed to make sure that we were both in a good place for welcoming a baby versus a baby "fixing" this unfortunate time in our life.

The week slowly drudged by and we kept talking about what we were expecting on Friday. Tom was already starting to feel guilt, and he didn't even know the answers. I was so worried about how he would take whatever news we received. The morning of the appointment, we both worked from home and hardly spoke. Work was a perfect distraction for us to avoid talking to each other about how we were feeling.

We left for the appointment and then suddenly we were sitting in the consultation room waiting for the doctor to come in. The days leading up had dragged on, and yet I don't quite remember getting to the doctor's office. We sat in the room in silence. I couldn't talk and thought I was going to throw up. I was having a very real physical reaction to everything I was feeling, and I could tell that Tom also felt helpless. My reaction was a rare one, and I know it freaked Tom out a bit because I was usually the strong, positive one who tried to make the best of our situation, but I couldn't do it that day.

Two fellowship doctors came in and had a quick chat with us about what to expect today and touched on the prostate blood test. Tom's levels were a little high for his age, so they wanted to keep an eye on it in the coming months, but in the meantime requested a quick prostate exam. Tom went a bit pale, as he knew what that meant, and I excused myself outside the consultation room for a moment while trying not to laugh. I heard Tom cracking jokes with the doctors and found myself chuckling in the hallway as I heard his commentary, it was the first time I laughed that day.

The fellows left the room and said they would be back shortly with the doctor. I went back in. Tom looked traumatized and I couldn't stop chuckling.

"It's a good thing you're not in charge of the childbirth in this relationship, or we'd be screwed," I said.

"Oh, I am the first to admit that too. Women are way stronger than men," he said.

We were interrupted as the doctor walked in to see us. He was a wonderful doctor and immediately apologized to Tom that he just had to experience his first prostate exam. He started talking about the tests and we didn't hear the answers we wanted. We would have to wait another year to know if we would be able to have kids. I felt like someone had ripped out my stomach and was jumping on it. The doctor explained in great details all of the different things he was considering and the most important one was that it was risky right now.

I felt heartbroken for many reasons, the biggest one being our continued lack of solid answers. We had both been under the impression, based on previous appointments, that we would get more concrete answers at this one-year appointment, and we had gotten the exact opposite, a longer wait. We asked several questions based on the information that he had just given us, and he patiently answered each one.

As he finished his explanations, he said to Tom that he would "throw the book at your testicles," meaning that he would try everything that the medical field recommends to make this happen for us.

I made a face as I replied, "Yikes, that sounds painful."

Tom didn't miss a beat. "I hope it's a paperback book."

The doctors paused and all laughed out loud as they realized we had taken their medical jargon literally.

"The only constant we've had in the last sixteen months is humor. Laughter is the best medicine!" I said.

They all agreed and started discussing our next steps. They would see us again in spring with hopes of better news going into the second part of the year.

After they left, Tom and I stared ahead as we waited for the nurse to come in with our discharge papers. Neither of us moved for several minutes, but Tom started to get very twitchy and I knew he was working himself up. I leaned over and put my head on his shoulder.

"This sucks," I said. "Are you okay?"

"I just didn't want the answer to be more waiting. But I also want nothing more than to have kids with you," he said.

I knew he was struggling between logic and immediate gratification. Of course we both wanted kids; we had wanted them for over two and a half years. But he was right, it was worth the wait if it was our ultimate goal.

The nurse walked in and we took care of the paperwork and headed out. It was a relatively quiet walk to the car. We tried to talk everything out on the way home, but there were still so many variables.

"I think what's upsetting me most is the fact that I was hoping for some answers so that we could continue our work towards moving on," I replied. It may sound ridiculous, but without answers we were about to embark on another year without any progress towards our family. Once again, that kept cancer very present in our everyday lives. Of course cancer would always be part of us now, but its overt impact was hard to handle day after day. To know another year of that void was ahead was a hard pill to swallow.

I hadn't cried like I thought I would though, because of the confusion of it all. I couldn't process all the different variables the doctor discussed with us; much less accept all those possibilities. I decided I needed to get some fresh air when I got home and took the dog for a walk. My sister called to see how things had gone, and I told her that we hadn't gotten much information. I started telling her that it made me sad that the doctors feel bad for us, and that's when it all hit me and I started to cry. I pulled myself together quickly, but the emotions had surprised me. I was walking down my block with tears running down my face and no real idea of what we were going to do.

From conversations with Dr. Crane, I tried to figure out what had triggered my tears, what had ultimately caused the emotion. What made me cry was picturing the doctors' faces in the consultation room. They all felt bad for us, and I hated that feeling. I hated the look that said we were too young for this to be happening or the look of sadness for us. We never projected that, so it was hard when it was projected on us because it required us to reconcile how we were choosing to deal with the dark reality of our situation. It would catch me off guard sometimes and create such sadness.

As anticipated, we added insult to injury when we woke up the next morning, the one-year anniversary of Tom being cancer-free. I had hoped it would be a joyous day, but I woke up and Tom had already been crying. I rolled over and gave him a hug.

"Happy One Year, babe – I'm so proud of you," I said.

"Thanks, but I don't get why you're proud," he said.

"Oh you know, just that whole beating cancer thing," I replied.

Proud didn't seem like a strong enough word, but I wasn't sure how else to describe it. We had both come so far. I was now running regularly, and Tom was slowly increasing his workouts too and planning to run a 5K in the spring. While you could physically see that, the deepest changes couldn't be seen from the outside. It was the ups and downs that broke us and then made us stronger. It was the survival of days that felt like an eternity. For me, it was the acknowledgement that as hard as this post-cancer struggle had been, it would have been a hundred times harder if the outcome had been different. If I was, instead, grieving the loss of my husband on my own. This milestone felt so real but also so strange.

When we woke up, we decided to celebrate by going to our favorite diner for breakfast.

"I don't know why I feel such sadness," he said as we were eating breakfast, "...and it's weird to me that I feel weird about how I feel...if that makes any sense."

"No, I get that, but you know what's great about that? That means you're feeling everything. That means you're not in shock and you can feel what you're feeling so we can continue to move on," I replied. I really believed that. We needed to force ourselves to feel everything, even if it wasn't fun, so that we had less of a chance of it derailing us next year.

As we ate our breakfast, we picked our lottery numbers. I figured it made sense to buy a lottery ticket on our way home because if ever there was a good day to buy a lottery ticket, the one-year anniversary seemed to be the one. I could tell Tom was having a harder day than he had anticipated and wanted him to be honest with me about what he wanted for his day.

"This is your day; do you still want to go to dinner? We can reschedule," I said.

Tom thought for a minute and then carefully replied, "I think we should do it another time. I'm just sad and I don't want to have to sit at a table and force myself to feel happy. I'd rather go another time," he replied.

"That's fine by me, babe. Today is your day. I want to do whatever you want to do. If that means sitting at home and hanging out, then so be it." I meant it too; I didn't want him to feel pressure on this day at all. That was the exact opposite of how I wanted him to feel.

To say the day was anticlimactic was an understatement. We ended up ordering takeout and catching up on our DVR, but it was perfect. In its simplest form we had done whatever we had wanted to do, and that was not our reality one year earlier, so to me that was a celebration in and of itself.

The year itself had passed quickly, but the days had been long, emotional, and trying. I often wondered how the first year of post-cancer life evolved for older people. When people are diagnosed later in life, it seems that there is a more renewed sense of life and appreciation, but they also don't have to deal with as many question marks. When young adults are diagnosed, there are so many additional factors to deal with, the biggest one often being the impact to a family. It makes moving on much harder and makes the months following the cancer-free diagnosis especially challenging.

The big day hadn't been a big day at all; it was a day full of strange feelings, of emptiness, of loss, of continued confusion. We had made it, and there were days that I didn't think we would. But it was a milestone, the first year cancer-free, and as Tom had so beautifully said at the beginning of the day, "It's the first of another fifty cancer-free anniversaries to come."

I Wish Books Could Play Dramatic "Last Chapter" Music

It had always been my intent to have a first draft of the book done by the one-year anniversary of Tom being cancer-free. In my head, I was going to be able to wrap up the book on a high note, when our luck had finally changed. I would leave readers with a joy of some kind that made the previous pages full of ups and downs worth the ending. I'm not sure that's how this book ends though, and yet that's the most real ending. There is no end to our cancer fight; it becomes less and less a part of our daily lives, but it's never going away. It forever changed us. We will always worry about it coming back, and that is the raw reality of this "ending". I'd imagine it's like having a child. The chapter starts but it really never has an end; they are always your child, and you continue to be part of their own chapters. If ever I wanted an end to a chapter of my life, this cancer fight would be it, but I have accepted that it's not the reality for this type of trauma. Don't get me wrong, life is better than it was a year ago, but we are still picking up the pieces of this massive explosion that occurred in our lives.

There are days where it doesn't seem fair, but there are more days that feel like we've been given additional purpose in our lives. There are days where we feel like we can't catch a break, but there are more days that remind us that we caught a lot of breaks during our fight. There are days where we just wanted to cry, but we smiled through it for the sake of our sanity and for others. There are days where I feel like we aren't making progress like we should, but we remind ourselves that progress is progress no matter how it looks or feels, and that we shouldn't have shame in how our story is playing out.

If there is one thing I know for sure it's that there was a critical moment in this post-cancer fight that occurred for us to make it this far. Tom shifted from people working on him to working on himself. During his initial treatments and surgery, Tom could do nothing but be a bystander to all of the treatments that were happening _to_ him. At some point – and I'm still unsure of the timing – he had to shift to work on himself. He could no longer be a bystander; he had to take ownership and participate in a different way physically, mentally, and emotionally. I think this is something that people often don't do when they've experienced a trauma like we did, and I find it to be one of the most critical factors to success.

Cancer has been the single hardest struggle of our lives, and we anticipate that the continued fertility struggles will top the list too. Cancer challenged our relationship and took a lot from us, but the only thing it took that we can't replace is time. It has given us more than we ever imagined too. We have an appreciation for life that is always top of mind; we have an even stronger belief in gratitude and acknowledgment; we have a relationship to be proud of, and we have more hope than ever before.

So the only ending I can provide revolves around one word – waiting. It's not ideal, but it's our reality. We have to wait to see if our dreams of a family can come true. We have to wait and see how Tom's recovery continues to evolve. We have to wait and see how life will settle, but as the saying goes, the best things in life are worth waiting for. I believe, and hope, that waiting will create a deeper appreciation for all the blessings in our life. I'm not naive enough to think it won't be hard, or that certain experiences won't upset us, but I hold onto hope that one day when I hold our kids in my arms, or make a life decision that, otherwise, we might not have made, that the waiting and this struggle suddenly makes sense.

But waiting doesn't mean we sit back and relax while everything happens around us. We are continuing to take an active role in helping others who are fighting this disease, donating our time and money, and doing everything we can to make our dreams a reality. I do hope we see the cure for cancer in our lifetime, and we will do our part, however we can, to ensure that everyone can be a survivor.

Equally as important, we continue to work on our own recoveries which are similar - but different. While we did this all together, our experiences, perspectives, memories and the impacts are very different. We've come too far to only come *this* far, and this adventure will continue whether we want it to or not. We can't hate the experiences that we've had to deal with because they are now a part of who we are. To disregard them would be disregarding a part of ourselves.

When I originally titled this book, it was titled "128 Days" because of the length of time he had active cancer. I soon realized that to box cancer into just the active cancer timeframe was naive and misleading. At the end of the 128 days, we were just starting. Cancer is part of our life every single day, and some days are much harder than others. The one-year anniversary marked 492 days since our lives changed, and we will continue to count our successes as time moves on. Count every day, count every small victory, and count our blessings.

As you read our story, I hope you recognized that every experience we had *before* cancer helped us make it *through* cancer. I know every moment of the cancer is somehow preparing us for the next thing that life hands us too. But there is no guarantee life will hand us anything at all and yet so many people worry about tomorrow like it's promised. It's not; it can change overnight. As an Irish proverb that hangs on our wall at home so beautifully states "Never for a moment take for granted the things that could be taken away from you in an instant."

-The End-